AF564586

NNF

NeoVentURE

Neonatal Ventilation pLus Respiratory CarE

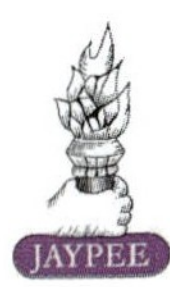

Jaypee Brothers Medical Publishers (P) Ltd

Headquarters
EMCA House, 23/23-B
Ansari Road, Daryaganj
New Delhi 110 002, India
Landline: +91-11-23272143, +91-11-23272703
+91-11-23282021, +91-11-23245672
e-mail: jaypee@jaypeebrothers.com

Corporate Office
4838/24, Ansari Road, Daryaganj
New Delhi 110 002, India
Phone: +91-11-43574357
Fax: +91-11-43574314
e-mail: jaypee@jaypeebrothers.com

Overseas Office
JP Medical Ltd
83 Victoria Street, London
SW1H 0HW (UK)
Phone: +44-20 3170 8910
e-mail: info@jpmedpub.com

EU GPSR Authorised Representative
Logos Europe, 9 rue Nicolas Poussin
17000, La Rochelle, France
Phone: +33 (0) 6 67 93 73 78
e-mail: contact@logoseurope.eu

Website: www.jaypeebrothers.com
Website: www.jaypeedigital.com

Inquiries for bulk sales may be solicited at: jaypee@jaypeebrothers.com

NNF NeoVentURE Neonatal Ventilation pLus Respiratory CarE

First Edition: **2026**

ISBN: 978-93-6616-435-9

Printed at: Samrat Offset Pvt. Ltd.

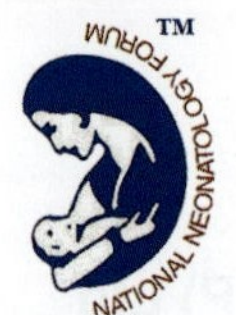

NNF NeoVentURE

Neonatal Ventilation pLus Respiratory CarE

Editors

Sushma Nangia
MD (Pediatrics) DM (Neonatology, AIIMS)
Director–Professor
Department of Neonatology
Lady Hardinge Medical College and
Associated Kalawati Saran Children
Hospital, New Delhi, India

Ashish Mehta
MD (Pediatrics) FNNF
Consultant Neonatologist
Department of Neonatology
Arpan Newborn Care Center
Ahmedabad, Gujarat, India

Surender Singh Bisht
MD (Pediatrics)
Head and Senior Specialist
Department of Pediatrics
Swami Dayanand Hospital
New Delhi, India

Amit Upadhyay
MD (Pediatrics) DM (Neonatology)
Director and Head
Department of Pediatrics and
Neonatology
Nutema Hospital
Meerut, Uttar Pradesh, India

Co-Editors

Tapas Bandyopadhyay
MD (Pediatrics) DM (Neonatology)
Professor
Department of Neonatology
Vardhman Mahavir Medical College and Safdarjung Hospital
New Delhi, India

Pratima Anand
MD (Pediatrics) DM (Neonatology)
Neonatologist
Department of Neonatology
Lady Hardinge Medical College and
Associated Hospitals
New Delhi, India

Kamal Arora
MD (Pediatrics) DM (Neonatolog
Professor and Neonatologi
Dayanand Medical College a
Hospital
Ludhiana, Punjab, India

Foreword

VC Manoj

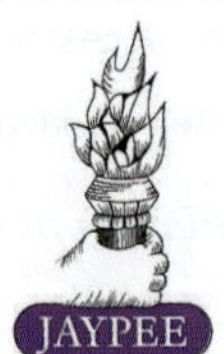

JAYPEE BROTHERS MEDICAL PUBLISHE

The Health Sciences Publisher

New Delhi | London

Dedication

This book is dedicated to all the newborns of our country—the tiniest warriors, who inspire us every day with their resilience and strength.

May NeoVentURE serve as a guiding light for healthcare professionals, helping them provide the best possible care to ensure that every newborn gets the healthiest start in life.

With hope, compassion, and commitment, we dedicate this work to the future—one newborn at a time.

The NeoVentURE Team

Contributors
(Alphabetical Order)

Aakash Pandita MBBS MD DNrB
Director
Department of Neonatology
Neonatology and Child Development Center
Medanta Hospital
Lucknow, Uttar Pradesh, India

Amanpreet Sethi
MD (Pediatrics) DM (Neonatology)
Associate Professor and Head
Department of Neonatology Division
Guru Gobind Singh Medical College
Faridkot, Punjab, India

Amit Upadhyay
MD (Pediatrics) DM (Neonatology)
Director and Head (Pediatrics and Neonatology)
Department of Pediatrics and Neonatology
Nutema Hospital
Meerut, Uttar Pradesh, India

Anish Pillai MD DrNB (Neo) Fellowship in Neonatal-Perinatal Medicine (Canada)
Lead Consultant
Department of Neonatology and Pediatrics
Motherhood Hospital
Navi Mumbai, Maharashtra, India

Archana Arumugom
MD DNB (Pediatrics) DrNB (Neonatology)
Neonatology Resident
Department of Neonatology
Kanchi Kamakoti CHILDS Trust Hospital
Chennai, Tamil Nadu, India

Ashish Mehta MD (Pediatrics) FNNF
Consultant Neonatologist
Department of Neonatology
Arpan Newborn Care Center
Ahmedabad, Gujarat, India

Bijan Saha MD DNB DM (Neonatology)
Professor
Department of Neonatology
Institute of Postgraduate Medical Education and Research (SSKM Hospital)
Kolkata, West Bengal, India

Chaitra Angadi DM
Assistant Professor
Department of Neonatology
Jawaharlal Institute of Postgraduate Medical Education and Research
Puducherry, India

Chandra Kumar Natarajan
MD DNB DM (AIIMS) DNB
Senior Consultant and Head
Department of Neonatology
Kanchi Kamakoti CHILDS Trust Hospital
Chennai, Tamil Nadu, India

Debashish Nanda
MBBS MD (Pediatrics) DM (Neonatology)
Professor
Department of Neonatology
Institute of Medical Sciences and SUM Hospital
Bhubaneswar, Odisha, India

Gunjana Kumar
MBBS MD DM (Neonatology, LHMC)
Associate Professor
Department of Neonatology
National Institute of Medical Sciences and Research
Jaipur, Rajasthan, India

Kamal Arora
MD (Pediatrics) DM (Neonatology)
Professor and Neonatologist
Dayanand Medical College and Hospital
Ludhiana, Punjab, India

Kiran More MD FRACP (Australia)
Head of Neonatology and Research Lead
MRR Children's Hospital
Thane, Maharashtra, India

Murugesan A DM
Assistant Professor
Department of Neonatology
Jawaharlal Institute of Postgraduate Medical Education and Research
Puducherry, India

Naveen Parkash Gupta MD DNB (Neonatology) Fellowship in Neonatology (BC Children's Hospital, Vancouver) Critical Care Ultrasound Trainee (CEURF, Paris)
Senior Consultant Neonatology
Madhukar Rainbow Children's Hospital
New Delhi, India

Neeraj Gupta
MD DM (Neonatology) MAMS
Professor and Head
Department of Neonatology
All India Institute of Medical Sciences
Jodhpur, Rajasthan, India

Pankaj Kumar Mohanty
MD Pediatrics (MAMC) DNB (Neonatology)
Additional Professor
Department of Neonatology
All India Institute of Medical Sciences
Bhubaneswar, Odisha, India

Pinaki Dutta DNB (Pediatrics)
NNF Fellowship in Neonatology
Associate Consultant Neonatology
Department of Neonatology
Madhukar Rainbow Children's Hospital
New Delhi, India

Pradeep Kumar Debata
DM (Neonatology)
Professor
Department of Pediatrics
Vardhman Mahavir Medical College and Safdarjung Hospital
New Delhi, India

Pradeep Sharma
MBBS MD DM (Neonatology)
Senior Consultant
Department of Neonatology
Deep Hospital
Ludhiana, Punjab, India

Prathik Bandiya MD DM (Neonatology)
Associate Professor
Department of Neonatology
Indira Gandhi Institute of Child Health
Bengaluru, Karnataka, India

Pratima Anand MD (Pediatrics)
DM (Neonatology)
Neonatologist
Department of Neonatology
Lady Hardinge Medical College and Associated Hospitals
New Delhi, India

Priyanka Gupta MBBS MD DNrB (Neonatology, Fernandez Hospital, Telangana)
Consultant Neonatologist
Department of Neonatology
Nutema Hospital
Meerut, Uttar Pradesh, India

Rohit Anand DM (Neonatology)
Assistant Professor
Department of Neonatology
All India Institute of Medical Sciences
Raipur, Chhattisgarh, India

Rohit Sasidharan MD DM (Neonatology) MRCPCH
Assistant Professor
Department of Neonatology
All India Institute of Medical Sciences
Guwahati, Assam, India

Shashi Kant Dhir MD IAP Fellowship of Neonatology DM (Neonatology)
Professor and Head
Department of Pediatrics
Guru Gobind Singh Medical College
Faridkot, Punjab, India

Sindhu Sivanandan
MD DNB DM (Neonatology)
Chief Neonatologist and Clinical Lead
Department of Neonatology
Kauvery Hospital
Chennai, Tamil Nadu, India

Surender Singh Bisht MD (Pediatrics)
Head and Senior Specialist
Department of Pediatrics
Swami Dayanand Hospital
New Delhi, India

Sushil Choudhary DM (Neonatology)
Associate Professor
Department of Neonatology
All India Institute of Medical Sciences
Jodhpur, Rajasthan, India

Sushma Nangia
MD (Pediatrics) DM (Neonatology, AIIMS)
Director–Professor
Department of Neonatology
Lady Hardinge Medical College
and Associated Kalawati Saran
Children Hospital
New Delhi, India

Tapas Bandyopadhyay
MD (Pediatrics) DM (Neonatology)
Professor
Department of Neonatology
Vardhman Mahavir Medical College
and Safdarjung Hospital
New Delhi, India

Tejo Pratap Oleti
MD (Pediatrics) DM (Neonatology)
Lead Consultant and Head
Department of Neonatology
Fernandez Hospitals
Hyderabad, Telangana, India

Umamaheswari B
MD MRCPCH (UK) FRCPCH (UK)
Head and Professor
Department of Neonatology
Sri Ramachandra Institute of Higher
Education and Research
Chennai, Tamil Nadu, India

Usha Devi R MD DM (Neonatology)
Assistant Professor
Department of Neonatology
Jawaharlal Institute of Postgraduate
Medical Education and Research
Puducherry, India

Viraraghavan Vadakkencherry Ramaswamy MD DM (Neonatology)
DNB (Neonatology) (LHMC)
Consultant Neonatologist and Head
Department of Neonatology
Ankura Hospital for Women
and Children
Hyderabad, Telangana, India

Reviewers
(Alphabetical Order)

Amit Tagare
MD DNB (Pediatrics) DCH DrNB (Neonatology)
Neonatal Fellow (Australia)
Associate Professor and Head of Neonatology
Department of Pediatrics
Bharati Vidyapeeth Deemed University Medical College
Sangli, Maharashtra, India

Anup Thakur
MD (Pediatrics) DNB (Neonatology)
Senior Consultant
Department of Neonatology
Sir Ganga Ram Hospital
New Delhi, India

Deepak Sharma
MD (Pediatrics) DrNB (Neonatology, Gold Medalist) MNAMS
Consultant and Head
Department of Neonatology
Hope Hospital
Jaipur, Rajasthan, India

Devadeep Mukherjee
DCH MRCPCH (UK) FRCPCH (UK) Fellowship in Neonatal and Pediatric Intensive Care (UK)
Senior Consultant
Department of Pediatrics and Neonatology
Healthworld Hospitals
Paschim Bardhaman, West Bengal, India

Gopal Agarwal DM (Neonatology)
Consultant
Department of Pediatrics and Neonatology
Cloudnine Hospitals
Gurugram, Haryana, India

Jafar Khan
MD (Pediatrics) DNB (Neonatology, Gold Medalist)
Assistant Professor
Department of Pediatrics
Ruxmaniben Deepchand Gardi Medical College
Ujjain, Madhya Pradesh, India

Jayasree Chandramathi
MD Fellowship in Neonatology
Associate Professor
Department of Neonatology/Division of Pediatrics
Amrita Institute of Medical Sciences
Kochi, Kerala, India

Kavita Sreekumar
MD (Ped) Fellowship in Neonatology
Associate Professor
Department of Pediatrics
Goa Medical College
Goa, India

Mayank Priyadarshi
DM (Neonatology)
Associate Professor
Department of Neonatology
All India Institute of Medical Sciences
Rishikesh, Uttar Pradesh, India

Rahul Illaparambath
MD (Ped) DNB (Ped) MNAMS MRCPCH (UK)
Fellowship in Neonatology (UK)
Senior Consultant and Head
Department of Neonatology
IQRAA International Hospital and Research Centre
Kozhikode, Kerala, India

Ruchi Rai MD (Pediatrics)
Professor and Head
Department of Neonatology
Postgraduate Institute of Child Health
Noida, Uttar Pradesh, India

Shajin T MBBS DCH MD DNB MRCPCH
Consultant
Department of Neonatology
Rosewalk by Rainbow Children's Hospital
New Delhi, India

Sheila Samanta Mathai
MD DNB DM (Neonatology)
Professor and Head
Department of Neonatology
Kasturba Medical College
Manipal, Karnataka, India

Shilpa Kalane DrNB (Neonatology)
Chief Neonatologist
Department of Neonatology
Deenanath Mangeshkar Hospital and Research Center
Pune, Maharashtra, India

Varun Sharma
MD (Pediatrics) Fellowship in Neonatology (RCPCH, UK)
Consultant Neonatologist
Department of Pediatrics and Neonatology
RHL Babylon Advanced Child Center
Jaipur, Rajasthan, India

Foreword

Esteemed Members,

The National Neonatology Forum (NNF) has always been at the forefront, leading the struggle of neonatologists to stay updated in knowledge and skills amidst continuously evolving treatment protocols of neonatal care worldwide, as neonatology has progressed in leaps and bounds.

Over the past few decades, advancements in neonatal respiratory care have dramatically reduced neonatal mortality and morbidity rates, with innovations focusing on more individualized, noninvasive, and less harmful approaches to respiratory support. From merely focusing on the survival and intact survival of the tiniest of babies, neonatology has now evolved to help these children reach their full potential and live adult lives free from lifestyle diseases.

Our respiratory care has also evolved in accordance with this principle. We have progressed from strategies aiming for normal blood-gas ventilation to those preventing ventilation-induced lung injury. Now, we aim to evolve neuroprotective ventilation strategies, understanding that "less is more" in respiratory care.

One of the most significant strides in the management of respiratory distress has been the development and refinement of noninvasive ventilation strategies. As neonatal respiratory care continues to evolve, prevention of ventilation-induced lung injury through strategies such as optimal oxygenation, volume-targeted ventilation in both conventional and high-frequency oscillatory ventilation (HFOV), and timely extubation in ventilated babies continue to remain significant. These approaches help make respiratory care less invasive, more precise, and tailored to the unique needs of each neonate. Novel diagnostic strategies such as lung ultrasound also hold potential to further improve outcomes for neonates worldwide.

This book is an excellent landmark in this regard, covering the basic principles in neonatal ventilation and providing an overview of the evolving techniques and strategies driving the future of respiratory management in neonatal care.

India has a very heterogeneous population, and one of the bottlenecks in the progress of neonatal care is our lack of a suitable protocol that fits each and every region of our country.

Friends, let us all endeavor to make new beginnings in these fields, together.

Warm regards,

VC Manoj
President, National Neonatology Forum (NNF), 2025

Preface

Advances in neonatal care have significantly improved survival rates and outcomes for premature and critically sick neonates. Among the cornerstones of this progress is the evolution of neonatal ventilation, which has become a life-saving intervention for countless neonates. Despite its widespread use, neonatal ventilation remains a complex and rapidly evolving field, requiring clinicians to possess a thorough understanding of physiology, technologies, and challenges to optimize care.

This book has been created to serve as a comprehensive resource for neonatologists, pediatricians, and nursing colleagues engaged in caring of neonates requiring respiratory support. It aims to bridge the gap between foundational knowledge and clinical application, offering insights into the physiology of neonatal respiration, the intricacies of various basic and advanced ventilatory modalities, and the latest innovations in the field.

Drawing upon the expertise of clinicians, researchers, and educators, this book covers topics ranging from basic respiratory mechanics and pathophysiology to advanced strategies in invasive and noninvasive ventilation in neonates, including the pharmacotherapy in respiratory disorders, and management of ventilation-associated complications. Special emphasis is placed on using tables, flowcharts, and figures to ease the understanding of bedside management of neonatal respiratory conditions.

We hope that this text will serve not only as a reference for seasoned practitioners but also as a learning tool for fellows and students seeking to master the art and science of neonatal ventilation. Through this work, we aim to empower clinicians to make informed, evidence-based decisions that enhance outcomes for our most vulnerable neonates.

We dedicate this book to the neonates who inspire our efforts, their families who demonstrate extraordinary strength, and the healthcare teams who tirelessly work to provide compassionate, state-of-the-art care in neonatal intensive care units (NICUs).

Sushma Nangia
Surender Singh Bisht
Ashish Mehta
Amit Upadhyay
Tapas Bandyopadhyay
Pratima Anand
Kamal Arora

Preface

Acknowledgments

The journey of NeoVentURE has been a collective effort, driven by the dedication and expertise of esteemed pediatricians, neonatologists, and fellows in neonatology. This book is the result of the collaborative spirit and shared commitment of all the authors, reviewers, and contributors who have worked tirelessly to create a comprehensive and algorithm-based management guide for neonatal ventilation.

We extend our sincere gratitude to all the authors for their invaluable contributions, which have made this book a rich source of knowledge. Their expertise and clinical insights have been instrumental in shaping each chapter, ensuring that the content remains practical and evidence based.

A heartfelt thank you to the reviewers from across various institutions and NNF Centers, whose meticulous evaluations and constructive feedback have enhanced the quality and accuracy of this book. Their dedication to refining the content and maintaining the highest standards of medical education is truly commendable.

We are deeply grateful to the National Neonatology Forum (NNF) for their unwavering support and encouragement throughout this endeavor. Their vision and commitment to neonatal care have provided a strong foundation for this project.

Finally, we acknowledge the collective efforts of all those involved in the editorial, design, and production processes. Their hard work and perseverance have transformed this initiative into a reality.

We hope NeoVentURE serves as a valuable resource for clinicians, guiding them in making informed and effective decisions in neonatal ventilation. This book stands as a testament to our shared mission of improving neonatal care and outcomes.

With heartfelt appreciation,

Sushma Nangia
Surender Singh Bisht
Ashish Mehta
Amit Upadhyay
Tapas Bandyopadhyay
Pratima Anand
Kamal Arora

Contents

SECTION 10: Nursing Care in Babies on Noninvasive and Invasive Ventilation, Transportation of Neonate on Assisted Ventilation

SECTION 11: Miscellaneous Topics

SECTION 12: Case Scenarios

SECTION

Respiratory Distress Overview and Assessment in Newborn, Pulmonary Physiology in Normal and Diseased States

CHAPTER

Hypoxic Respiratory Failure, Clinical Features, and Assessment of Severity

Shashi Kant Dhir

INTRODUCTION

Hypoxic respiratory failure (HRF) in the neonates is defined as either inability of maintenance of normal oxygenation or removal of carbon dioxide from the blood and may result from a number of underlying conditions **(Table 1)**.

National Neonatal Perinatal Database of India defines respiratory distress as the presence of any two of the three essential features, viz., tachypnea (respiratory rate counted for 60 seconds >60 breaths/min), retractions (intercostal and/or subcostal), and expiratory grunting. HRF is clinically suspected when the neonate is having signs of severe respiratory distress (score of >6, described later). Laboratory wise HRF is defined as the presence of ≥2 of the following with a fraction of inspired oxygen (FiO_2) of 100% and pH <7.25 in arterial blood gas analysis:

- Partial pressure of arterial carbon dioxide ($PaCO_2$) >60 mm Hg
- Partial pressure of arterial oxygen (PaO_2) <50 mm Hg or
- O_2 saturation <80%

TABLE 1: Common causes of hypoxic respiratory failure.

Respiratory causes:	*Nonrespiratory causes:*
• Respiratory distress syndrome • Meconium aspiration syndrome • Other aspiration syndromes • Congenital pneumonia • Persistent pulmonary hypertension • Congenital pulmonary arterial malformation • Bronchopulmonary dysplasia spells • Pulmonary hemorrhage • Worsening pneumonia • Pulmonary hypoplasia • Pleural effusion • Pneumothorax	• Critical cyanotic heart diseases • Severe congenital heart diseases • Neuromuscular conditions • Congenital diaphragmatic hernia • HIE • Maternal medications leading to CNS depression

(CNS: central nervous system; HIE: hypoxic-ischemic encephalopathy)

CLINICAL MONITORING OF RESPIRATORY DISTRESS IN NEONATES

Assessing and monitoring of presence of respiratory distress remains a cornerstone in the management of the neonate in the neonatal intensive care unit (NICU). A detailed physical examination of the respiratory system helps in timely initiation of the respiratory support and early diagnosis of impending respiratory failure. All neonates with impending HRF will be having different levels of respiratory distress evident by increased respiratory rates, retractions, flaring of alae nasi, and expiratory grunting. Two validated scoring systems, Silverman–Anderson score **(Table 2)** and Downes Vidyasagar score **(Table 3),** are commonly used to assess the

TABLE 2: Silverman–Anderson scoring system for assessment of respiratory distress.

Score	*Method of evaluation*	*0*	*1*	*2*
Upper chest retractions (to be seen tangentially from the side)	Observe the synchrony of the upper chest with abdomen movement during inspiration	Equal upper chest synchronized with abdomen	• Respiratory lag • Upper chest lags compared to abdomen	• See-saw respiration • See-saw movement of the chest and abdomen (both moving in opposite direction)
Lower chest retractions	Observe the retractions between the ribs below the midaxillary line	None	Minimal	Marked
Xiphoid retractions	Retraction below the xiphoid process	None	Minimal	Marked
Nasal flaring	Observe the nasal flaring before application of nasal interface	None	Minimal	Marked
Expiratory grunt		None	Audible with stethoscope	Audible without stethoscope

Score less than 3: Oxygen alone; *Score 4–6:* Continuous positive airway pressure (CPAP); *Score >7:* Ventilation

Source: Silverman WA, Andersen DA. A controlled clinical trial of effects of water mist on obstructive respiratory signs, death rate and necropsy findings among premature infants. Pediatrics. 1956;17(1):1-10.

TABLE 3: Downes Vidyasagar scoring system for assessment of respiratory distress.

Score	*0*	*1*	*2*
Retractions	None	Mild	Severe
Grunting	None	Audible with stethoscope	Audible without stethoscope
Air entry	Clear	Decreased	Barely audible
Cyanosis of lips and oral mucosa	None	In room air	In 40% FiO_2
Respiratory rate	Under 60	60–80	Over 80 or apnea

Score less than 3: Oxygen alone; *Score 4–6:* Continuous positive airway pressure (CPAP); *Score >7:* Ventilation

(FiO_2: fraction of inspired oxygen)

Source: Downes JJ, Vidyasagar D, Boggs TR, Morrow GM. Respiratory distress syndrome of newborn infants. I. New clinical scoring system (RDS score) with acid–base and blood-gas correlations. Clin Pediatr. 1970;9:325-31.

respiratory distress in neonatal population. The signs of respiratory distress are assigned a numerical value (0 indicating normal and 2 indicating the worst).

RESPIRATORY MONITORING OF NEONATES ON RESPIRATORY SUPPORT

The basic principles remain the same as in neonates without support. Same scores as mentioned earlier can also be used in neonates who are on respiratory support. Appearance of signs of respiratory distress in neonates who are already on respiratory support imply that hiking of support may be needed after ruling out correctable causes. Low threshold should always be used to increase respiratory support in such neonates and all efforts should be made to establish the cause of new-onset respiratory distress.

ASSESSMENT OF SEVERITY OF RESPIRATORY DISTRESS

The assessment of severity can be done by clinical examination, noninvasively as well as by invasive methods. The clinical examination includes the assessment of the signs of respiratory distress using validated scores and do not require advanced equipment. The pulse oximetry is one of the most common tools being used in the monitoring of the neonates with respiratory distress. A-a DO_2, oxygenation index, and a/A ratio are the three most common oxygenation indices used in the neonates. Transcutaneous CO_2 monitoring, capnography, and pulmonary graphics (discussed elsewhere) are also used to monitor respiratory distress in centers having advanced equipment. **Table 4** summarizes the salient features of the common assessment methods.

TABLE 4: Different methods used for assessment of respiratory failure in neonates.

Clinical monitoring		
Silverman Anderson score and Downes scoring system	• Serial monitoring can be done by nurses and residents • Easy to use • Validated	• *Score 0:* None • *Score 1–3:* Mild respiratory distress • *Score 4–6:* Moderate respiratory distress • *Score >6:* Impending respiratory failure
Pulse oximetry		
Oxygen saturation (SpO_2)	• Primary tool for noninvasive continuous oxygen monitoring • Based upon relative absorption of light by saturated and unsaturated hemoglobin • Preductal saturation should be checked for best assessment • SET technology should be used wherever possible • Excessive movement, light, low perfusion states, and abnormal hemoglobin may give aberrant values	*Age and gestation-specific saturation targets are to be followed:* *Gestation wise target SpO_2** ***GA*** / ***Target SpO_2*** / ***Alarm limits*** <32 / 89–94% / 88–95 32–37 / 90–94% / 89–95% >37 / 95–98% / 94–99%
Oxygen indices		
Alveolar–arterial oxygen gradient (A-aDO_2)	• Reflects the degree of V/Q mismatch or diffusion impairment • Depends upon FiO_2 • $PAO_2 - PaO_2$ (i.e., *p* Alveolar – P arterial *oxygen tension*) $= [(P_B - P_W) \times FiO_2 - PaCO_2/RQ] - PaO_2$ $= [(760 - 47) \times FiO_2 - PaCO_2/RQ] - PaO_2$	• *Normal range in a newborn:* 5–15 • *Abnormal:* 15–40 • *Definitely abnormal:* >40 Values more than 600 for 6 hours is associated with high mortality
a/A ratio	• Ratio of PaO_2 to PAO_2 • Ratio is less affected oy changes in FiO_2 • Considered to be a better indicator of gas exchange in patients breathing higher FiO_2 • Commonly used index in surfactant therapy and inhaled nitric oxide therapy	• *Greater than 0.9:* Normal • *Less than 0.6:* Need for O_2 therapy • *Less than 0.15:* Severe hypoxemia

Contd…

Contd...

Oxygenation index (QI)	Suitable for ventilated babies as MAP is included in calculation OI = (MAP × FiO_2) × 100/PaO_2 Gives intermittent measurement	• *OI >15:* Indicates a ventilation–perfusion mismatch • *OI 15–25:* Moderate respiratory failure • *OI 25–40:* Severe respiratory failure with mortality risk of 50–60% • *OI >40:* Mortality risk is >80%, also an indication of ECMO
PaO_2/FiO_2 ratio	• Simple measure of oxygenation • Most often employed in ventilated patients	• *Normal:* 300–500 mm Hg • *Abnormal gas exchange:* <300 mm Hg (ALI) • *Severe hypoxemia:* <200 mm Hg (ARDS)

(ALI: acute lung injury; ARDS: acute respiratory distress syndrome; ECMO: extracorporeal membrane oxygenation; FiO_2: fraction of inspired oxygen; GA: gestational age; MAP: mean airway pressure; V/Q: ventilation/perfusion)

Source: *Cloherty JP, Eichenwald EC, Hansen AR, Stark AR, eds. Cloherty and Stark's Manual of Neonatal Care. 9th ed. South Asian Edition. Gurgaon: Wolters Kluwer Health (India); 2021.

CONCLUSION

Hypoxic respiratory failure in neonates is a life-threatening condition resulting from varied pulmonary and extrapulmonary causes. Early recognition using validated clinical scores, combined with continuous monitoring through pulse oximetry, oxygenation indices, and blood gas analysis, is essential for timely diagnosis and intervention. A structured approach with prompt initiation and escalation of respiratory support, guided by objective assessment tools, remains the cornerstone of management to reduce morbidity and mortality in this vulnerable population

SUGGESTED READING

1. AIIMS Protocols in Neonatology. Approach to Respiratory Distress in the Newborn. 2nd edition. New Delhi: All India Institute of Medical Sciences; 2019.
2. Downes JJ, Vidyasagar D, Boggs TR, Morrow GM. Respiratory distress syndrome of newborn infants. I. New clinical scoring system (RDS score) with acid-base and blood-gas correlations. Clin Pediatr. 1970;9:325-31.
3. Kumar P. Hypoxic respiratory failure. In: Rajiv PK, Vidyasagar D, Lakshminrusimha. Essentials of Neonatal Ventilation. New Delhi: Relix India Pvt Limited; 2021. pp. 81-101.

4. NNPD Network. (2005). South East Asia Regional Neonatal Perinatal Database: Report 2002–2003. [online] Available from: www.newbornwhocc.org/pdf/nnpd_report_2002-03.PDF. [Last accessed January, 2025].
5. Rhein LM. Blood Gas and Pulmonary Function Monitoring. In: Jain N (Ed). Cloherty and Stark Manual of Neonatal Care. South Asian Edition. Gurgaon: Wolters Kluwer Health (India); 2021. pp. 427-36.
6. Silverman WA, Andersen DA. A controlled clinical trial of effects of water mist on obstructive respiratory signs, death rate and necropsy findings among premature infants. Pediatrics. 1956;17(1):1-10.

CHAPTER

Applied Physiology in Normal and Diseased States

Umamaheswari B

INTRODUCTION

A good understanding of the unique physiology and pathophysiology of neonatal respiratory system is necessary to provide individualized care that optimizes pulmonary and neurodevelopmental outcomes.

STAGES OF LUNG DEVELOPMENT AND IMPLICATIONS

With the wide spectrum of gestational ages being cared for, one must be mindful of the stage of lung development of the individual **(Table 1)**. The lung vulnerabilities of a full-term grown neonate suffering from meconium aspiration syndrome (MAS) are different from those of a 25-week ELGAN (extremely low gestational age neonates) being managed for respiratory distress syndrome (RDS).

SALIENT FEATURES OF NEWBORN ANATOMY AND PHYSIOLOGY

The salient features of anatomy and physiology in neonates are summarized in **Table 2**.

MECHANICS OF NEWBORN LUNG

Mechanics is the result of an interesting interplay between compliance, resistance, time constant, work of breathing (WOB), gas transport, and oxygenation.

TABLE 1: Phases of lung development and its clinical implication.

Phases of lung development	*Birth and initiation of spontaneous or mechanical ventilation during the terminal sac phase may result in*
• Embryonic phase (weeks 3–6) • Pseudoglandular phase (weeks 6–16) • Canalicular phase (weeks 16–26) • Terminal sac phase (weeks 26–36) • Alveolar phase (weeks 36 to 3 years)	• Pulmonary insufficiency of prematurity • Respiratory distress syndrome (RDS) • Pulmonary interstitial emphysema (PIE) • Bronchopulmonary dysplasia (BPD)

TABLE 2: Unique anatomy and physiology in neonates.

	Unique anatomy/physiology	*Clinical implication*
Airway	• Small mandible • Large tongue • Superior laryngeal position • Soft, narrow, short trachea	Intubation is difficult
Airway resistance	Bronchi are smaller and lung volumes are smaller	Respiratory resistance is increased at birth
Lung volumes and spirometry variables	• Functional residual capacity (FRC) is similar to adult • Tidal volume (VT) is similar to adult • Minute volume is increased • Respiratory rate is increased • Expiratory reserve volume (ERV) is reduced • Closing capacity is increased • Anatomical dead space is increased (3.0 mL/kg)	• Smaller the neonate, higher the anatomical dead space and hence require higher VT to maintain ventilation • Constant distending pressure and positive end-expiratory pressure (PEEP) to maintain alveolar collapse
Compliance	• Lung compliance is decreased (less surfactant) • Chest wall compliance is increased (cartilaginous ribs) • Cylindrical thorax with horizontal ribs • Shorter course of intercostal muscles	Increased work of breathing and fatigue
Gas exchange	• Increased shunt (10–25%, due to patent ductus arteriosus) • Fetal hemoglobin = left shift of the oxygen dissociation curve (ODC) [poor affinity for 2,3-DPG (diphosphoglycerate)] • Postnatal increase in 2,3-DPG = right shift of the ODC • High oxygen-carrying capacity of blood because of higher Hb and hematocrit	• Variable tissue oxygen delivery • Preductal and postductal saturation difference posing challenge in monitoring oxygenation • Oxygen toxicity includes retinopathy
Control of respiration	Immature respiratory center, rhythmogenesis, and reflex responses: • Decreased response to hypercapnia • Paradoxical response to hypoxia	Periodic apneas and cyclical oscillating respiratory rate
Respiratory energetics	• The total oxygen consumption of the neonate is increased (6–10 mL/kg/min) • Work of breathing is increased • Ideal efficiency is at respiratory rates between 30 and 50 breaths/min • Diaphragm is more susceptible to fatigue (fewer type 1 fibers)	High respiratory rate triggered by underlying pathophysiology, resulting in fatigue and increased work of breathing

Compliance

Compliance is a measure of the change in volume (V) resulting from a given change in pressure (P) **(Table 3 and Fig. 1)**. There are two types of compliance—static (measured under static condition) and dynamic compliance (measured under clinical condition).

Preterm neonates have smaller lungs, resulting in lower compliance. Specific compliance is a measure of compliance corrected to lung volume and identical for term and adult. During transition immediately after birth,

TABLE 3: Compliance and resistance.

	Compliance	*Resistance*	*Time constant*
Definition	Change in volume of lung resulting from a unit change in pressure: C = ΔP/ΔV	Impediment of airflow offered by respiratory system: R = ΔP/Q	Time taken for the proximal airway pressure to equilibrate to the alveolar pressure
Clinical application	• Measure of distensibility of lung • Awareness of dynamic compliance is essential to alter the ventilatory parameters	• Resistance of respiratory system = Resistance of airways (60%) + Resistance of lung tissue (viscous) (40%) • Airways resistance = Resistance by nares + glottis + proximal bronchi	Knowledge of Tc can help clinicians determine the appropriate inspiratory time (I-time) and respiratory rate that will permit lung inflation and deflation to be fully complete with every breath

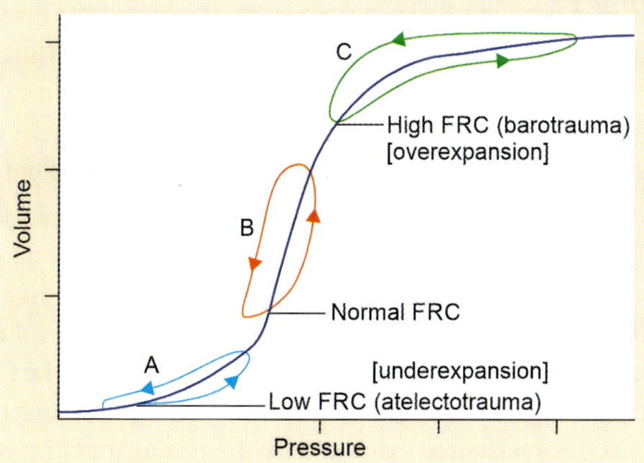

Fig. 1: Compliance curve: *Curve A:* Low FRC and atelectatic state; *Curve B:* Optimal lung recruitment; *Curve C:* High FRC and overdistended state. (FRC: functional residual capacity)

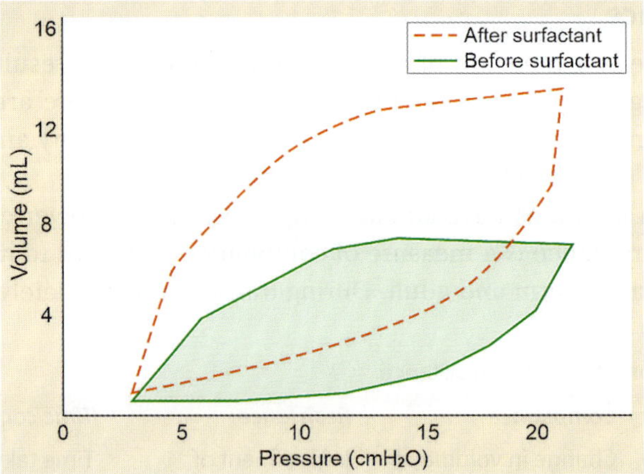

Fig. 2: Change in compliance before and after surfactant. As compliance improves for the same pressure, the volume delivered is greater; unless the pressure is reduced or volume-targeted ventilation is used, barotrauma ensues.

specific compliance is low. As the lung fluid gets absorbed, the specific compliance normalizes resulting in establishing normal FRC. However, in preterm neonates, due to poor lung compliance and highly compliant chest wall, specific compliance remains low resulting in low FRC. As a result, lung collapses, ventilation/perfusion (V/Q) mismatch ensues. A constant distending pressure is required to maintain FRC and gas exchange. Usage of compliance curve in ventilation graphs helps in optimizing positive end-expiratory pressure (PEEP) and peak inspiratory pressure (PIP), understanding the effect of surfactant use and effect of volume-targeted ventilation **(Fig. 2)**.

Clinical Connect

Recruitment of lungs and early rescue surfactant results in reducing atelectotrauma (trauma due to repeated collapse and reopening of air sacs) and oxygen induced injury. Use of volume guarantee (whenever invasive ventilation is needed) results in reduction of volutrauma and barotrauma.

Resistance

Airway resistance (R) is defined as the pressure gradient needed for the movement of gas through the airways at a constant flow rate (volume per unit of time). Inverse of resistance is conductance, and the specific conductance (conductance per unit volume) is low in neonates. There are two types of resistance—viscous resistance exhibited by the tissue, and airway resistance exhibited respiratory airways.

The radius of the tube is the most significant determinant of resistance, and Poiseuille's law states that resistance is directly proportional to the length of the tube and viscosity of the gas but inversely proportional to the fourth power of the radius in laminar flow and fifth power of radius in turbulent flow. Therefore, a reduction in the radius by half results in a 16-fold increase in resistance.

Clinical Connect

Mild airway constriction such as secretion results in significant increase in resistance. Lung recruitment reduces resistance to airflow by reducing viscous resistance. Length of endotracheal tube (ET) tube can be cut to optimize the resistance.

Time Constant

The time constant (TC) is the time taken for equilibrating proximal airways and distal alveoli. TC depends on compliance **(Box 1)** and resistance.

BOX 1: Key concepts related to compliance.

- *C20/C ratio:* Compliance of last 20% upon the total compliance and should be >0.8. This is a good measure of adequacy of PIP. Lower C20/C ratio results in beaking in lung compliance curve **(Fig. 3)**
- *Opening pressure:* During the initial phase of breathing, there is hardly any change in the volume for unit change in pressure. The alveoli tends to collapse till the pressure reaches the critical opening pressure, beyond which the compliance curve is steep
- *Closing pressure:* During the expiratory phase, as the pressure gets reduced there is little change in the volume till the pressure reaches the critical closing pressure. Beyond the closing pressure, the volume drops steeply. Pressure at critical closing pressure is always lower than the critical opening pressure due to Laplace law Laplace law states that pressure (required to keep a spherical structure open) depends on twice the surface tension divided by the radius **(Figs. 4A and B)** Radius of the alveoli is higher during expiration compared to inspiration
- *How to move the pressures from inspiratory to expiratory phase:* Optimal recruitment of lung followed by optimal PEEP to prevent collapse of alveoli moves the pressure from inspiratory to expiratory phase **(Fig. 4B)**. Recruitment depends on the inflating pressure/volume not on PEEP. PEEP is an expiratory phenomenon, which helps in preventing alveolar collapse after recruitment
- *Alveolar recruitment:* Pressure required for opening up the collapsed alveoli resulting in optimizing V/Q (ventilation/perfusion)
- *Alveolar distension:* Pressure is applied on already opened up alveoli, and this does not result in change in V/Q
- *Alveolar overdistension:* Pressure is applied on already opened up and distended alveoli, and this results in decreasing V/Q **(Figs. 5A to D)**
- *How to differentiate between alveolar recruitment and distension*: Oxygenation is the only tool which helps in differentiating alveolar recruitment and overdistension. As the pressure (MAP) is increased, at one point FiO_2 starts dropping. MAP when FiO_2 reaches 30% is the optimal MAP and indicates optimal recruitment. Once this is achieved, further increase in MAP results in impaired venous return, increase in CO_2, and increase in FiO_2 need indicating overdistension phase **(Fig. 6)**. Although the majority of lung conditions in neonates is heterogeneous, the lung recruitment strategy is protective

(FiO_2: fraction of inspired oxygen; MAP: mean airway pressure; PIP: peak inspiratory pressure; PEEP: positive end-expiratory pressure)

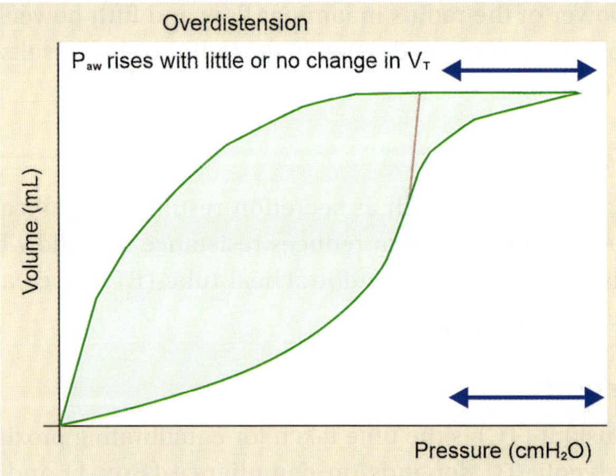

Fig. 3: C20/C: Compliance of last 20% of compliance loop/total compliance; overdistension results in beaking and lower C20/C ratio.

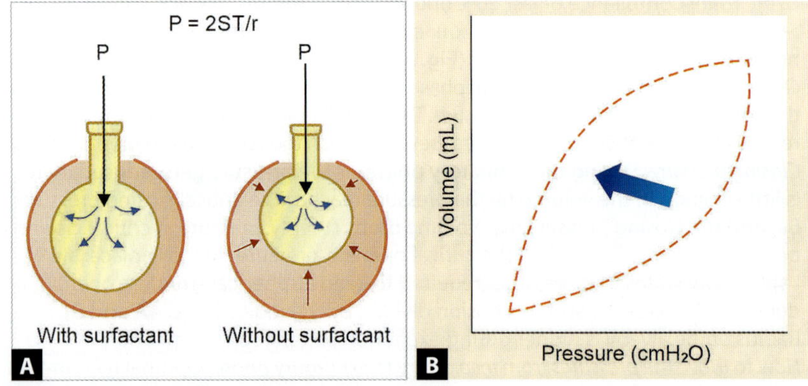

Figs. 4A and B: (A) Diagrammatic representation of the Laplace equation and the influence of (A) surfactant film and (B) alveolar radius on wall or surface tension. The magnitude (indicated by the size of the blue arrows) of airway or intra-alveolar pressure (P) required to counterbalance the propensity of alveoli to collapse (illustrated by the brown arrows) is directly proportional to twice the wall or surface tension (ST) and inversely proportional to the radius (r). Constant distending pressure is compared to "pneumatic splint." (B) Lung recruitment strategy enables ventilating with lower pressure by moving the pressure from inspiration to expiration.

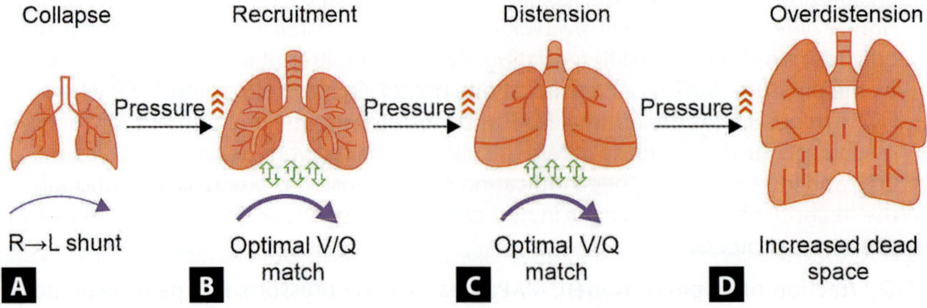

Figs. 5A to D: Effect of optimal recruitment. (V/Q: ventilation/perfusion)

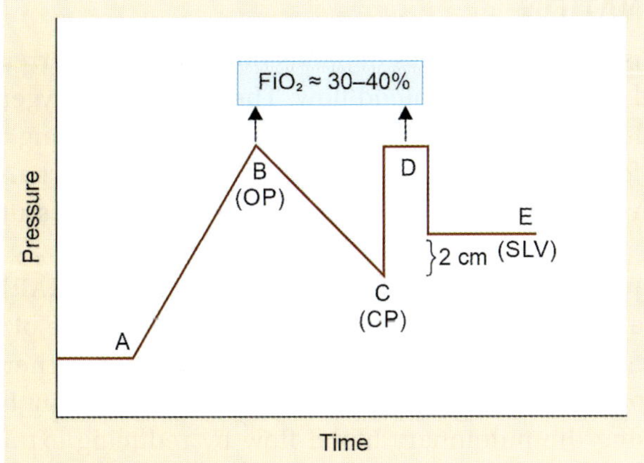

Fig. 6: Lung recruitment strategy.

- *Point A:* Lung collapsed and V/Q mismatch with high FiO_2 need
- *Point B:* Opening pressure where V/Q is optimal with lowest FiO_2
- *Point C:* Closing pressure beyond which further reduction results in MAP results in higher FiO_2
- *Point D:* Known opening pressure; MAP is increased to known opening pressure
- *Point E:* MAP 2 cm above closing pressure, which results in stabilized lung volume

(CP: closing pressure; FiO_2: fraction of inspired oxygen; MAP: mean airway pressure; OP: opening pressure; SLV: stabilized lung volume; V/Q: ventilation/perfusion)

Inspiratory time (iTime) and expiratory time (eTime) can be decided by understanding the concept of TC and in general is three times of TC. Flow graph helps in understanding the appropriate iTime and eTime.

Clinical Connect

In RDS, the lungs are stiff and poorly compliant, the time taken to equilibrate is faster, and hence the TC is less and hence requiring lower iTime and higher rate. If the resistance is high as in MAS, eTime should be kept long as TC is prolonged. Highly compliant lungs with high resistance such as bronchopulmonary dysplasia (BPD) lungs require higher iTime and a lower rate.

Work of Breathing

Work of breathing is proportional to the force generated to overcome the frictional resistance (resistance exhibited mainly by airways) and static elastic forces (compliance and elastance) that oppose lung expansion.

Clinical Connect

Resting oxygen consumption is increased in conditions such as RDS, MAS, and BPD. Mechanical ventilation reduces the WOB by reducing oxygen consumption.

OXYGENATION

Oxygen transport to the tissues depends on the oxygen-carrying capacity of the blood and the rate of blood flow. The amount of oxygen in arterial blood is called oxygen content (CaO_2) **(Box 2)**. Optimal lung recruitment is essential for efficient gas exchange and the ambient partial pressure of oxygen in alveolar space must be greater than the partial pressure of oxygen in blood.

Oxygenation depends on mean airway pressure (MAP), which in turn depends on the PIP and PEEP (area under the curve of pressure in **Figure 7**) and fraction of inspired oxygen (FiO_2). Other measures include optimizing ventilation to perfusion matching, optimizing hemoglobin, and increasing the pulmonary blood flow by reducing extrapulmonary shunts.

BOX 2: Important formula related to applied physiology.

- Compliance $C = V/P$
- Resistance $R = (P\ 1 - P\ 2)/V$
- Laplace law $P = 2 \times ST/r$
- Poiseuille's law $R\ \alpha\ L \times \eta / r^4$
- $TC = C \times R$
- WOB = Pressure (force) × Volume (displacement)
- $CaO_2 = (1.34 \times Hb \times SaO_2) + (0.003 \times PaO_2)$

(C: compliance; CaO_2: oxygen content; Hb hemoglobin; L: length; P: pressure; PaO_2: partial pressure of oxygen; R: resistance; r: radius; SaO_2: arterial oxygen saturation; ST: surface tension; TC: time constant; V: volume; WOB: work of breathing; η: viscosity)

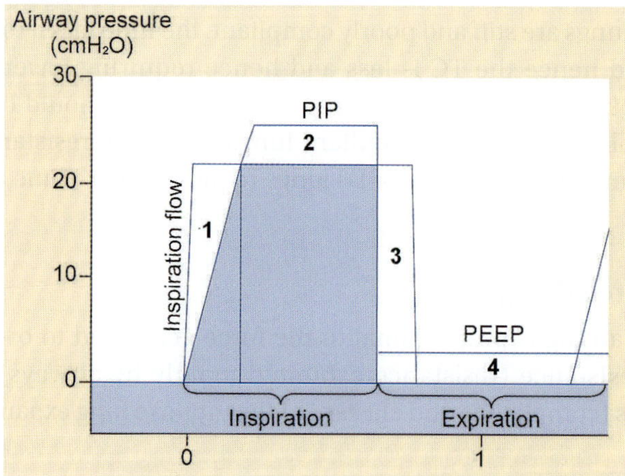

Fig. 7: Maneuvers to improve oxygenation. *Methods to improve oxygenation:* (1) Increase flow converting sine wave to square wave; (2) Increase in PIP; (3) Increase in iTime; and (4) Increase in PEEP.

Clinical Connect

Optimizing PEEP in poorly compliant lung improves oxygenation. Improvement in oxygenation can be achieved by increasing flow rate, increasing iTime (not in all conditions), increasing PIP, and PEEP.

Measures of Oxygenation

Oxygen saturation level by pulse oximetry is a simple tool, and saturation is targeted between 91 and 95%. Measures of oxygenation is summarized in **Box 3**.

VENTILATION

Ventilation is ability to wash out carbon dioxide, and it occurs due to diffusion. CO_2 exchange is 20 times more efficient than oxygen exchange. For gas exchange to occur efficiently, ventilation and perfusion must be well matched. Ventilation in healthy lungs is determined by gravity-dependent differences in interpleural or transpulmonary pressure, whereas in the sick lung, it is determined by local differences in compliance and airway resistance (TC). Key concepts are summarized in **Table 4**.

BOX 3: Measures of oxygenation.

- $A\text{-}aDO_2 = (700 \times FiO_2) - (PaCO_2 + PaO_2)$
- PF ratio = PaO_2/FiO_2
- Oxygenation index = $(MAP \times FiO_2)/PaO_2$
- Saturation index = $(MAP \times FiO_2)/SpO_2$

($A\text{-}aDO_2$: alveolar arterial diffusion gradient of oxygen; MAP: mean airway pressure; FiO_2: fraction inspired oxygen; $PaCO_2$: partial pressure CO_2; PaO_2: partial pressure of oxygen; SpO_2: pulse oximetry saturation)

TABLE 4: Key concepts on ventilation.

Parameters	*Definition*	*Normal value*
Minute ventilation (MV)	Product of VT and frequency	0.2–0.3 L/min/kg
Tidal volume (VT)	Amount of gas inspired in a single spontaneous breath or delivered through an endotracheal tube during single mechanical inflation	4–6 mL/kg
Anatomical dead space	Airways and other anatomical structure not involved in ventilation/ gas exchange	1–2 mL/kg
Anatomical and alveolar dead space	Alveolar regions not involved in gas exchange either due to disease status or due to perfusion mismatch	Variable

Clinical Connect

Minimal pressure needed to achieve the required tidal volume must be used to minimize ventilation-induced lung injury. Clinician should be mindful of changing lung compliance (e.g., postsurfactant therapy) to optimize ventilation as hypocarbia can induce cerebral hypoperfusion and ischemia. Volume-targeted ventilation is the better modality of invasive ventilation in neonates. In extreme preterm neonate, the volume target should be kept higher (6 mL/kg) to account for higher anatomical dead space.

PERFUSION

Rapid reduction in pulmonary resistance and increase in blood flow occur following delivery as the lung expands and low resistance placental circulation is terminated. Optimal lung recruitment and adequate oxygenation increases the pulmonary blood flow, whereas atelectasis as well as overdistension and hypoxia decreases the pulmonary blood flow **(Fig. 8)**. Two types of pulmonary vessels include: Alveolar vessels comprised of capillaries influenced by hydrostatic pressure and extra-alveolar vessels comprised of arteries and veins influenced by lung volume.

Clinical Connect

Optimal lung recruitment and avoidance of hypoxia are the key factors in influencing PPHN (persistent pulmonary hypertension). Whenever there is deterioration following improvement postsurfactant therapy, optimize

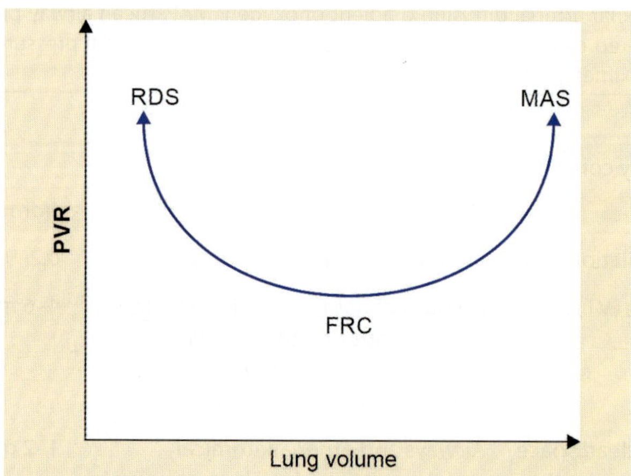

Fig. 8: Relation between FRC and PVR. The vascular architecture of the lung is designed such that PVR is minimized at FRC and increases when lung volume is diminished below FRC (respiratory distress syndrome) or augmented over FRC (MAS). (FRC: functional residual capacity; MAS: meconium aspiration syndrome; PVR: pulmonary vascular resistance)

the lung expansion as increase in pulmonary pressure occurs due to overexpansion of lungs.

CONTROL OF RESPIRATION

The respiratory control center in neonates is immature, and the ability to respond to hypoxia and hypercarbia is blunted. Factors which affect include acid-base status, temperature, sleep state, hypoxia, and medications. During rapid eye movement (REM) sleep, reduction in tone of intercostal muscles results in paradoxical movement and results in increase in WOB and muscle fatigue leading to apnea.

Clinical Connect

Methylxanthines such as caffeine acts through central stimulation, thereby optimizing ventilation. Distending pressure (invasive/noninvasive ventilation) stabilizes the compliant chest wall by providing pneumatic splint.

CARDIOPULMONARY INTERACTION

There is a continuous significant interaction between cardiac and pulmonary system in neonates **(Table 5)**. Inappropriately high MAP/PEEP results in impaired venous return and increase the pulmonary vascular resistance (PVR). Inappropriately low MAP also increases PVR.

Clinical Connect

Peak inspiratory pressure and PEEP used for optimization of lung recruitment does not cause any hemodynamic instability.

TABLE 5: Cardiopulmonary interaction.

Component	*Respiratory alteration*	*Resultant effect*
Preload	High mean arterial pressure	↓ RV preload
	High PVR secondary to overdistension/atelectasis	↓ LV preload
Contractility	High PVR secondary to overdistension/atelectasis	↓ RV contractility
	Acidosis secondary to permissive hypercapnia	• ↓ Contractility • *Additional effect:* Cerebral reperfusion injury
Afterload	High PVR secondary to overdistension/atelectasis	↑ RV afterload
	Positive intrathoracic pressure	↓ LV afterload, improves left atrial return

(LV: left ventricle; PVR: pulmonary vascular resistance; RV right ventricle)

PHYSIOLOGICAL PRINCIPLES AND MECHANISM IN NONINVASIVE VENTILATION

Primary Mechanism in Noninvasive Ventilation

The primary mechanism of action of noninvasive ventilation (NIV) **(Flowchart 1)** in neonates includes improvement in FRC, reduce WOB, and dead-space washout.

Physiological Reflexes in Respiratory Support

Physiological reflexes involved in NIV include the following:

Hering–Breuer Reflex Mechanism

The Hering-Breuer reflex is a defensive mechanism that inhibits excessive lung expansion. Upon stimulation of lung stretch receptors by expansion, inhibitory signals are transmitted to respiratory centers through the vagus nerve, facilitating exhale.

Clinical connect: In continuous positive airway pressure (CPAP), positive pressure maintains alveolar patency and moderate inflation, facilitating the Hering-Breuer reflex, which can regulate respiratory patterns and avert excessive lung inflation.

Head's Paradoxical Reflex Mechanism

Head's paradoxical reflex functions as the antithesis of Hering-Breuer reflex. Stimulation of lung stretch receptors facilitates further inhalation rather than cessation, enabling a more profound breath.

Clinical connect: Nasal intermittent positive pressure ventilation (NIPPV) can enhance this reflex, promoting alveolar recruitment, enhancing lung expansion, and augmenting oxygenation.

Flowchart 1: Mechanism of NIV.

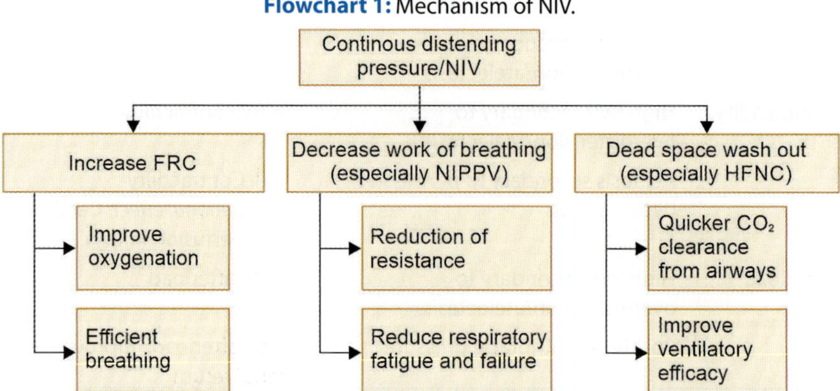

(FRC: functional residual capacity; HFNC: high-flow nasal cannula; NIV: noninvasive ventilation; NIPPV: nasal intermittent positive pressure ventilation)

Principles of Fluid Dynamics in Continuous Positive Airway Pressure and Noninvasive Ventilation

Principles of fluid dynamics in NIV include the following:

Coandă Effect

Mechanism: Coandă effect refers to the propensity of a fluid stream, such as airflow, to cling to adjacent curved surface. When airflow is channeled along a curved surface, it generates a low-pressure zone that attracts the stream toward the surface, enabling precise airflow direction.

Clinical connect: Coandă effect in CPAP and high-frequency ventilation can effectively direct airflow to targeted lung regions, minimizing turbulence and enhancing gas delivery to areas with partial collapse or increased ventilation–perfusion mismatch.

Fluidic flip: The fluidic flip utilizes the Coandă effect to redirect a fluid stream among multiple stable paths by inducing minor alterations in the surrounding pressure **(Figs. 9A and B)**.

Clinical connect: In flow-driven CPAP, the fluidic flip mechanism facilitates swift transitions between inspiratory and expiratory phases without the use of mechanical valves. This delivers regular, short breaths at elevated frequency, facilitating accurate and efficient ventilation while reducing the risk of lung injury.

A good understanding of fundamental principles on mechanics of respiration is needed for ventilating a neonate successfully. Lung mechanics can be different according to the disease and highly heterogeneous in different regions, especially during disease states.

Various lung mechanics in diseased status are summarized in **Table 6**.

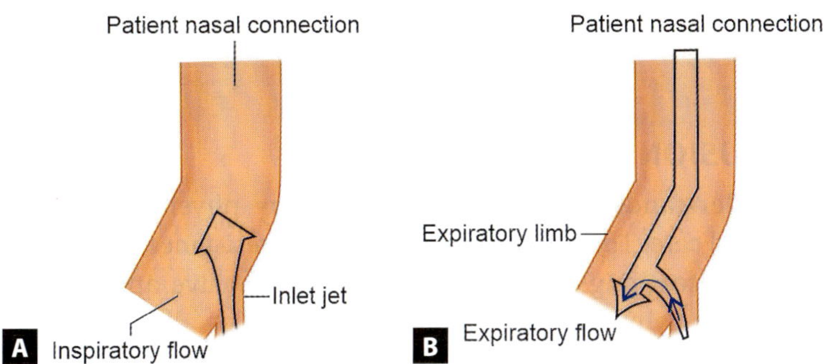

Figs. 9A and B: Coandă effect and fluidic flip. (A) During inspiration, if the infant inhales additional gas, the mechanism draws gas from the exhaust channel via the Venturi effect; (B) During exhalation, the device employs the Coandă effect and the fluidic-flip mechanism to redirect the gas jet to the exhaust channel.

TABLE 6: Summary of lung mechanics in various diseased status.

Diseased states	*Compliance*	*Resistance*	*Time constant*	*Clinical implications in invasive ventilation*	*Applied physiologic principles in noninvasive*
Respiratory distress syndrome	Reduced	Normal	Reduced inspiratory time constant	Rapid respiratory rates, ↑ PEEP	Laplace law Hering–Breuer reflex
Meconium aspiration syndrome	Reduced	Increased	Increased expiratory time constant	Air trapping, air leak, lower rates, adequate Te	
TTN (transient tachypnea of newborn)	Reduced	Normal	Normal	Adequate pressures [positive end-expiratory pressure (PEEP)] to drive out the fluid	Hering–Breuer reflex
BPD (broncho-pulmonary dysplasia)	Reduced lung compliance and increased airway compliance	Increased	Increased time constant	Lower respiratory rates, ↑ PEEP	
Apnea of prematurity/ central nervous system (CNS) pathology	Normal	Normal	Normal		Heads paradoxical reflex

CONCLUSION

A clear understanding of neonatal respiratory physiology is vital for individualized care. The interplay of compliance, resistance, time constants, and work of breathing guides optimal use of invasive and noninvasive ventilation. Applying these physiological principles allows clinicians to minimize lung injury, maintain hemodynamic stability, and improve both immediate and long-term outcomes in sick newborns.

SUGGESTED READING

1. Chakkarapani AA, Adappa R, Mohammad Ali SK, Gupta S, Soni NB, Chicoine L, et al. "Current concepts of mechanical ventilation in neonates" - Part 1: Basics. Int J Pediatr Adolesc Med. 2020;7(1):13-8.
2. Cheifetz IM: Cardiorespiratory interactions: the relationship between mechanical ventilation and hemodynamics. Respir Care. 2014;59:1937-45.
3. Keszler M, Suresh GK (Eds). Goldsmith's Assisted Ventilation of the Neonate: An Evidence-based Approach to Newborn Respiratory Care. Elsevier; 2022.
4. Neumann, Roland P, Britta S. von Ungern-Sternberg. "The neonatal lung–physiology and ventilation." Pediatr Anesth. 2014;24.1:10-21.
5. Ryan DP, Mychaliska GB. Neonatal pulmonary physiology. Semin Pediatr Surg. 2013;22(4).

SECTION

Noninvasive Respiratory Support

CHAPTER

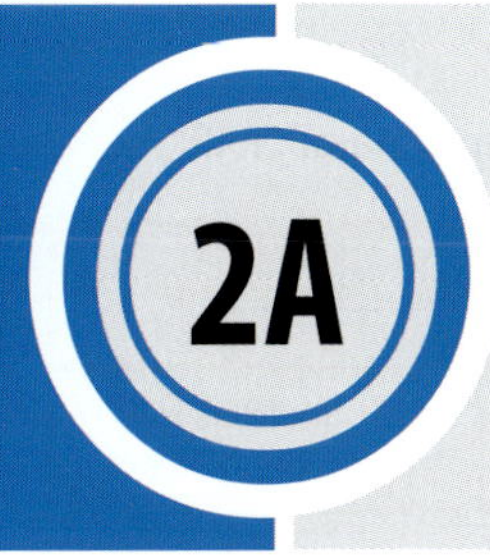

Art of Using Continuous Positive Airway Pressure

Rohit Sasidharan, Neeraj Gupta

INTRODUCTION

Nasal continuous positive airway pressure (nCPAP) is a commonly used form of noninvasive respiratory support in neonates. It has become the standard care in preterm neonates with respiratory distress. With the advancement of technology and a better understanding of the physiology behind respiratory diseases in neonates, there is a shift toward a noninvasive form of ventilation and earlier initiation of nCPAP in the delivery room (DR).

MECHANISM OF ACTION

It is the application of continuous pressure during both inspiration and expiration in a spontaneously breathing neonate. It keeps the alveoli open and recruits them, resulting in improved functional residual capacity (FRC) apart from splinting the airways and the chest wall. This decreases the work of breathing and improves gas exchange at the alveolar level. It also enhances the production and cycling of surfactants **(Flowchart 1)**.

EVIDENCE OF CLINICAL USE

The three distinct indications of nCPAP in neonates are as shown follows:
1. Primary treatment of respiratory distress
2. Apnea of prematurity (AOP)
3. Postextubation support

Primary Treatment of Respiratory Distress Syndrome

CPAP versus No CPAP (Supportive Care/Hood Oxygen)

A meta-analysis evaluating CPAP versus spontaneous breathing with supplemental oxygen if necessary, using head box oxygen or low flow nasal cannula for respiratory distress syndrome (RDS) among preterm infants has demonstrated a reduced risk of treatment failure, mortality, combined mortality and treatment failure with an increased risk for pneumothorax. **Table 1** depicts the results of the Cochrane review regarding using nasal CPAP as a primary mode of respiratory support.

Flowchart 1: Physiology behind the mechanism of action of nasal CPAP.

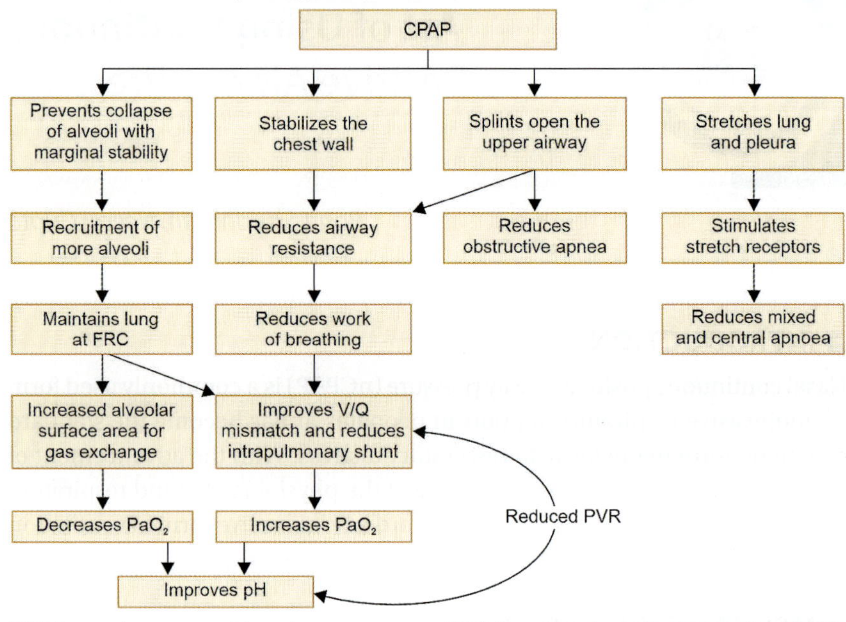

(CPAP: continuous positive airway pressure; FRC: functional residual capacity; $PaCO_2$: partial pressure of arterial carbon dioxide; PaO_2: partial pressure of arterial oxygen; PVR: pulmonary vascular resistance)

Source: Sankar MJ, Sankar J, Agarwal R, Paul VK, Deorari AK. Protocol for administering continuous positive airway pressure in neonates. Indian J Pediatr. 2008;75(5):471-8.

TABLE 1: CPAP for respiratory support in preterm infants.

Outcome measures	*Effect size with 95% CI*	*Remarks*
CPAP versus supplemental oxygen alone as a primary support for respiratory distress in preterm neonates		
Treatment failure (death/use of additional ventilatory support)	RR 0.64 (0.50–0.82)	Five studies, 322 infants, very low certainty of evidence
Mortality	RR 0.53 (0.34–0.84)	Five studies, 322 infants, moderate certainty of evidence
Need for assisted ventilation	RR 0.72 (0.54–0.96)	Five studies, 322 infants, very low certainty of evidence
Pneumothorax	RR 2.91 (1.38–6.13)	Four studies, 274 infants, low certainty of evidence
BPD (oxygen dependency at 28 days)	RR 1.04 (0.35–3.13)	Two studies, 209 infants, very low certainty of evidence

Contd...

Contd...

Outcome measures	*Effect size with 95% CI*	*Remarks*
Delivery room/very early initiation of CPAP versus supplemental oxygen by oxygen hood/prongs		
Treatment failure	RR 0.60 (0.49–0.74)	Four studies, 765 infants, very low certainty of evidence
BPD at 36 weeks	RR 0.76 (0.51–1.14)	Three studies, 683 infants, moderate certainty of evidence
Mortality	RR 1.04 (0.56–1.93)	Four studies, 765 infants, moderate certainty of evidence
Combined mortality or BPD	RR 0.69 (0.40–1.19)	One study, 256 infants, low certainty of evidence
Pneumothorax	RR 0.75 (0.35–1.16)	Three studies, 568 infants, low certainty of evidence
Grade 3 or 4 IVH	RR 0.96 (0.39–2.37)	In two studies, 468 infants, moderate certainty of evidence
Delivery room/very early initiation of CPAP versus mechanical ventilation		
Treatment failure	RR 0.49 (0.45–0.54)	In two studies, 1,042 infants, moderate certainty of evidence
BPD at 36 weeks	RR 0.89 (0.80–0.99)	Three studies, 2,150 infants, moderate certainty of evidence
Mortality	RR 0.82 (0.66–1.03)	Three studies, 2,358 infants, moderate certainty of evidence
Combined mortality or BPD	RR 0.89 (0.81–0.97)	Three studies, 2,358 infants, moderate certainty of evidence
Pneumothorax	RR 1.24 (0.91–1.69)	Three studies, 2,357 infants, low certainty of evidence
Grade 3 or 4 IVH	RR 1.09 (0.86–1.39)	Three studies, 2,301 infants, moderate certainty of evidence
Nasal CPAP versus no CPAP for postextubation respiratory support		
Extubation failure	RR 0.62 (0.51–0.76)	Nine studies, 726 infants, low certainty of evidence
Endotracheal reintubation	RR 0.79 (0.64–0.98)	Nine studies, 726 infants, very low certainty of evidence
BPD	RR 0.89 (0.47–1.68)	One study, 92 infants, very low certainty of evidence

(BPD: bronchopulmonary dysplasia; CI: confidence interval; CPAP: continuous positive airway pressure; IVH: intraventricular hemorrhage; RR: relative risk)

Delivery Room/Very Early CPAP

Recent guidelines (European Consensus Guidelines on the Management of Respiratory Distress Syndrome, 2022 update) recommend early initiation of nasal CPAP as early as in the DR. Applying early CPAP (DR CPAP) prevents alveolar collapse and promotes surfactant production and recycling, thereby reducing lung injury. Many landmark trials have compared DR CPAP with conventional approaches (intubation, prophylactic surfactant, and mechanical ventilation) among extreme preterm neonates, such as the COIN trial (2008), SUPPORT trial (2010), and VON DRM trial (2011). Most of these studies concluded that early stabilization of preterm neonates with DR CPAP can lessen the need for surfactant administration and mechanical ventilation by almost 40–50%. The results of a Cochrane meta-analysis that compared DR CPAP (prophylactic/within 1 hour CPAP) with supportive care (supplemental oxygen delivered by head box or standard nasal cannula) or mechanical ventilation among preterm neonates with respiratory distress are depicted in **Table 1**.

Apnea of Prematurity

Nasal CPAP is widely used for the management of AOP among preterm infants, along with methylxanthines as an adjuvant therapy. By splinting the upper airways, preventing them from collapsing and stretching the upper airways, and stimulating various receptors for respiration, CPAP has been found effective in managing AOP. In a small single center cross over trial comparing nasal intermittent positive pressure ventilation (NIPPV) via a conventional ventilator, NIPPV and nCPAP via a variable flow device, and nCPAP delivered via a constant flow underwater bubble system concluded that variable flow devices are better than underwater bubble CPAP systems in reducing the risk of AOP with median [interquartile range (IQR)] event rates per hour being 2.8 (1.5–7.7) and 5.4 (3.0–9.8) in variable flow CPAP and constant flow bubble CPAP, respectively. A recently published Cochrane review could not find any randomized controlled trials (RCTs) that directly compared nasal CPAP with supportive care alone for the management of apnea, and it would be ethically not possible to conduct such a study in the current era.

Postextubation Failure

Nasal CPAP has been used routinely in preterm neonates postextubation to prevent extubation failure. It acts by preventing postextubation atelectasis and apneas and has been found effective in decreasing extubation failure. **Table 1** depicts the latest evidence from a recent Cochrane review on nasal CPAP versus no CPAP for postextubation respiratory support.

CONTINUOUS POSITIVE AIRWAY PRESSURE AND SURFACTANT

Early initiation of CPAP with selective surfactant administration for preterm neonates with signs of RDS has been recommended in preterm neonates. The "Intubation-Surfactant-Extubation (INSURE)" technique in which surfactant is administered as a bolus into the trachea through an endotracheal tube followed by brief bag ventilation and rapid extubation to CPAP has been practiced widely and seemed to reduce lung injury. However, newer, less invasive surfactant administration (LISA) or minimally invasive surfactant technique (MIST) using thin catheters and in small aliquots, without the need for bag ventilation while maintaining spontaneous breathing on a CPAP has been associated with a lesser need for mechanical ventilation and reduction in the combined outcome of death/bronchopulmonary dysplasia (BPD) on head-to-head comparison with INSURE technique. **Table 2** depicts the latest evidence comparing the use of a thin catheter for surfactant administration with the standard INSURE technique.

COMPONENTS OF CONTINUOUS POSITIVE AIRWAY PRESSURE DEVICE

The physiological purpose behind CPAP is similar to the mechanism of grunting in newborns with respiratory distress. By exhaling against a closed glottis, the neonate tends to prevent the alveoli from collapse, thus maintaining FRC. There are many sophisticated devices available which can be used to provide CPAP in neonates. The components required to provide nasal CPAP for neonates are tabulated in **Table 3** and **Figure 1**.

TABLE 2: Less invasive surfactant administration (LISA) versus INSURE for respiratory distress syndrome.

Outcome measures	*Effect size*	*Remarks*
Mechanical ventilation within 72 hours	RR 0.60 (0.47–0.76)	Fourteen studies, 1,599 infants
BPD among survivors	RR 0.65 (0.51–0.82)	Thirteen studies, 1,758 infants
Pneumothorax	RR 0.60 (0.38–0.96)	Nine studies, 1,093 infants
PIVH	RR 0.77 (0.54–1.10)	Thirteen studies, 1,776 infants
Death during hospitalization	RR 0.76 (0.58–1.00)	Thirteen studies, 1,588 infants

(BPD: bronchopulmonary dysplasia; INSURE: Intubation-Surfactant-Extubation; PIVH: peri/intraventricular hemorrhage; RR: relative risk)

TABLE 3: Components of continuous positive airway pressure (CPAP).

Component	*Remarks*
Source of air and oxygen	A source of a continuous flow of warm, humidified blended air-oxygen mixture is required for delivering nasal CPAP. This can be achieved either from a compressed source or centralized source of air and oxygen
Air oxygen blender	This can be achieved by an air-oxygen blender to mix the pressured gases to get the desired level of oxygen concentration [fraction of inspired oxygen (FiO_2)]
A servo-controlled humidifier	For warming and humidification, i.e., by passing the blended mixture of gases through a servo-controlled humidifier to achieve a temperature of 37°C and 100% relative humidity for the inspired mixture of gases
Pressure generator	This component generates the pressure. These are of two types: 1. Constant flow devices 2. Variable flow devices The commonly used constant flow devices are the bubble CPAP and ventilatory CPAP devices • *Ventilator CPAP:* Here the expiratory valve generates the continuous CPAP pressure in the circuit • *Bubble CPAP:* Here the positive pressure is offered by the far end of the expiratory limb immersed in a column of water. The pressure is adjusted by altering the height of the immersed water column Variable flow devices provide a differential flow of incoming gases, which depends on the respiratory cycle phase of the spontaneously breathing neonate • Flow-driven CPAP devices have an integrated nasal interface and pressure generator and use higher gas flow than other devices. These devices allow variable flow and a fluid-flip mechanism, allowing greater gas flow during inspiration than expiration, thereby decreasing the work of breathing
Nasal interface	The following interfaces are commonly used in neonates: • Short binasal prongs • Nasal masks • Nasal cannula with long and narrow tubing (RAM cannula) Traditionally, short binasal prongs used to be the most commonly used interface. Due to their effectiveness, they replaced the older interfaces, namely, single nasal and nasopharyngeal prongs. Recently, nasal masks have emerged as the most favored interface devices due to their efficacy and less association with nasal injury **(Table 4)**. Rotation of nasal interfaces has also been shown to be effective in decreasing nasal injury

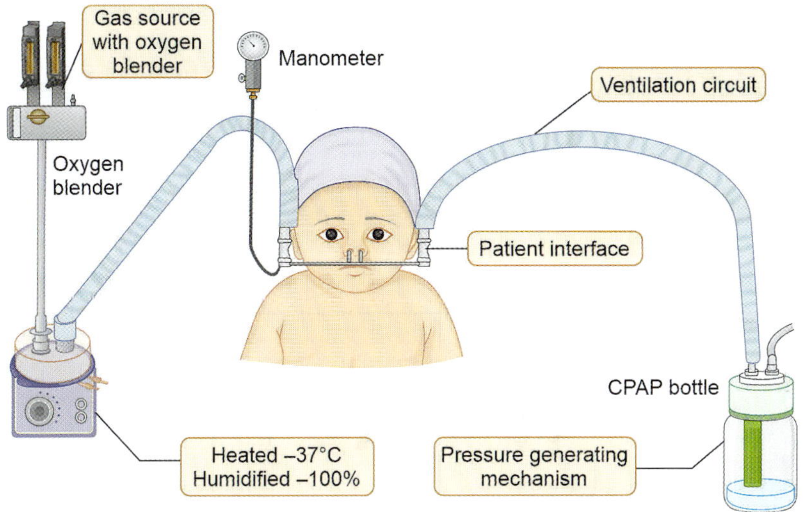

Fig. 1: Components of bubble continuous positive airway pressure (CPAP).

TABLE 4: Comparison of nasal mask versus nasal prongs for CPAP delivery in neonates.

Outcome measures	*Effect size*	*Remarks*
Treatment failure	RR 0.72 (0.58–0.90)	Eight trials, 919 infants, low certainty of evidence
Mortality during hospitalization	RR 0.83 (0.56–1.22)	Seven trials, 814 infants, low certainty of evidence
Moderate to severe nasal injury	RR 0.55 (0.44–0.71)	Ten trials, 1,058 infants, low certainty of evidence
Pneumothorax	RR 0.93 (0.45–1.93)	Five trials, 625 infants, low certainty of evidence
BPD among survivors	RR 0.69 (0.46–1.03)	Seven trials, 843 infants, very low certainty of evidence

(BPD: bronchopulmonary dysplasia; CPAP: continuous positive airway pressure; RR: relative risk)

PRACTICAL ASPECTS OF NASAL CONTINUOUS POSITIVE AIRWAY PRESSURE

The CPAP is initiated in neonates with moderate to severe respiratory distress as shown in **Figure 2** (Silverman Anderson score >3). While applying nasal CPAP, maintaining an adequate seal is essential for effectively delivering the CPAP pressure. Use the appropriately sized nasal mask, prongs or cannula as per the manufacturer's instructions using the various job aid kits provided. As discussed earlier, start CPAP early, preferably in the DR. The "rule of 5" gives a reasonable direction to start the bubble CPAP with a flow of 5 L/min, water

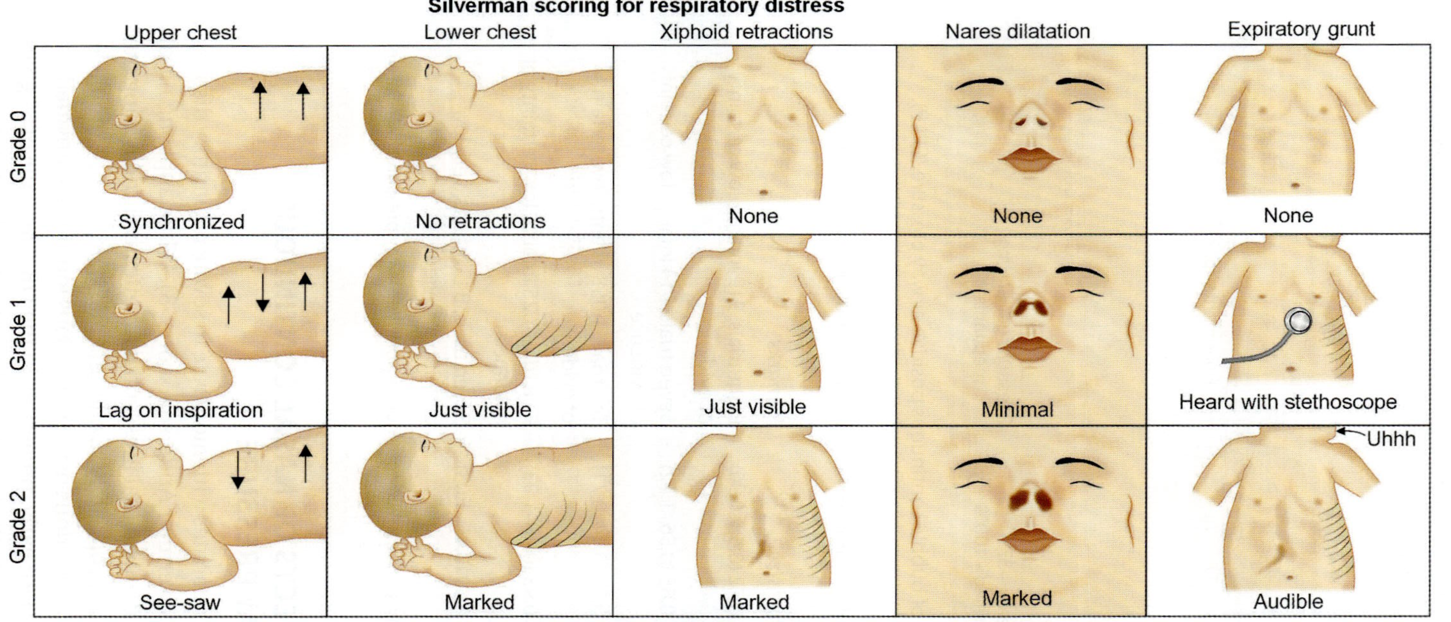

Downe's score for respiratory distress

Score	0	1	2
Respiratoy rate	<60	60–80	>80
Central cyanosis	None	None of FiO_2 of 40%	None of 40% FiO_2
Retractions	None	Mild	Severe
Grunt	None	Minimal	Obvious
Air entry	Good	Fair	Poor

Fig. 2: Clinical monitoring of respiratory distress in neonates. (FiO_2: fraction of inspired oxygen)
Source: Deorari A, Kumar P, Murki S (Eds). Workbook on CPAP Science, Evidence and Pratice Learner's Guide, 5th edition. India: Noble Vision (Medical Book Publishers); 2020.

column of 5 cm height as a primary support for neonates with respiratory distress. The usual initial fraction of inspired oxygen (FiO_2) is between 25 and 30% in most of the cases. The flow is adjusted in a bubble CPAP to ensure minimal continuous bubbling during both inspiratory and expiratory phase and is automatically set in the ventilator CPAP. The need for flow >7 L/m to ensure bubbling in the water chamber usually suggests a leak in the circuit or at the interface level. The FiO_2 is adjusted between 21 and 60% to maintain the oxygen saturation (SpO_2) target of 90–95%. Further bedside titration and algorithmic approach for escalation and weaning of CPAP support have been illustrated in **Figure 3**.

NURSING AND SUPPORTIVE CARE

Nursing care for neonates on nasal CPAP is very important for favorable outcomes. Any newborn supported on CPAP needs three-phased monitoring: (1) Monitoring of the patient for the adequacy of CPAP settings and for assessing the complications, (2) monitoring of the CPAP machine for leaks, water condensation, the water level in the bubble chamber, and the humidifier, and (3) the interface for nasal injury, nasal block, and appropriateness of CPAP and interface size and fixation. Supportive care during CPAP includes providing developmentally supportive care, orogastric tube insertion for stomach decompression and feeding, and monitoring for clinical distress and complications related to CPAP **(Figs. 4A to C)**.

COMPLICATIONS OF NASAL CONTINUOUS POSITIVE AIRWAY PRESSURE

Administration of CPAP may be associated with the following complications as shown in **Table 5**.

IMPROVING CONTINUOUS POSITIVE AIRWAY PRESSURE SUCCESS RATE

The following steps and precautions have been associated with improved outcome of neonates with respiratory distress:

- Use of antenatal steroids
- Initiate CPAP early, preferably in the DR
- Use of selective surfactant therapy for preterm neonates with RDS
- Use less invasive methods of surfactant administration whenever possible
- Optimize the FRC using CPAP pressure up to 7–8 cm while managing a preterm neonate with respiratory distress to recruit the alveoli
- Use nasal prongs or mask as an interface and ensure adequate seal
- Diligent nursing care to ensure proper application of CPAP interface, clinical monitoring of the patient, machine and nasal interface, and good supportive care
- Doing “audits” and undertaking quality improvement initiatives to fix the problems by taking care of contextual issues.

Application of bubble CPAP for newborn

Indications:
Respiratory distress:
- Preterm infants (Gestation <35 weeks): SAS score >3
- Term infants (Gestation >35 weeks): SAS score >5
- Recurrent apneas in a preterm infant
- Postextubation in VLBW infant

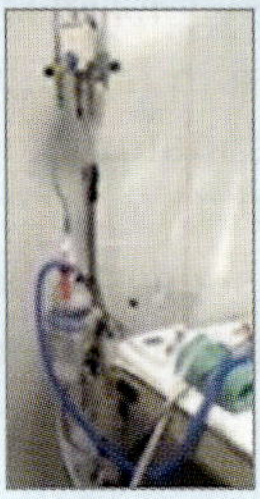

Contraindications:
- Poor respiratory efforts
- Nasal seal poor (Cleft Palate)
- Tracheoesophageal fistula and congenital diaphragmatic hernia
- Pnuemothorax and other air leaks

Preparation of machine and interface:
- Assemble the sterile circuit
- Fill distilled water in humidifier and clean water in bubble chamber
- Connect air and oxygen to blender, switch on the humidifier
- Fix the cap to the baby and appropriated size prongs to the cap
- Connect interface to the sterile circuit

Initiation of CPAP

	Preterm infants with RD	Recurrent apnea	Postextubation
Initial setting	CPAP: 5 cm FiO_2: 25–30% Flow: 5 liter/min	CPAP: 4 to 5 cm FiO_2: <25% Flow: 5 liter/min	CPAP: 5 cm FiO_2: As on MV Flow: 5 liter/min

Adjustment of FiO_2 and CPAP pressure

Increase CPAP in steps of 1 cm:
- If retractions++ and SpO_2 <90% and chest X-ray (1/2 hour after starting) <6 spaces

Increase FiO_2 in steps of 5%:
- If mild or no retractions and SpO_2 <90%
- For every 10% increase in FiO_2 assess the need for increase in CPAP pressure by 1 cm

No change in CPAP or FiO_2 is required if baby is comfortable, minimal or no retractions, CFT and BP are normal, SpO_2 between 90 to 95%, bubbling is good and breath sounds are heard

Nursing care and monitoring
- Ensure correct size and fixation of nasal prongs
- Ensure gap between columella and nasal prongs
- Fix the prongs to cap and cover ears with cap
- Remove prongs, inspect nostrils, use saline drops if needed and do gentle massage in each shift
- Ensure water level in bubble chamber and Humidifier
- Record depth of immersion of expiratory limb
- Maintain monitoring sheet

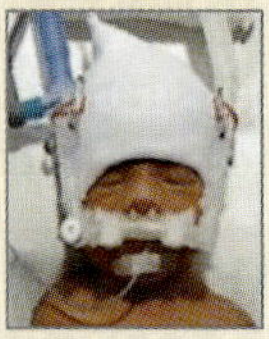

Weaning of CPAP

CPAP and FiO_2:
- Reduce FiO_2 if SpO_2 >95% in steps of 59%
- If FiO_2 reduced by 10% and retractions are mild or absent, reduce CPAP pressure by 1 cm till CPAP is 5 cm and FiO_2 is 50%
- Subsequently reduce FiO_2 in steps of 5% till FiO_2 <30% before reducing CPAP pressure from 5 cm to 4 cm of water
- Remove CPAP if FiO_2 is <25% and CPAP is 4 cm

Failure of CPAP or need for MV
- SpO_2 <90% on FiO_2 >70% and CPAP >7 cm
- Moderate to severe retractions on CPAP >7 cm
- Recurrent apneas
- Shock or multiorgan dysfunction
- Poor respiratory efforts or $PaCO_2$ >60 mm Hg

Fig. 3: Practical aspects of application of CPAP. (BP: blood pressure; CPAP: continuous positive airway pressure; FiO_2: fraction of inspired oxygen; MV: mechanical ventilation; $PaCO_2$: partial pressure of arterial carbon dioxide; RD: respiratory distress; SpO_2: oxygen saturation; VLBW: very low birth weight)

Source: Deorari A, Kumar P, Murki S (Eds). Workbook on CPAP Science, Evidence and Pratice Learner's Guide, 5th edition. India: Noble Vision (Medical Book Publishers); 2020.

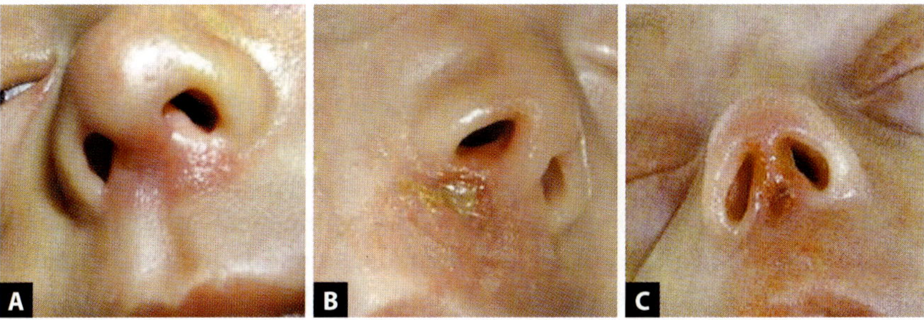

Figs. 4A to C: Staging of nasal injury. (A) Grade 1; (B) Grade 2; (C) Grade 3.
Source: Gautam G, Gupta N, Sasidharan R, Thanigainathan S, Yadav B, Singh K, et al. Systematic rotation versus continuous application of 'nasal prongs' or 'nasal mask' in preterm infants on nCPAP: a randomized controlled trial. Eur J Pediatr. 2023;182(6):2645-54.

TABLE 5: Complications and preventive solutions of using nasal continuous positive airway pressure (nCPAP).

Complication	*Remarks*	*Prevention*
Nasal injury	Continuous pressure over the skin of the nose can damage the skin and columella region	• Use of appropriately sized nasal interfaces • Using a nasal mask interface over nasal prongs or alternate rotation of interfaces may be helpful • Use of barrier protection material at the point of contact • Coconut oil applications can also be used as a strategy to prevent it
Air leaks	There is an increased incidence of air leaks compared to supportive care alone	Avoid excessive pressures and flow
CPAP belly	Abdominal distention secondary to gaseous distention of the intestine can present as feed intolerance	Decompress the stomach with an orogastric tube and allow the tube to be kept open for some time in between feeds
Cardiac	Excess CPAP pressure can decrease the cardiac output and can cause shock	Avoid excessive pressures and monitor for signs of hemodynamic instability
Sepsis	Data suggests that even nCPAP can also lead to infection	Follow all aseptic precautions

CONCLUSION

India contributes to a major chunk of preterm births in this world and respiratory distress is one of the most common reasons for mortality among this cohort. This is compounded by lack of antenatal supervision, poor antenatal steroid coverage, home deliveries, delayed resuscitation, lack of intensive care unit (ICU) facilities and issues with neonatal transportation. A holistic approach is required for the management of preterm neonates, and providing adequate respiratory support at birth is important to improve the outcomes. The use of antenatal steroids, early initiation of nasal CPAP for preterm infants with respiratory distress, selective surfactant administration, and good nursing care can go a long way in optimizing the outcomes among preterm neonates.

SUGGESTED READING

1. Ho JJ, Subramaniam P, Davis PG. Continuous positive airway pressure (CPAP) for respiratory distress in preterm infants. Cochrane Database Syst Rev. 2020;10(10):CD002271.
2. Ramaswamy VV, Abiramalatha T, Bandyopadhyay T, Shaik NB, Pullattayil S AK, Cavallin F, et al. Delivery room CPAP in improving outcomes of preterm neonates in low-and middle-income countries: A systematic review and network meta-analysis. Resuscitation. 2022;170:250-63.
3. Silveira RC, Panceri C, Munõz NP, Carvalho MB, Fraga AC, Procianoy RS. Less invasive surfactant administration versus intubation-surfactant-extubation in the treatment of neonatal respiratory distress syndrome: a systematic review and meta-analyses. J Pediatr (Rio J). 2024;100(1):8-24.
4. Subramaniam P, Ho JJ, Davis PG. Prophylactic or very early initiation of continuous positive airway pressure (CPAP) for preterm infants. Cochrane Database Syst Rev. 2021;10(10):CD001243.
5. Sweet DG, Carnielli VP, Greisen G, Hallman M, Klebermass-Schrehof K, Ozek E, et al. European Consensus Guidelines on the Management of Respiratory Distress Syndrome: 2022 Update. Neonatology. 2023;120(1):3-23.

CHAPTER

Art of Using Nasal Intermittent Positive Pressure Ventilation

Bijan Saha

INTRODUCTION

Respiratory distress is the most common encountered disease presentation in newborns and employing optimal ventilation strategies is crucial for effectively managing these infants. Over the past few decades, noninvasive ventilation (NIV) has progressively replaced invasive mechanical ventilation (IMV). Early initiation of nasal continuous positive airway pressure (CPAP) for respiratory distress syndrome (RDS) is now recommended. Despite the physiological and clinical advantages, the rate of CPAP failure remains around 50% during the first week of life in extremely preterm infants necessitating additional support. Consequently, there has been growing interest in other modes of noninvasive respiratory support.

DEFINITION

Noninvasive intermittent positive pressure ventilation (NIPPV) is a noninvasive mode of respiratory support that provides intermittent increases in pressure levels, known as peak inspiratory pressure (PIP), superimposed on a baseline positive end-expiratory pressure (PEEP), which is similar to CPAP, with or without synchronization with neonatal breaths and delivered using nasal masks or short nasal bi prongs. In simple words, if endotracheal tube (ET) tube is replaced with a mask or prong, it mimics invasive ventilation.

The NIPPV serves as an intermediate approach between invasive ventilation with an ET and noninvasive CPAP. The other terminologies for NIPPV are nasal intermittent mandatory ventilation (N-IMV) or noninvasive pressure support ventilation (NI-PSV).

SYNCHRONIZED VERSUS NONSYNCHRONIZED NASAL INTERMITTENT POSITIVE-PRESSURE VENTILATION

The NIPPV can be administered in two different ways in relation to synchronizing with an infant's spontaneous breaths:

1. *Nonsynchronized NIPPV (nsNIPPV):* The additional airway pressure is not coordinated with the infant's spontaneous breaths. In nsNIPPV, asynchronous breaths delivered late in the inspiratory phase or during the

patient's expiratory phase can disrupt the spontaneous breathing pattern and may even cause glottic closure, potentially redirecting gas flow to the stomach. Studies indicate that only 10–15% of breaths delivered during nsNIPPV are synchronous with patients' efforts.

2. *Synchronized NIPPV (sNIPPV):* The additional peak airway pressure is coordinated with the baby's spontaneous breaths, similar to synchronization in a ventilator. Four types of triggering devices are employed to achieve synchronization in NIPPV as mentioned in **Table 1**.

Clinical data directly comparing sNIPPV and nsNIPPV are scarce. While some studies have indicated physiological advantages of sNIPPV compared to nsNIPPV, critical clinical outcomes remain lacking. Surveys indicate that the majority of centers employing NIPPV utilize the nonsynchronized mode. **Table 2** enumerates the devices commonly used to deliver NIPPV.

TABLE 1: Triggering devices used for synchronized NIPPV.

Abdominal capsule (Graseby capsule)	• Detects spontaneous efforts by sensing abdominal movements • High spontaneous breathing rates, frequently seen in premature infants, are linked to trigger delays and decreased consistency in trigger response
Pressure trigger devices	• These devices deliver a breath in response to a decrease in pressure that accompanies a patient's inspiratory effort • Pressure trigger devices are unsuitable for use in preterm neonates because of their weak respiratory drive
Flow trigger device	• A pneumotachograph (placed between the nasal prongs and Y-piece), when attached to software can detect sudden changes in flow during inspiratory efforts • Not considered entirely reliable for noninvasive ventilation in neonates due to the potential impact of variable leaks at the mouth and nose on its effectiveness • The device requires frequent calibration and changes in gas temperature, humidity, and water condensation can affect performance
NAVA trigger device	• In NIV-NAVA, respiratory assistance is triggered by the detection of the diaphragmatic electrical signal, recorded by a specialized catheter (nasogastric tube with embedded electrical sensors) • The level of pressure support provided is adjusted breath-by-breath. Compared to other noninvasive respiratory support modes, NIV-NAVA may offer improved patient-ventilator synchrony and respiratory drive monitoring, regardless of leaks • It requires nasogastric insertion, and its sensors are expensive

(NAVA: neurally adjusted ventilatory assist; NIPPV: noninvasive intermittent positive pressure ventilation; NIV: noninvasive ventilation)

TABLE 2: Ventilators used for delivering noninvasive intermittent positive pressure ventilation (NIPPV) in neonates.

nsNIPPV	*sNIPPV*
• Any ventilator that can provide IMV modes • *Ventilators with software for nsNIPPV:* SLE 6000, UK VN 600, Germany Servo-N, Sweden	• *Giulia V3 neonatal ventilator (Ginevri, Italy):* Pneumotachograph • Comen NV8 neonatal ventilator (Shenzhen Comen Medical Instruments Co., Ltd., China) • Sophie (Stephan Medizintechnik, Germany) • SLE 6000 (UK) • Freedom Advance Optimedics (India) • Neurally adjusted ventilatory assist (NAVA) in the Servo-i ventilator (Maquet Critical Care AB from Getinge, Sweden)

(IMV: invasive mechanical ventilation; NIPPV: noninvasive intermittent positive pressure ventilation; nsNIPPV: nonsynchronized NIPPV; sNIPPV: synchronized NIPPV)

NASAL INTERMITTENT POSITIVE PRESSURE VENTILATION: MECHANISM(S) OF ACTION

Several proposed explanations have been suggested for the effectiveness of NIPPV:

- Increasing pharyngeal dilation
- Improving the respiratory drive
- Inducing Head's paradoxical reflex
- Increasing mean airway pressure allowing recruitment of alveoli
- Increasing functional residual capacity
- Increasing tidal and minute volume.

Indications

The NIPPV is used in neonates for a number of clinical conditions as has been enlisted in **Table 3**.

Nasal Interface

Although, there is no head-to-head comparison of different nasal interfaces to deliver NIPPV in neonates, the evidence is largely derived from the studies conducted for nasal CPAP delivery in preterm infants as shown in **Table 4**.

Settings

The initial and the maximum settings to deliver NIPPV in neonates when using as primary and secondary mode of respiratory support is as shown in **Table 5**.

TABLE 3: Clinical indications for noninvasive intermittent positive pressure ventilation (NIPPV).

Preterm neonates with respiratory distress syndrome (RDS)	NIPPV can be used as the primary mode of respiratory support in place of continuous positive airway pressure (CPAP). A recent Cochrane review suggest NIPPV likely reduces the rate of respiratory failure [risk ratio (RR) 0.65, 95% confidence interval (CI) 0.54 to 0.78] and needing endotracheal tube ventilation (RR 0.67, 95% CI 0.56 to 0.81) in very preterm infants (gestational age of 28 weeks and above) with RDS or at risk for RDS. NIPPV may also reduce the risk of developing chronic lung disease (CLD) compared to CPAP (RR 0.70, 95% CI 0.52 to 0.92)
Prevention of postextubation failure	Compared to nasal continuous positive airway pressure (NCPAP), NIPPV likely reduces the risk of respiratory failure postextubation (RR 0.75, 95% CI 0.67 to 0.84); and endotracheal reintubation (RR 0.78, 95% CI 0.70 to 0.87) and may reduce pulmonary air leaks (RR 0.57, 95% CI 0.37 to 0.87)
Treatment of apnea of prematurity	Beneficial effects in short-term outcomes, namely the incidence of apnea, desaturations, and bradycardia episodes
CPAP failure	NIPPV may be tried as a bridge before shifting to intubation and mechanical ventilation

TABLE 4: Evidence on nasal interface.

Best prong type	Short binasal prongs
Mask versus prong	• Low certainty evidence suggest that mask decrease failure rate and injury • Mask has least pressure drop and least resistance

Monitoring

Monitor respiratory rate, Silverman score, oxygen saturation (SpO_2), and heart rate. Blood gas and chest X-ray should be done if there is worsening respiratory distress. The clinical, ventilator, and blood gas parameters to define NIPPV failure is as shown in **Table 6**.

One should look for leak in the interface. In NIPPV there will be lot of leak. One should always see the measured PIP in the screen. If measured PIP is less than set PIP, flow need to be adjusted in case of NIPPV machine where software is not available. Nowadays in most of the machine flow is auto adjustable. To deflate the stomach, a bigger size orogastric (OG) tube 8 FG is to be used especially in case of nsNIPPV.

TABLE 5: NIPPV settings when used as primary and secondary mode of respiratory support.

Parameters	*Primary mode*	*Secondary mode*
PIP	15–20 cmH_2O (maximum 30 cmH_2O)	2–4 cmH_2O more than PIP of ventilator at the time of extubation
PEEP	5–6 cmH_2O (maximum 8 cmH_2O)	Same as PEEP of ventilator at time of extubation
Rate	10–40/min	20–30/min
Inspiratory time (Ti)	0.3–0.5 seconds	0.3–0.5 seconds
Flow	8–12 L/min to deliver the set PIP	8–12 L/min
FiO_2	Titrate to maintain SpO_2 of 91–95%; maximum FiO_2 of 60%	Titrate to maintain SpO_2 of 91–95%; maximum $FiO_2$of 60%

(FiO_2: fraction of inspired oxygen; NIPPV: noninvasive intermittent positive pressure ventilation; PIP: peak inspiratory pressure; PEEP: positive end-expiratory pressure; SpO_2: oxygen saturation)

TABLE 6: noninvasive intermittent positive pressure ventilation (NIPPV) failure criteria (indication for reintubation).

Clinical	Severe and recurrent apnea (>4 apnea/h requiring tactile stimulation or >2 episodes requiring bag and mask ventilation in a day), Silverman score >6 despite maximum NIPPV settings, and shock requiring inotropes
Ventilator	The maximum NIPPV ventilation settings as has been enlisted in **Table 5**
Blood gas	pH <7.2 with partial pressure of arterial carbon dioxide ($PaCO_2$), >60 mm Hg

Weaning

Step 1: Gradually decrease fraction of inspired oxygen (FiO_2) by 5% while maintaining target SpO_2 in the range of 91–95% until it reaches 30%

↓

Step 2: If there is no worsening of distress, taper PIP by 1–2 cm of H_2O till PIP is 13–15 cmH_2O

↓

Step 3: Then decrease rates in steps to 20/min

↓

Wean to nasal CPAP if settings are PIP 13–15 cmH_2O, PEEP 5 cmH_2O, rate 20 bpm, and FiO_2 30%

CONCLUSION

The NIPPV operates through multiple physiological mechanisms. Evidence suggests that NIPPV is superior to CPAP both as primary mode in preterm infants with RDS and postextubation respiratory support for preventing respiratory failure. For both indications, ventilator-generated, synchronized NIPPV is physiologically more logical and most effective in preventing respiratory failure. No significant harm has been noted with NIPPV use in neonates. However, utmost care should be taken in selection and use of nasal interfaces to prevent nasal injury.

SUGGESTED READING

1. Anne RP, Murki S. Noninvasive respiratory support in neonates: a review of current evidence and practices. Indian J Pediatr. 2021;88(7):670-8. doi: 10.1007/s12098-021-03755-z
2. Chandrasekaran A, Deorari (Chairperson) AK, Gupta N, Murki S, Sankar MJ, Sivanandan S. Noninvasive respiratory support for newborns. J Neonatol. 2020;34(3):118-52. doi: 10.1177/0973217920974573
3. Kumar J, Kumar P, Bhandari V. Noninvasive ventilation strategies in neonates. Indian Pediatrics. 2025;62:451-60. The article provides recommendations based on NNF guidelines, including delivery room and NICU NIV approaches and surfactant administration.
4. Ramaswamy VV, Devi R, Kumar G. Non-invasive ventilation in neonates: a review of current literature. Front Pediatr. 2023;11:1248836. doi: 10.3389/fped.2023.1248836

CHAPTER

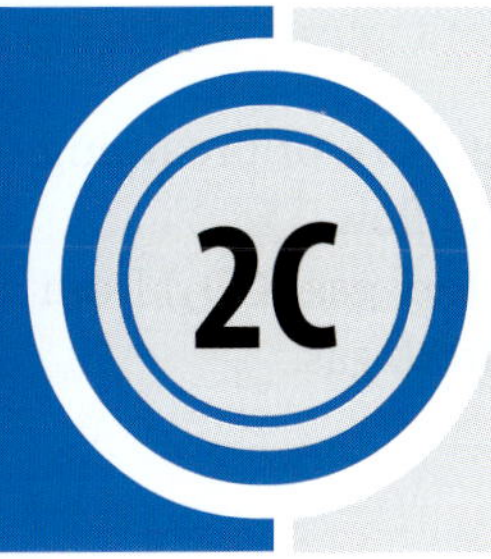

Heated Humidified High-flow Nasal Cannula

Pradeep Kumar Debata

INTRODUCTION

Heated humidified high-flow nasal cannula (HHHFNC) is used very often in neonates for respiratory support as an alternative to nasal continuous positive airway pressure (nCPAP). It has become popular due to its ease of application, better tolerance, and lesser nasal trauma. It is basically administration of blended oxygen at a rate of >1 L/min.

DEVICE

- *Gas source:* Oxygen and air
- *Blender:* To mix the oxygen and air to get the required fraction of inspired oxygen (FiO_2)
- *Flow meter:* To regulate the flow of the blended oxygen to generate optimal pressure (2 L/min to maximum of 8 L/min)
- *Humidifier:* To deliver gas at an optimal temperature 33–34°C and relative humidity (RH) of close to 100%. At higher flow rate, it becomes difficult to maintain the optimal temperature and RH
- *Circuit:* To deliver the blended heated humidified gas to the distal end maintaining the temperature and humidity without rainout
- *Interface:* The cannula which is fitted to the circuits and to patient's nostrils
- *Water for humidification:* Distilled water [normal saline (NS), dextrose in normal saline (DNS), or other intravenous (IV) fluids are not used].

MECHANISM OF ACTION

- Splinting the upper airways along with the pharynx providing distending pressure.
- Decreases the metabolic work of breathing by providing heated and humidified gas.
- The distending positive pressure recruits alveoli, helps preventing them to collapse at end expiration and thus maintains the functional residual capacity (FRC).

- This prevents collapse of alveoli, so decreases the work of breathing improving oxygenation providing adequate inspiratory flow.
- The high flow of humidified gas removes the expiratory gas (CO_2) from the nasopharyngeal dead space and replaces it with fresh gas.

INDICATIONS

- *For postextubation support (as an alternative to CPAP):* Though the failure rate is similar in both high-flow nasal cannula (HFNC) and CPAP, the nasal trauma rate reduces significantly. However, there is insufficient evidence for extreme preterm neonates in this regard.
- *For apnea of prematurity:* Can be used to prevent apnea in preterm in place of CPAP.
- *For primary respiratory support:* Can be used as a primary respiratory support in very/moderate/late preterm neonates. However, CPAP should be available for back up. For extreme preterm neonates, HFNC should not be used as a primary respiratory support as failure rate is higher.
- *As a weaning mode from CPAP:* Weaning from CPAP is usually done directly to room air. Sometimes can be weaned to HFNC if nasal trauma is there or for Kangaroo mother care (KMC). However it does not improves the success of weaning.

CONTRAINDICATION

- *Congenital anomalies:* Cannot be used with anomalies such as choanal atresia and cleft palate
- *Severe respiratory pathology:* Severe respiratory distress syndrome (RDS), recurrent apnea requiring higher mode of support, and pneumothorax
- Hemodynamically unstable neonates
- *Encephalopathy:* Having no spontaneous breathing or nonsustainable breathing.

INITIAL SETTINGS

- The neonate needs to be put in a thermoneutral environment.
- *Cannula size:* An appropriate size cannula is chosen to cover 50% of the nostril which helps in removal of expired air and not snugly fitting as in CPAP which may create inadvertently high pressure.
- The cannula is attached to the circuit and then the circuit is attached to the humidifier.
- *Setting of flow rate:*
  - For a 1–2 kg neonate the flow rate is 3 L/min
  - For a 2–3 kg neonate the flow rate 4 L/min
  - For a >3 kg neonate the flow rate would be 5 L/min
  - A general flow rate may be 4–6 L/min

- *FiO_2*:
  - Same as the previous noninvasive mode of ventilation
  - 5–10% higher if used for postextubation
  - For use in primary mode FiO_2 can be set at 30–40%
  - The target saturation is to be maintained between 90 and 95%.

TITRATION OF SETTINGS

The increment is by 1 L/min at a time and should not go beyond 8 L/min. Before increasing the flow rate, must check the cannula is attached to the nostrils, the circuit is in place and the humidifier is working properly.

- No improvement/increase in respiratory distress
- No adequate lungs expansion in X-ray
- Increase in requirement of FiO_2 by 10%
- Increase in partial pressure of carbon dioxide (PCO_2) in blood gas by 10%.

MONITORING OF THE PATIENT

- For clinical response (work of breathing) objectively by using Silverman/Downes scores.
- The baby must be put on with monitor with oxygen saturation (SpO_2) to be maintained between 90 and 95%.
- Blood gas is to be done as indicated (not as routine).
- X-ray chest to look for lungs expansion if no anticipated response obtained.
- Every 4 hourly (at least in each shift) the nares are to be looked for erythema (nasal trauma).
- If the baby is on tube feeding then to keep the outer end of the tube open for at least 30 minutes after each feed.
- Monitor the baby's temperature continuously particularly if the baby is in KMC.
- Look for the displacement of the interface.
- Temperature, water level, and the attachment of sensors in the humidifier time to time.

WEANING

Once the neonate is stable for 24 hours one can consider for weaning considering the disease pathology and severity.

- The FiO_2 is reduced first by a decrement of 5 to <25%
- The flow rate is decreased by 1 L/min up to 2 L/min.

These decrements would be guided by work of breathing and the FiO_2 requirement to maintain a saturation of 90–95%.

FAILURE OF HIGH-FLOW NASAL CANNULA

- FiO_2 requirement of >40% or;
- Respiratory acidosis of pH <7.2 or PCO_2 >60 mm Hg or;
- Recurrent apnea (>3 per hour or requiring positive pressure ventilation) or;
- If the neonate becomes hemodynamically unstable.

In these conditions, the neonate needs to be put on CPAP or higher modes of respiratory support.

SIDE EFFECTS

- *Gastric distension:* Placement of an orogastric tube is mandatory and the outer end is to be kept open after 30 minutes of feeding.
- *Air leak:* Common with unregulated high flow rate. The flow rate should not go beyond 8 L/min. In the condition of any deterioration after an improvement, air leak may be looked for.
- *Nasal trauma:* Though the incidence is less than CPAP, close monitoring is required to prevent it.

SUMMARY AND CHECKLIST

- The interface must be in place.
- The inflow gas should be 37°C and the RH should be 100%.
- The flow rate should be 4–6 L/min to start with and should not go beyond 8 L/min.
- The increase in flow rate should be according to the work of breathing and FiO_2 requirement. Blood gas should not be done routinely. In case of failure, one can do a blood gas.
- Decrease the FiO_2 first to <25% in weaning (decrement by 5%).
- The flow rate is decreased when the FiO_2 requirement is <25% and there is no increased work of breathing.
- Stop HFNC when FiO_2 requirement is <25%, flow rate is 2 L/min, and there is no work of breathing.
- Consider failure if FiO_2 requirement remains >40% along with increased work of breathing despite on a flow rate of 8 L/min or recurrent apnea persists.
- Monitoring for nasal trauma is mandatory when the neonate is on HFNC.
- Do not forget to put an orogastric tube to vent out the gastric air.
- The setting up of HHHFNC circuit is as shown in **Figure 1**.

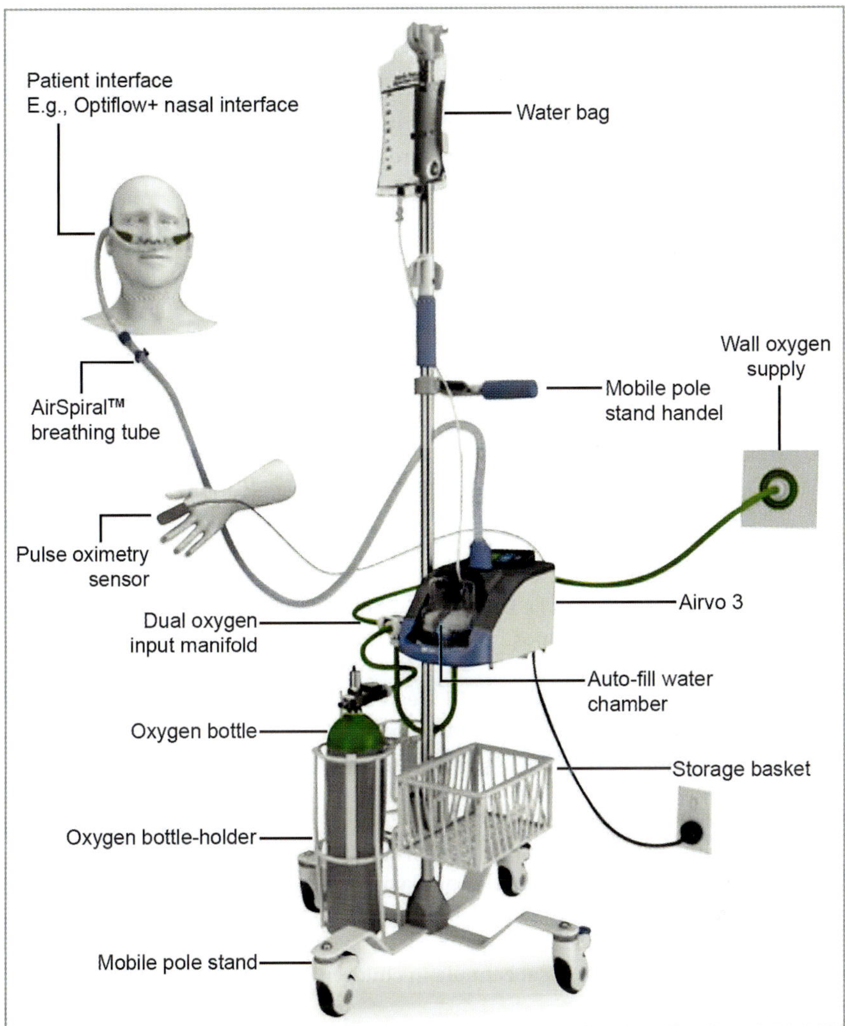

Fig. 1: Setting up of heated high-flow nasal cannula circuit.

CONCLUSION

Heated humidified high-flow nasal cannula (HHHFNC) is a simple, effective, and well-tolerated noninvasive respiratory support modality in neonates. By delivering blended, warmed, and humidified gases at high flows, it reduces the work of breathing, improves alveolar recruitment, and facilitates CO_2 washout from the upper airway. It is useful as post-extubation support, in apnea of prematurity, and in selected preterm and term infants as an alternative to CPAP, with the advantage of less nasal trauma and greater comfort. However, it should be avoided in extreme prematurity or severe respiratory compromise where failure rates are higher. Appropriate patient selection, careful titration of flow and FiO_2, vigilant monitoring, and timely escalation to higher modes of support are critical for safe and effective use of HHHFNC.

SUGGESTED READING

1. Alanazi MM, Algarni SS. Use of a high flow nasal cannula in extremely premature infants: benefits and drawbacks. Global Pediatr. 2004;7:100092.
2. Balharetha Y, Razak A. High flow nasal cannula for weaning nasal continuous positive airway pressure in preterm infants: a systematic review and meta-analysis. Neonatology. 2024;121:359-69.
3. Cresi F, Maggiora E, Lista G, Dani C, Borgione SM, Spada E, et al. Effect of nasal continuous positive airway pressure vs heated humidified high-flow nasal cannula on feeding intolerance in preterm infants with respiratory distress syndrome: The ENTARES randomized clinical trial. JAMA Netw Open. 2023;6(7):e2323052.
4. Hodgson KA, Wilkinson D, De Paoli AG, Manley BJ. Nasal high flow therapy for primary respiratory support in preterm infants. Cochrane Database Syst Rev. 2023;5(5):CD006405.
5. Hutchings FA, Hilliard TN, Davis PJ. Heated humidified high-flow nasal cannula therapy in children. Arch Dis Child. 2015;100:571-5.
6. Liew Z, Fenton AC, Harigopal S, Gopalakaje S, Brodlie M, O'Brien CJ. Physiological effects of high-flow nasal cannula therapy in preterm infants. Arch Dis Child Fetal Neonatal Ed. 2020;105:87-93.
7. Li J, Deng N, He WJA, Yang C, Liu P, Albuainain FA, et al. The effects of flow settings during high-flow nasal cannula oxygen therapy for neonates and young children. Eur Respir Rev. 2024;33:230223.
8. Venanzi A, Filippo PD, Santagata C, Pillo SD, Chiarelli F, Attanasi M. Heated humidified high-flow nasal cannula in children: State of the Art. Biomedicines. 2022;10:2353.

SECTION

Evaluation and Monitoring

CHAPTER

Pulmonary Graphics

Amanpreet Sethi

INTRODUCTION

Bedside pulmonary graphics in intubated neonates provide vital information regarding pulmonary pathophysiology, the effect of various respiratory medicines including surfactant and the effect of change in ventilator settings on pulmonary mechanics. Neonatal respiratory diseases cause certain pathophysiological alterations that result in precise ventilator graphic patterns. Pediatricians should be aware of these patterns so that better clinical care can be provided to sick neonates. Lung function monitoring as pulmonary graphics has never been evaluated in randomized controlled trials in neonates to reduce neonatal mortality, chronic lung disease, or long-term neurodevelopmental impairment.

The pulmonary graphics is real time visualization of three most commonly utilized signals: Pressure (cmH_2O), volume (mL), and flow (mL/s). These signals are specifically captured by flow sensors (hot wire anemometers or pneumotachometers). Most of the neonatal ventilators display pulmonary graphics as Waveforms and loops, which are explained here:

1. *Waveforms:* These show how respiratory parameters (pressure, flow, and volume) and time relate to one another on a breath-by-breath basis. By convention, the respiratory parameters are kept on Y-axis and time on X-axis. So, waveforms are time based. Three waveforms (pressure, volume, and flow waveforms) are shown in **Figure 1**.
2. *Loops:* These are formed when pressure, flow, and volume respiratory parameters are displayed in relation to each other. The pressure-volume (P-V) and flow-volume (F-V) loops are the two most commonly utilized loops in clinical practice shown in **Figure 2**.

ROLE OF PULMONARY GRAPHICS IN EVALUATION AND MONITORING

- *To optimize ventilator settings:* Mean airway pressure (Paw), which determines oxygenation in a given neonate, can be ascertained from the pressure waveform as the area under the curve (AUC). Alterations in peak

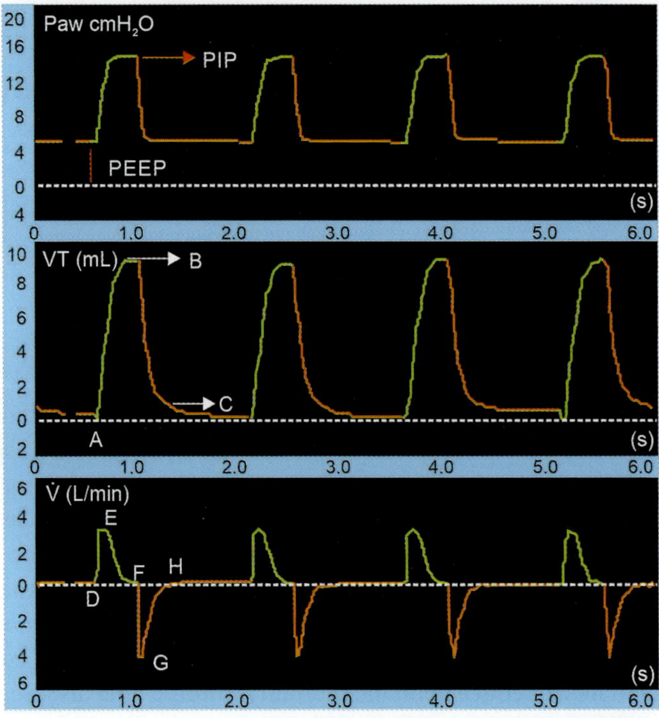

Fig. 1: Pressure, volume, and flow waveforms against time (seconds): Point A shows the beginning of inspiration, point B represents the maximum volume, and point C represents the end-expiratory volume. Point D indicates the start of the accelerating inspiratory flow phase, point E indicates the peak inspiratory flow rate (PIFR), point F represents zero flow rate at the end of inspiration, point G indicates peak expiratory flow rate (PEFR), and point H represents zero flow rate at the end of expiration.

inspiratory pressure (PIP) and positive end-expiratory pressure (PEEP) can change the AUC as shown in **Figures 3A to C**. Similarly, changes in inspiratory time (Ti) and rates can lead to an increase or decrease in mean Paw. We can also ascertain the optimum PEEP level (lower inflection point) in the lungs with poor compliance as shown in **Figures 4A and B**. Similarly, lung hyperinflation can also be ascertained as characterized by the typical "penguin beak" appearance at the end of inspiration in the P-V loop as shown in **Figure 5**.

- *Objective assessment of a respiratory therapy or medication:* Pulmonary graphics can provide valuable insights on the effect of various respiratory medications on pulmonary mechanics. For example, changes in compliance (P-V loop) after surfactant therapy **(Figs. 6A and B)** and changes in flow volume loops after bronchodilator therapy in a preterm infant with bronchopulmonary dysplasia **(Figs. 7A and B)**.
- *Early identification of ventilation errors such as endotracheal tube leaks, obstructions, displacements, excessive water condensation in the circuit,*

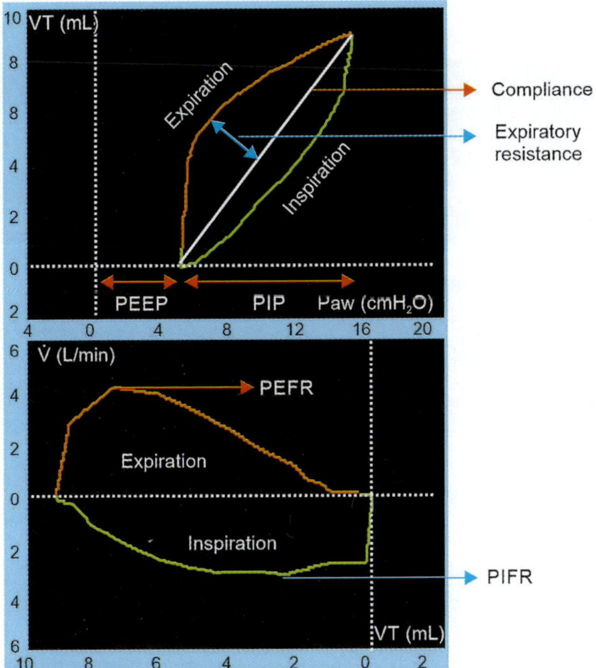

Fig. 2: Pressure-volume (P-V) and flow-volume (F-V) loops. (*Note:* Orientation of loops varies from ventilator to ventilator).

autotriggering, and air trapping: Pulmonary graphics have a vital role in the early detection of these mishaps. Typical graphical patterns for leaks, obstruction, displacement, auto triggering, and air trapping as mentioned above are shown in **Figures 8 and 9**.

- *Understanding the course of a disease and its effect on pulmonary mechanics:* Respiratory conditions in newborns have diverse pathophysiology, and the addition of mechanical ventilation further complicates the management. Pulmonary graphics help us to better understand the interaction of spontaneous breathing of the neonate with mechanical ventilator breaths **(Fig. 10)**. This allows us to evaluate patient-ventilator synchrony more objectively and modify ventilator settings to suit the neonate's specific needs depending on the underlying pathophysiology. Moreover, analyzing the past trends in pulmonary graphics can guide us whether the respiratory condition is improving or worsening.
- *Understanding different modes of ventilation:* In neonatal intensive care, there are basically four types of ventilation modes: Pressure support ventilation (PSV), assist control ventilation (A/C), synchronized intermittent mandatory ventilation (SIMV), and intermittent mandatory ventilation (IMV). Moreover, they can be volume or pressure controlled

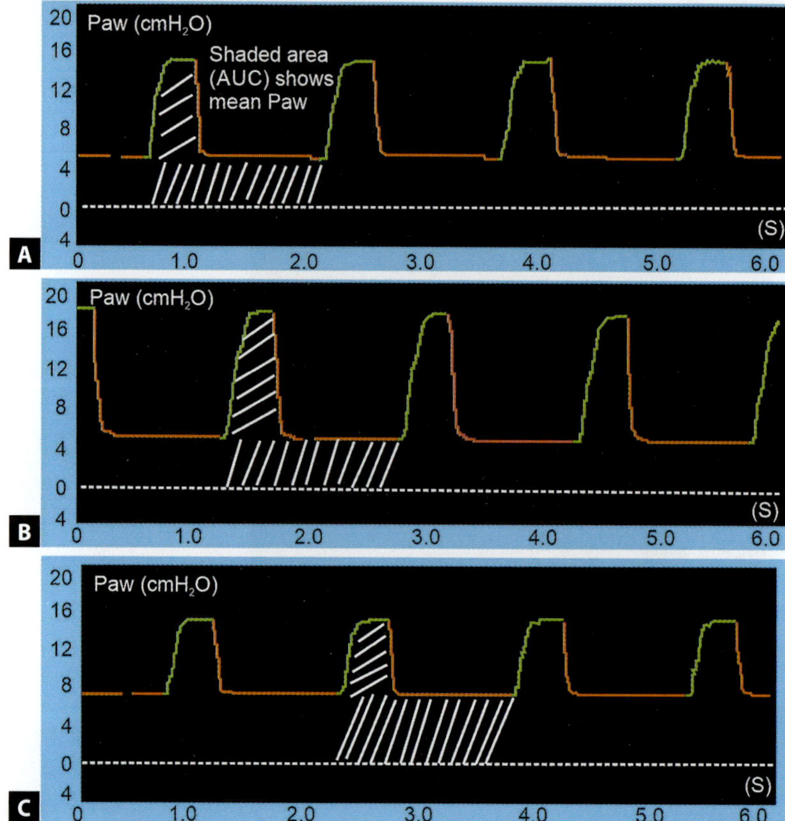

Figs. 3A to C: Effect of increase in peak inspiratory pressure (PIP) and positive end-expiratory pressure (PEEP) on mean airway pressure (Please note the increase in AUC in **Figs. 3B and C**). (A) Mean Paw with PIP of 15 cm of H_2O; (B) Mean Paw with an increase of PIP from 15 to 18 cm of H_2O; (C) Mean Paw with an increase of PEEP from 5 to 7 cm of H_2O.

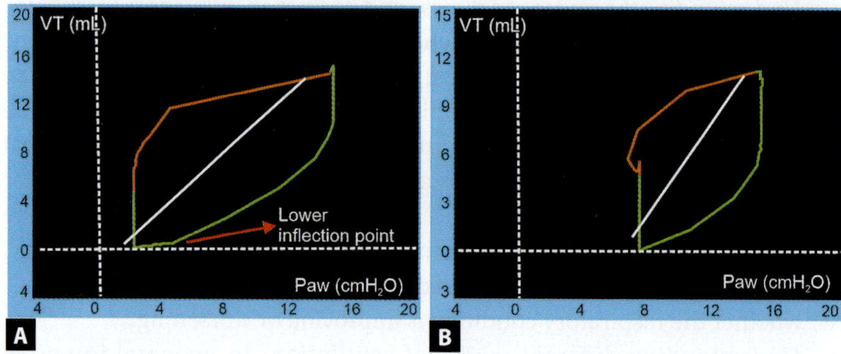

Figs. 4 and B: (A) P-V loop with positive end-expiratory pressure (PEEP) of 2 cm: There is minimal change in volume as pressure is increased from 2 to 6 cm. At around 6 cm (lower inflection point—red arrow), there is an adequate increase in volume with an increase in pressure. Also, note the right-sided shift in the slope of the P-V loop indicating poor compliance; (B) P-V loop with PEEP of 7 cm: There is a left-sided shift in the slope of the P-V loop indicating better compliance.

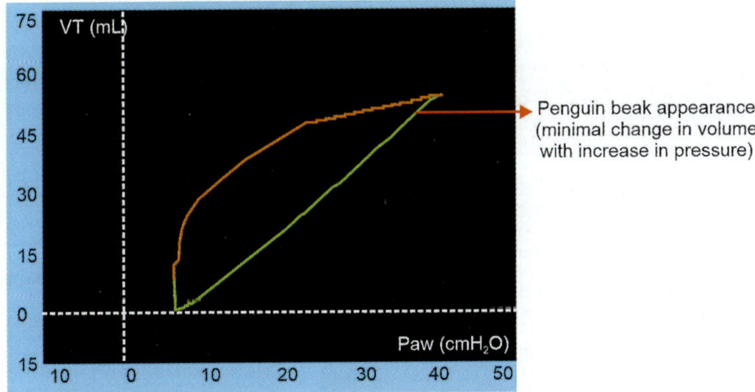

Fig. 5: P-V loop showing hyperinflation (Penguin beak) at the end of inspiration.

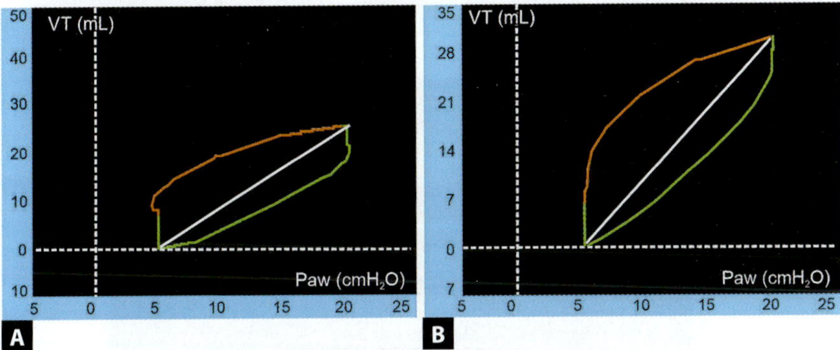

Figs. 6A and B: Response to surfactant therapy: (A) Presurfactant P-V loop: Note the slope of the compliance curve; (B) Postsurfactant P-V loop: Note the improvement in compliance curve.

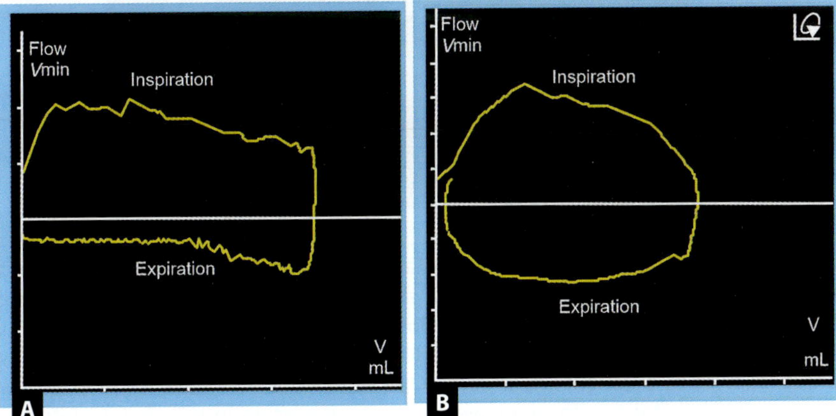

Figs. 7A and B: Response to bronchodilator therapy in neonates with bronchopulmonary dysplasia (BPD): (A) F-V loop with compressed inspiratory and expiratory phase; (B) F-V loop after bronchodilator therapy.

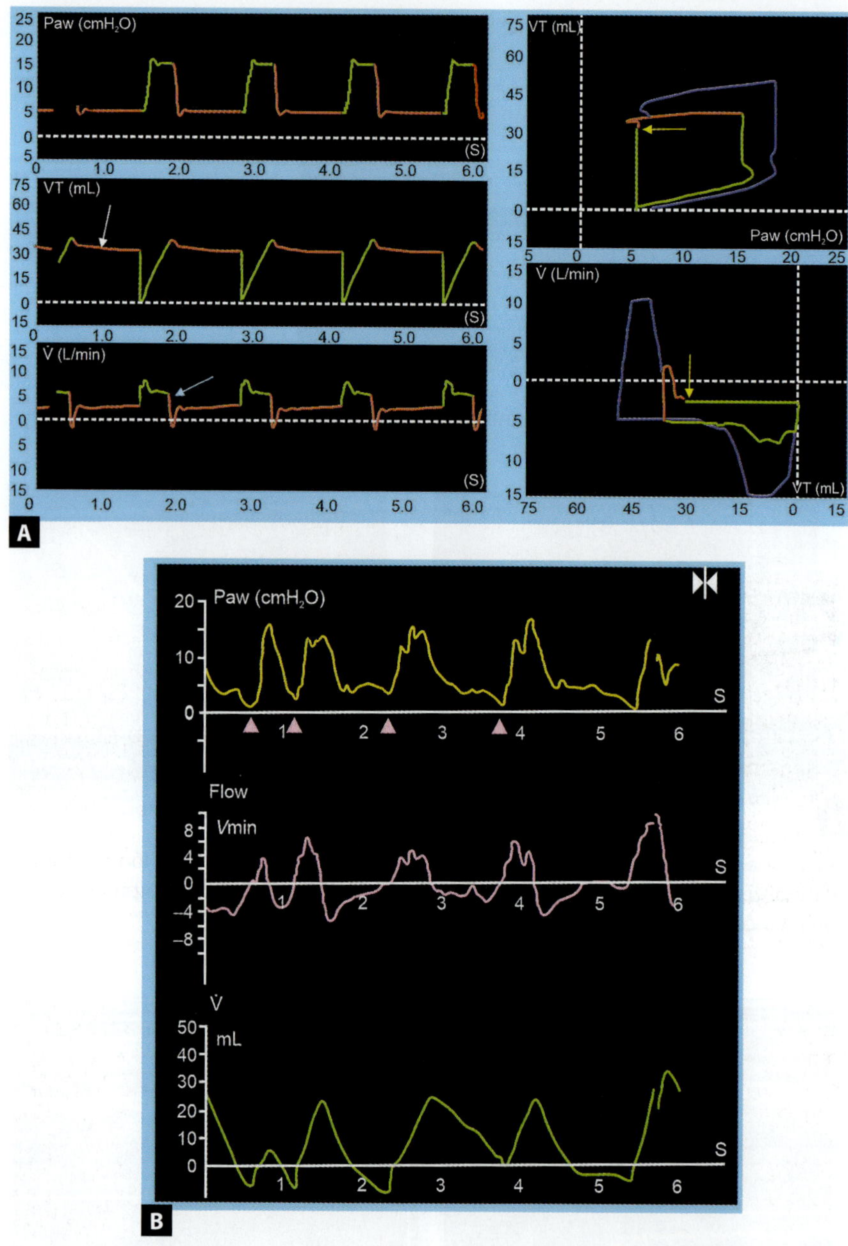

Figs. 8A and B: Errors in ventilation: (A) Massive endotracheal tube leak: On the left side, the volume waveform in the middle shows no volume in the expiratory phase (white arrow). The flow waveform in the lower panel has no expiratory component (blue arrow). On the right side, F-V and P-V loops show an abrupt end in the expiratory phase followed by a straight line artifact by the ventilator to complete the loop (yellow arrows); (B) Waveform with excessive water condensation in the circuit: Note the turbulence in the waveforms.

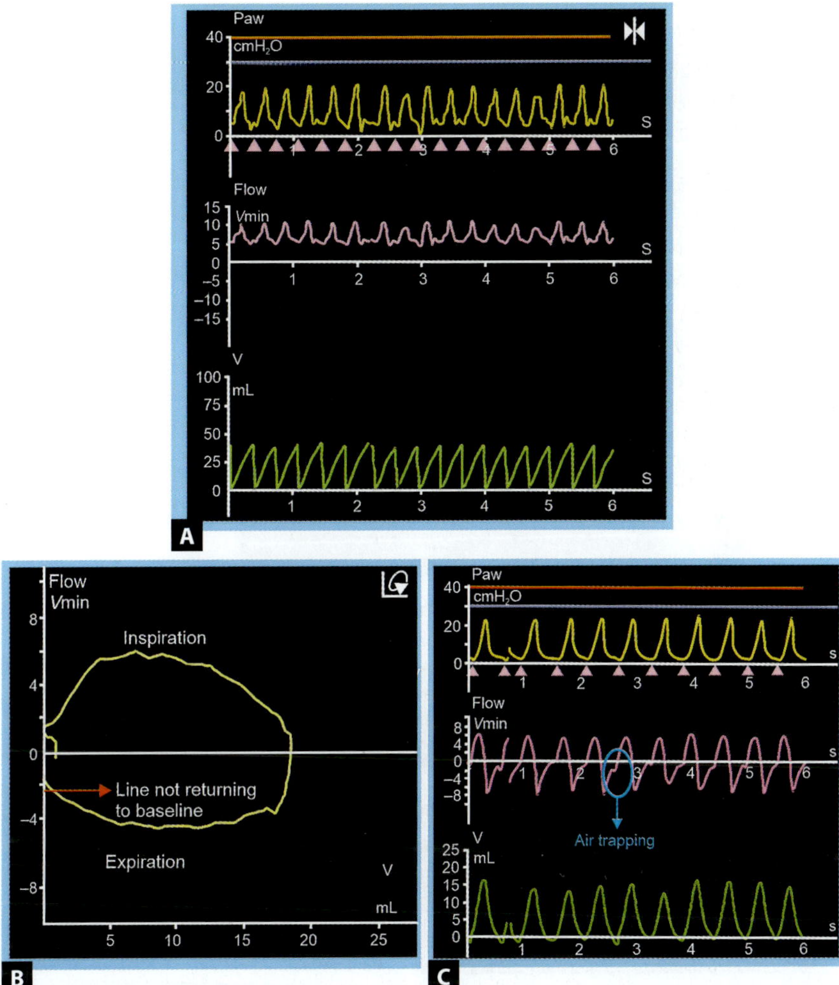

Figs. 9A to C: Errors in ventilation: (A) *Autotriggering:* In patient-triggered ventilation, sometimes due to leaks or water in the circuit, there is repetitive delivery of breaths by a mechanical ventilator. Note the characteristic uniformly spaced breaths in autotriggering; (B and C) *Air trapping:* In the F-V loop on the left side, the red arrow shows that the expiratory flow is unable to reach the baseline before the next breath is started. In the flow waveform on the right side, the blue circle in the middle panel indicates air trapping as explained above.

(Figs. 11A and B). All these ventilation modes are diverse due to differences in trigger and cycling mechanisms, thus forming typical waveforms as shown in **Figure 12**.

A deep understanding of the pulmonary graphics helps us to better comprehend respiratory physiology and how a sick neonate and ventilator interact with each other. Thus, its judicial use can help us to customize mechanical ventilation according to the needs of the neonate. However,

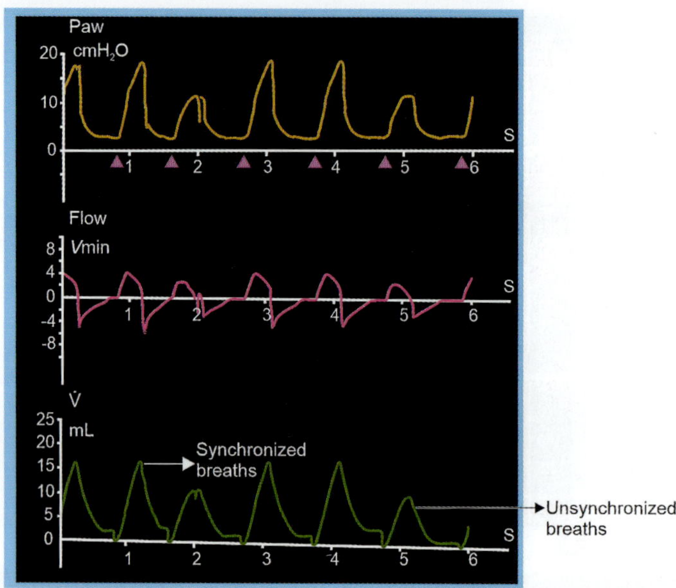

Fig. 10: Effect of spontaneous breathing on Mechanical ventilation: Note the increased tidal volume in the synchronized ventilator breaths.

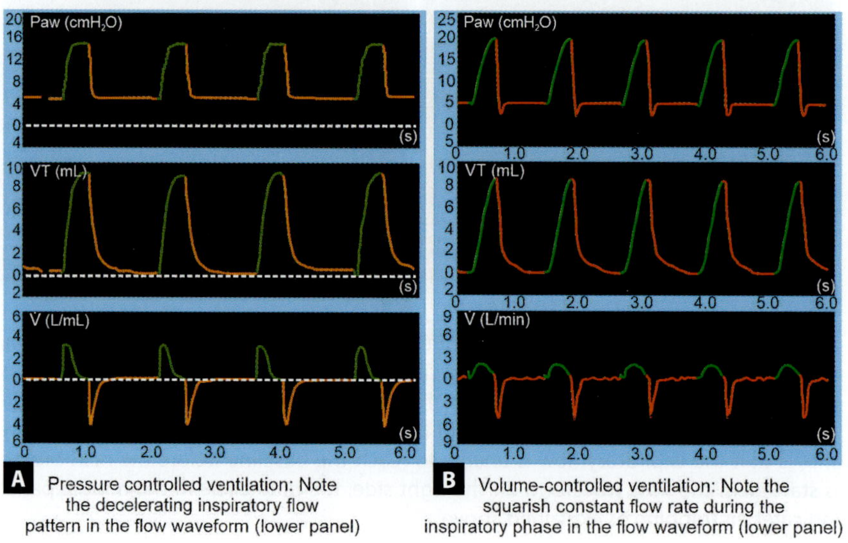

Figs. 11A and B: Difference between pressure and volume-controlled ventilator breaths.

we should understand that the pulmonary graphic signals are recorded by specialized flow sensors, and we must confirm that these sensors are operational before we can begin depending on them.

The only pitfall of the pulmonary graphic display is that it is just a simplified snapshot of the respiratory system and does not give the entire picture, especially in nonhomogeneous lung diseases such as meconium

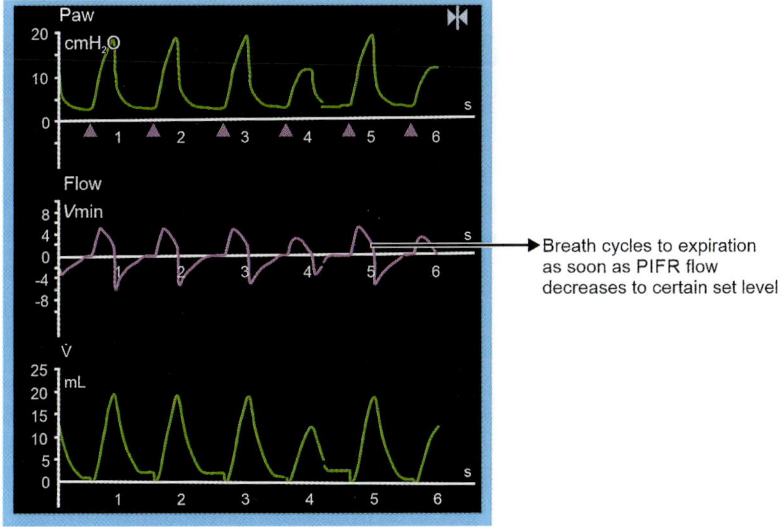

Fig. 12: Flow cycling in pressure support ventilation.

aspiration syndrome, bronchopulmonary dysplasia (BPD), and pneumonia. Hence, information obtained from the pulmonary graphics must be corroborated with history, physical examination, arterial blood values, and chest X-rays.

CONCLUSION

Pulmonary graphics offer a valuable real-time window into neonatal respiratory physiology, enabling optimization of ventilator settings, assessment of therapeutic interventions, and early detection of ventilation errors. They enhance understanding of patient–ventilator interaction and disease progression, thereby supporting individualized care. Nevertheless, as they provide only a simplified representation of pulmonary function, interpretation must always be integrated with clinical examination, blood gas analysis, and imaging to ensure safe and effective neonatal respiratory management.

SUGGESTED READING

1. Becker MA, Donn SM. Real-time pulmonary graphic monitoring. Clin Perinatol. 2007;34:1-17.
2. Donn SM, Mammel MC. Neonatal Pulmonary Graphics: A Clinical Pocket Atlas. Springer; 2015.
3. Mammel MC, Donn SM. Real-time pulmonary graphics. Semin Fetal Neonatal Med. 2015;20(3):181-91.
4. Schmolzer G, Hummler H. Pulmonary Function and Graphics. In: Keszler M, Suresh GK, (Eds). Goldsmith's Assisted Ventilation of the Neonate, 7th edition. Philadelphia: Elsevier; 2025. pp. 124-43.

CHAPTER

Blood Gas Technical Aspects and Interpretation

Chandra Kumar Natarajan, Archana Arumugom

INTRODUCTION

Blood gas analysis is an indispensable tool in the neonatal intensive care unit (NICU) for the assessment of respiratory and metabolic status. Given the unique physiological characteristics of neonates, understanding the technical aspects of blood gas interpretation, particularly through an algorithmic approach, is vital. This chapter focuses on the comprehensive evaluation of blood gas results, including mixed disorders and compensatory mechanisms in acid-base balance, ultimately aiding clinicians in optimizing neonatal care.

TECHNICAL ASPECTS OF BLOOD GAS ANALYSIS

Sample Collection

Site selection:

- *Arterial Samples:* Common sites include the radial artery, femoral artery, and umbilical arteries. The radial artery is often preferred for its ease of access and lower risk of complications. Femoral arteries may be used in more critical situations where other sites are not viable.
- *Capillary samples:* These samples can be obtained from the heel, particularly in stable neonates or for point-of-care testing. However, capillary samples may be less reliable than arterial samples due to potential contamination and variability.

Collection technique:

- *Aseptic technique:* Strict adherence to aseptic techniques is essential to prevent infections, especially in vulnerable neonates.
- *Heparinized syringe:* Use of a heparinized syringe helps prevent clotting, preserving the integrity of the sample.

Sample handling:

- *Timeliness:* Samples should be analyzed within 30 minutes to avoid metabolic changes that can skew results.
- *Storage:* If delayed analysis is unavoidable, samples should be placed on ice to reduce metabolic activity.

Equipment

Blood gas analyzer:

- *Calibration and maintenance:* Accurate results depend on regular calibration of the analyzer with known control solutions. Routine maintenance is critical to ensure optimal performance.
- *Parameters measured:* Standard measurements include pH, partial pressure of carbon dioxide (pCO_2), partial pressure of oxygen (pO_2), bicarbonate (HCO_3^-), and base excess.
- *Quality control:* Implement rigorous quality control protocols, including periodic checks with control samples to validate the accuracy of the analyzer.

APPROACH TO INTERPRETATION

Initial Assessment

The interpretation of blood gas results should follow a systematic approach as shown in **Flowchart 1**:

- *pH:* Evaluate for acid-base status (normal range: 7.35–7.45).
- *pCO_2:* Assess for respiratory function (normal range: 35–45 mm Hg).
- *pO_2:* Determine oxygenation (normal range: 60–100 mm Hg).
- *HCO_3^-:* Assess metabolic status (normal range: 22–26 mEq/L).

BLOOD GAS INTERPRETATION

- *Check pH:*
  - *pH <7.35:* Acidosis
    - *Check pCO_2:*
      - pCO_2 >45 mm Hg: Respiratory acidosis
      - pCO_2 <35 mm Hg: Metabolic acidosis
  - *pH > 7.45:* Alkalosis
    - *Check pCO_2:*
      - pCO_2 <35 mm Hg: Respiratory alkalosis
      - pCO_2 >45 mm Hg: Metabolic alkalosis
- *Compensation assessment:*
  - *In acidosis:* Evaluate for respiratory compensation (increased ventilation) or metabolic compensation (increased HCO_3^-).
  - *In alkalosis:* Evaluate for respiratory compensation (decreased ventilation) or metabolic compensation (decreased HCO_3^-).

MIXED DISORDERS

Mixed acid-base disorders occur when two or more primary acid-base disturbances coexist. Recognizing these disorders is essential for appropriate management.

Flowchart 1: Approach to acid-base disorders.

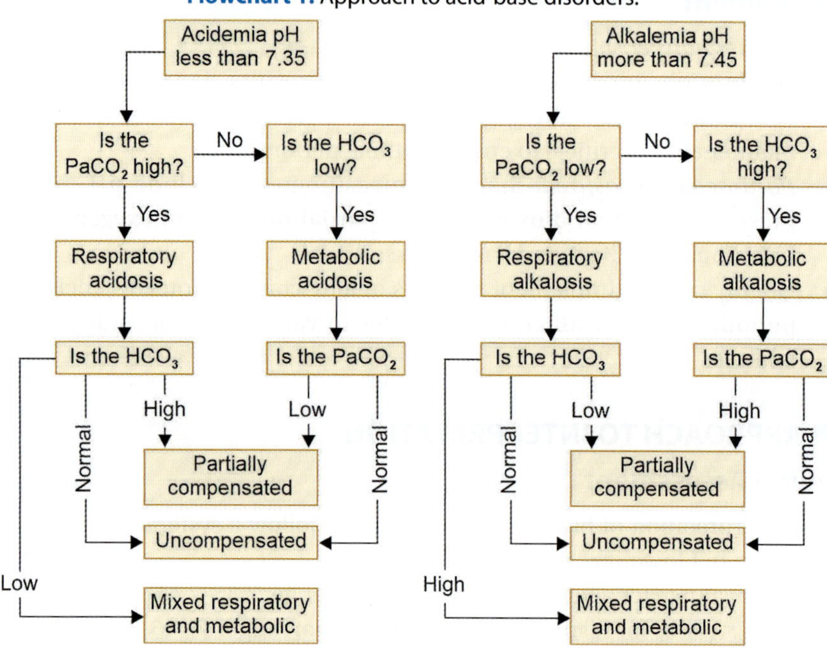

Common Mixed Disorders

- *Respiratory and metabolic acidosis:*
  - *Example:* In a septic infant, hypoventilation (increased pCO_2) may co-occur with lactic acidosis (decreased HCO_3^-). The blood gas analysis might show low pH, high pCO_2, and low HCO_3^-.
  - *Management:* Immediate ventilation support and treatment of the underlying infection are crucial.
- *Respiratory and metabolic alkalosis*:
  - *Example*: Hyperventilation from overventilation (decreased pCO_2) alongside vomiting (increased HCO_3^-) can result in high pH, low pCO_2, and high HCO_3^-.
  - *Management*: Addressing the cause of hyperventilation and restoring fluid balance are critical.

Diagnostic Approach to Mixed Disorders

- *Evaluating each component:* Assess pH, pCO_2, and HCO_3^- individually to identify the primary disturbances.
- *Compensation check:* Evaluate whether compensation is appropriate. For instance, in a case of acidosis, if HCO_3^- is high, this may indicate a compensatory metabolic response or a mixed disorder.

Clinical Examples

Respiratory Acidosis

Common causes in neonates:

- *Respiratory distress syndrome (RDS):* Due to surfactant deficiency, leading to inadequate alveolar ventilation and CO_2 retention
- *Meconium aspiration syndrome:* Blockage of airways by meconium can impair gas exchange and lead to CO_2 buildup.
- Congenital diaphragmatic hernia (CDH)
- *Upper airway obstruction:* Conditions such as choanal atresia or laryngeal clefts can obstruct the upper airway, causing CO_2 retention.
- *Severe apnea:* Intermittent cessation of breathing can reduce ventilation and cause CO_2 retention.

Respiratory Alkalosis

Common causes in neonates:

- *Hyperventilation due to hypoxia:* Neonates, especially preterm infants, may exhibit hyperventilation in response to hypoxia (e.g., from patent ductus arteriosus, persistent pulmonary hypertension, or pulmonary edema).
- *Pain or stimulation:* Neonates undergoing painful procedures (e.g., intubation and chest tube insertion) may experience transient hyperventilation.
- *Mechanical ventilation:* Overventilation, especially in premature infants, can lead to respiratory alkalosis.
- *Central nervous system (CNS) causes:* CNS depression or irritation, such as from perinatal asphyxia, intraventricular hemorrhage (IVH), or metabolic encephalopathy, can cause altered breathing patterns, leading to hyperventilation.

Metabolic Acidosis

Classified based on anion gap:

- Anion gap = Na - (Cl + HCO_3)
- Normal value = 12 to 16

Common causes in neonates:

- *High anion gap metabolic acidosis:*
  - *Perinatal asphyxia:* Inadequate oxygen delivery during labor and delivery leads to anaerobic metabolism and accumulation of lactic acid.
  - *Sepsis:* Systemic infections can lead to tissue hypoxia, producing lactic acidosis, or through the accumulation of other metabolic byproducts.

- *Renal failure:* Neonates with renal insufficiency or acute kidney injury may be unable to excrete acids, leading to acidosis.
- *Inborn errors of metabolism:* Disorders such as organic acidemias (e.g., propionic acidemia and methylmalonic acidemia) result in the buildup of organic acids.
- *Shock:* Decreased perfusion to tissues leads to anaerobic metabolism, with subsequent accumulation of lactic acid.

- *Normal anion gap metabolic acidosis:*
  - *Diarrhea*: Loss of bicarbonate due to gastrointestinal fluid loss
  - Stoma losses

Metabolic Alkalosis

Common causes in neonates:

- *Vomiting:* Loss of gastric contents rich in hydrochloric acid (HCl) can lead to a decrease in hydrogen ions, thereby increasing blood bicarbonate.
- *Diuretic use:* Diuretics, especially in neonates with conditions like congenital heart failure, can lead to electrolyte imbalances, including hypokalemia and alkalosis.
- *Congenital adrenal hyperplasia (CAH):* In this disorder, aldosterone excess leads to renal bicarbonate retention and hydrogen ion loss.
- *Excessive sodium bicarbonate administration:* Overcorrection of acidosis with sodium bicarbonate in neonatal resuscitation can result in alkalosis.

Blood gas analysis, combined with clinical context and additional diagnostic tests (e.g., electrolyte levels, and lactate), is essential to determining the precise cause of the acid-base disturbance. The pattern of respiratory or metabolic compensation observed in the blood gas (e.g., a normal bicarbonate in respiratory acidosis or respiratory compensation in metabolic acidosis) can also help in identifying the underlying condition.

COMPENSATION MECHANISMS

Compensatory mechanisms are physiological responses that help restore acid-base balance.

Compensation in acidosis:

- *Respiratory compensation:*
  - Increased ventilation occurs in response to elevated pCO_2 (e.g., respiratory acidosis). This process happens rapidly within minutes to hours.
  - In chronic respiratory acidosis, the kidneys compensate by increasing bicarbonate retention.
- *Metabolic compensation:*
  - In acute metabolic acidosis (e.g., lactic acidosis), the respiratory rate increases to blow off CO_2, thereby raising pH.

- In chronic cases, the kidneys will retain bicarbonate to counteract acidosis, leading to increased HCO_3^- levels.

Compensation in alkalosis:

- *Respiratory compensation:*
  - In respiratory alkalosis, the body decreases the respiratory rate to retain CO_2, which can take hours to days to achieve a balance.
  - In acute cases, this response may not be fully effective.
- *Metabolic compensation:* In metabolic alkalosis, the kidneys may excrete bicarbonate to lower HCO_3^- levels. This response can also take days to normalize pH.

Formulae for calculating expected pCO_2 and HCO_3^- in neonatal acid-base disturbances:

- *Metabolic acidosis:* Expected $pCO_2 = 1.5\ [HCO_3] + 8 + 2$
- *Metabolic alkalosis:* Expected $pCO_2 = 0.9\ [HCO_3] + 16$
- *Respiratory acidosis:*
  - *Acute:* For every 10 increase in pCO_2, pH decreases by 0.08.
  - *Chronic:* For every 10 increase in pCO_2, pH decreases by 0.03.
- *Respiratory alkalosis:*
  - *Acute:* For every 10 decrease in pCO_2, pH increases by 0.08.
  - *Chronic:* For every 10 decrease in pCO_2, pH increases by 0.03.

Clinical correlation:

- Always correlate blood gas results with the clinical picture, including signs of distress, vital signs, and other laboratory values.
- Treatment plans should be adjusted based on a comprehensive evaluation of the neonate's clinical status rather than solely relying on blood gas results.

Calculation of delta ratio:

- Delta ratio is used to assess the contribution of unmeasured anions to metabolic acidosis.
- Delta ratio = Delta anion gap/delta HCO_3

Interpretation of delta ratio:

- <0.4 = Normal anion gap metabolic acidosis
- 0.4 to 0.8 = High and normal anion gap metabolic acidosis
- 0.8 to 2 = High anion gap metabolic acidosis
- >2 = Mixed high anion gap metabolic acidosis and metabolic alkalosis.

CONCLUSION

Blood gas analysis is a cornerstone of neonatal care, facilitating the assessment and management of complex respiratory and metabolic disorders. A thorough understanding of technical aspects, an algorithmic approach to interpretation, and insights into mixed disorders and compensatory mechanisms enhance clinicians' ability to make informed decisions. Ultimately, this knowledge is crucial for optimizing outcomes in the neonatal population.

SUGGESTED READING

1. Alabed M, Omer O. Blood Gas Analysis: A Neonatologist's Perspective. J Pediatr Intensive Care. 2022;15(4):230-9.
2. Miller AH, Calkins H. Blood Gas Management in the NICU. J Neonat Respir Care. 2023;18(2):102-9.
3. Roberts DJ, McKinlay C. Algorithmic Approach to Blood Gas Interpretation in Neonates. Clin Pediatr Emerg Med. 2020;21(3):267-76.
4. Roberts JL, Green JM. Clinical Guidelines for Blood Gas Monitoring in Neonates. Neonatology Today. 2021;16(1):14-22.
5. Sood P, Paul G, Puri S. Interpretation of arterial blood gas. Indian J Crit Care Med. 2010;14(2):57-64. doi: 10.4103/0972-5229.68215.
6. Tan RN, Mulder EE, Lopriore E, Te Pas AB. Monitoring Oxygenation and Gas Exchange in Neonatal Intensive Care Units: Current Practice in the Netherlands. Front Pediatr. 2015;3:94. doi: 10.3389/fped.2015.00094.
7. Wong DT, Singhal N. Neonatal Blood Gas Analysis: A Comprehensive Review. Pediatr Clin North Am. 2020;67(3):511-25.
8. Zimmerman JJ, Clark RSB, Fuhrman BP, Rotta AT, Kudchadkar SR, Relvas, MS, Tobias JD. Fuhrman & Zimmerman's Pediatric Critical Care. 6th edition. Philadelphia, PA: Elsevier; 2022.

CHAPTER

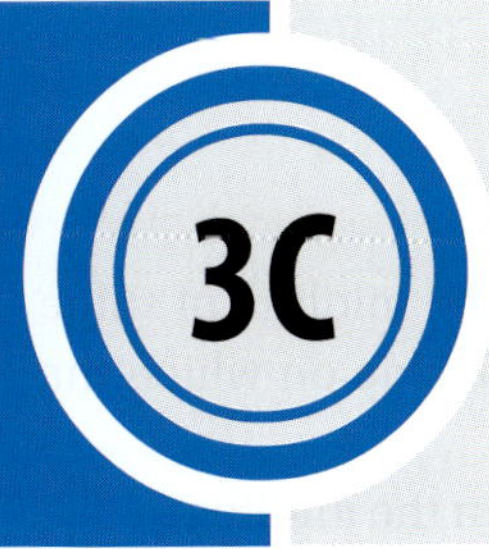

Lung Imaging—Evaluation and Monitoring

Amit Upadhyay, Priyanka Gupta

INTRODUCTION

Lung imaging, which includes plain radiography and lung ultrasound, is crucial in managing neonatal respiratory distress. Neonatal respiratory distress can be caused by various conditions, such as respiratory distress syndrome (RDS), transient tachypnea of the newborn, meconium aspiration syndrome, pneumothorax, and congenital heart diseases.

INDICATIONS OF LUNG IMAGING IN NEWBORNS

The following are the indications of lung imaging in newborns:

- Respiratory distress
- Sudden worsening of respiratory distress in a newborn
- Evaluation of cyanosis
- For suspected cardiac disease
- Confirmation of position of endotracheal tubes (ETTs), central lines, and chest tubes

The dose of radiation exposure from a single chest X-ray (CXR) is approximately 0.008–0.03 mSv. When combined with an abdominal radiograph, the dose is 1.5–2 times higher.

NEONATAL CHEST X-RAY

The plain chest radiograph [anteroposterior (AP)] is the most widely used imaging modality in the neonatal intensive care unit (NICU). Appropriate positioning of the infant is essential to interpret a radiograph correctly. Lateral CXRs can aid in assessing retrocardiac lung fields, small air leaks (affected side up), location of the pleural drain, and sometimes free air under the diaphragm. The cross-table view is better for assessing abdomen in suspected necrotizing enterocolitis (NEC). Abdomen erect view is surgeon's view for suspected perforation.

ROTATION

A film is said to be rotated if:

- The distance of the anterior ends of the ribs from the midline of spine is unequal on either side. The film is rotated to that side on which the distance appears greater, and/or
- The medial end of the clavicles is not equidistant from the midline.

A "rotated" CXR may lead to a false diagnosis of cardiomegaly, mediastinal shift, atelectasis, or abnormal central line location. The infant's arms should be extended from the chest to prevent the scapulae from obscuring the upper lung fields **(Figs. 1A and B)**.

EXPOSURE (FIGS. 2A AND B)

- If the retrocardiac vertebrae are easily seen, the X-ray film is overexposed.
- If long bones appear very dark, the X-ray film is overexposed.

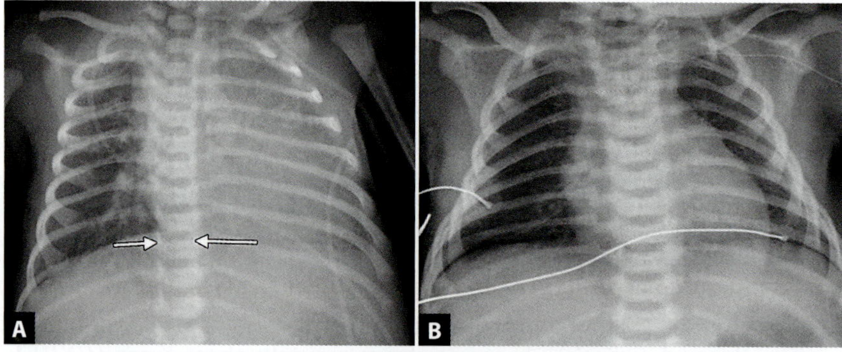

Figs. 1A and B: (A) Rotated versus (B) nonrotated chest X-ray films.

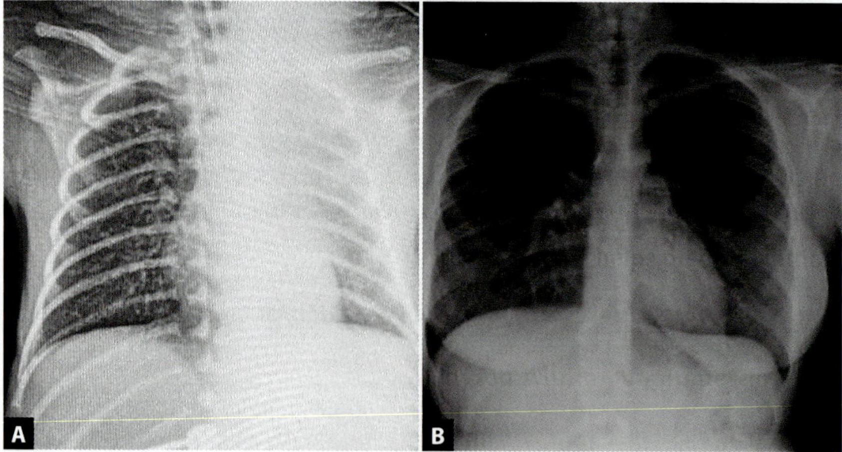

Figs. 2A and B: (A) Underexposed and (B) overexposed films. Underexposed films accentuate the parenchymal abnormalities.

In a normal, correctly positioned AP CXR, the neonatal chest appears trapezoid in shape with horizontal ribs **(Fig. 3)**. The diaphragm lies at the level of the sixth to eighth rib **(Figs. 4A and B)**. Both lungs are symmetrically aerated with uniform radiolucency soon after birth. Air bronchograms in the lung bases, particularly in the lower left lobe behind the cardiac border, are normal. Pulmonary vascular markings are visualized centrally and become less prominent toward the periphery. The transverse cardiothoracic ratio should not exceed 60–65%. The thymus may occupy majority of the upper chest, especially during the first few days of life.

One often concentrates on the lungs in the CXRs, but other structures in chest are equally important to be looked at. A systemic approach using the "ABCDEFG" (A: airway trachea and its branches, B: bones, C: cardiac structures including vessels, D: diaphragm, E: effusions, F: fields and fissures, and G: gastric fundus and other visible intrabdominal structures) approach may help the clinician to evaluate it systematically and not miss important findings in other structures **(Fig. 3)**.

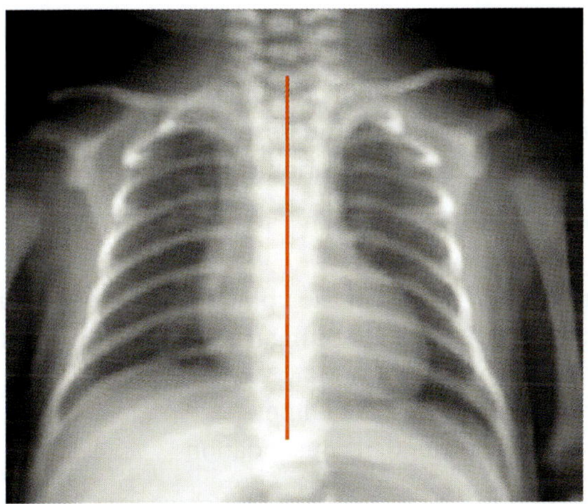

Fig. 3: Normal X-ray.

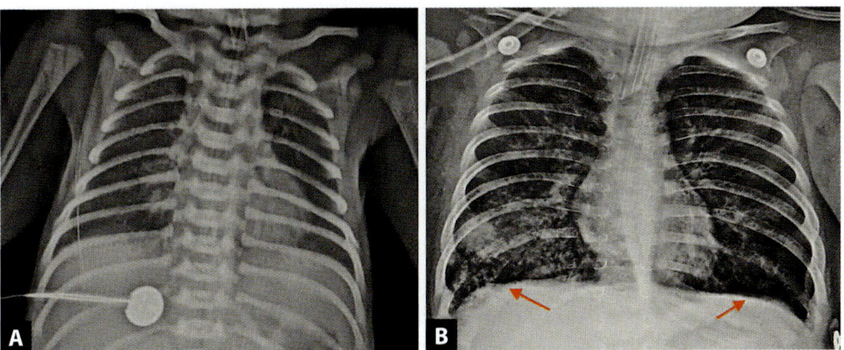

Figs. 4A and B: (A) Normal expansion versus (B) hyperexpansion. Note the flattening of the diaphragm and small heart [marked by red arrows (B)].

Decreased pulmonary blood flow (oligemia) is diagnosed by relative blackness of lung fields such as tricuspid atresia, Ebstein anomaly, pulmonary stenosis, tetralogy of Fallot, and pulmonary atresia. Increased blood flow/ vascularity is seen when the pulmonary vessels are seen in the lateral third of the film such as atrial septal defect (ASD), ventricular septal defect (VSD), patent ductus arteriosus (PDA), transposition of great arteries, total anomalous pulmonary venous connection, persistent truncus arteriosus, and single ventricle.

Lung ultrasonography (USG): The advantages of USG include its ready availability in NICU, relative ease of use by trained personnel, noninvasive "real-time" point-of-care imaging capabilities, and lack of ionizing radiation. Lung USG is used for multiple indications including RDS severity assessment, diagnosis of pulmonary air leak in acutely deteriorating baby, management of pleural effusion, diagnosis of pneumonia, assessment of diaphragmatic movement, evaluation of congenital lung lesions (CLLs), and confirmation of ETT and vascular catheter tip location. A linear high-frequency probe >9 MHz or a hockey stick probe is preferred for lung imaging. Each side is divided into three areas:

1. Anterior area between sternum and anterior axillary line
2. Lateral area between anterior and posterior axillary line
3. Posterior area between the posterior axillary line and the spine

Lung USG score for RDS **(Fig. 5)***:*

- *Score 0:* Presence of only A lines
- *Score 1:* Presence of A lines in the upper part of the lung and coalescent B lines in the lower part of the lung (pattern A) or at least three B lines (pattern B)
- *Score 2:* Presence of coalescent B lines
- *Score 3:* Presence of extended consolidation

Lung USG score in transient tachypnea of the newborn (TTNB):

- *Type 1:* Fluid retention appears as compact B lines
- *Type 2:* Confluent B lines, pleural line are seen
- *Type 3:* Full aeration, pleural line clear, and A lines

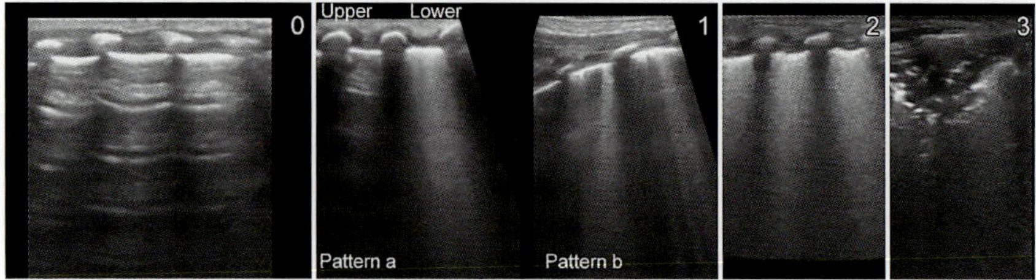

Fig. 5: Neonatal lung ultrasonography (USG) score ≥5 showed a sensitivity of 86% and a specificity of 88% in predicting the need for surfactant.

Note: When severe RDS is observed in more mature infants and fails to respond to conventional management, clinicians should consider congenital etiologies such as surfactant deficiencies and alveolar capillary dysplasia.

Table 1 summarizes the characteristic appearances of common neonatal conditions on X-ray and USG.

TABLE 1: Characteristic appearance of common respiratory disease conditions.

Disease conditions	*X-ray findings*	*USG findings*
Respiratory distress syndrome **(Figs. 6A to C)**	• Low lung volumes • Fine granular or ground glass appearance • Air bronchograms • White-out lungs • Cardiac borders are difficult to identify	• Thick (>0.5 mm)/irregular pleural line • Absence of A lines • Confluent B lines • Consolidation (subpleural/most often in the posterior parts) • Air bronchograms
Transient tachypnea of newborn **(Figs. 7 and 8)**	• Mildly overexpanded lungs • Prominent interlobar fissure • Increased interstitial streaky shadowing extending to periphery • Small pleural effusion	• Bilateral confluent B lines in the dependent regions • Normal pattern in the superior regions • There should be no lung consolidation • Double lung point • Mild pleural effusion
Meconium aspiration syndrome	• Heterogenous lungs—hyperexpanded ± heterogenous infiltrates to complete opacification of thorax • Pneumothorax	• Nonspecific • Shred sign • Pleural is abnormal • Disappearance of A lines • B lines visible in the nonconsolidated zone
Pneumonia **(Figs. 9A to C)**	• Early onset pneumonia—normal or hyperexpansion with heterogeneously distributed densities • Late onset—diffusely hazy, may be similar to RDS	• Irregular hypoechoic areas • Fragmented pleural line • Air bronchograms/fluid bronchograms in the area of consolidation • Shred sign • Bigger consolidation—dynamic air bronchogram is visible • More commonly observed in posterior lower regions • Ecostructural liver pattern (hepatization of lung) • Dynamic air bronchogram in pneumonic consolidation due to the possibility of observing the air move back and forth with the breaths • A static air bronchogram, in which air movement is not observable, is seen in atelectasis

Contd...

Contd...

Disease conditions	*X-ray findings*	*USG findings*
Pneumothorax/air leak **(Figs. 10A to D)**	• Air in the pleural space with compression of the affected lung • Flattening of diaphragm • Shift of the mediastinum to the contralateral side	• *B-mode:* – Presence of lung points – Absence of lung sliding – No B lines – Absence of lung pulse • *M-mode:* – Barcode sign/stratosphere sign – Seashore sign—normal
Pneumomediastinum **(Fig. 11)**	• Presence of air adjacent to the heart, outlining and elevating it • *Spinnaker sign:* In a left anterior oblique view, in which air is seen surrounding the thymus above the cardiac shadow	
Pneumopericardium **(Fig. 12)**	Air surrounds the cardiac border that does not extend beyond the reflection of the aorta or the pulmonary artery. The presence of air under the heart is also diagnostic	
Pulmonary interstitial emphysema **(Fig. 13)**	• Appears as small cystic/linear translucencies extending from the hilum to the periphery • Increased lung volumes	• Noncoalescent (confluent) B lines in affected areas • Unaffected areas look normal, with normal A lines
Pulmonary hemorrhage **(Fig. 14)**	Variable findings that range from patchy infiltrates to complete opacification of one or more lungs	• Shred sign • Consolidation with air bronchograms • Pleural line abnormalities • Disappearing A lines
Pleural effusion **(Figs. 15A to D)**	• Blunting of costophrenic angle • Large pneumothorax—progressive opacification of the pneumothorax on the same side and shift of the mediastinum toward the opposite side	• Hypoechoic collection between parietal and visceral pleura (empyema/blood may show particulate matter in the effusion) • Sinusoid sign—M-mode • Quad sign

Contd...

Contd...

Disease conditions	*X-ray findings*	*USG findings*
Lung abscess	• Cavity containing a gas–fluid level • Round in shape • All margins are equally seen	Appears as a well-demarcated capsular structure surrounding a hypoechoic core without internal vascularity on color Doppler
BPD **(Fig. 16)**	Norway, et al.: • *Stage 1*: Air bronchogram, reticulogranular pattern • *Stage 2*: Opacification, coarse irregular densities • *Stage 3*: Small generalized radiolucent cystic areas, hyperinflated lung cysts • *Stage 4*: Dense fibrotic strands, generalized	Nonspecific
Diaphragmatic palsy	• Usually, right diaphragm is elevated slightly compared to the left side – This right side elevation is further elevated in diaphragmatic palsy of right side – More acute costophrenic angle	• On lung USG, the diaphragms appear as bright curved lines that move with respiration • Excursion of <4 mm and a difference of >50% between the excursion of one hemidiaphragm compared to other (B-mode) • M-mode can also show the paradoxical movement of the paralyzed diaphragm
Congenital lung lesions		
CPAM **(Fig. 17A)**	• Multiple air-filled cysts • Collapse of the surrounding parenchyma	A large hypoechogenic cystic single lesion, small communicating cystic lesions, and consolidations
Bronchopulmonary sequestration	Dense mass, usually in the medial basal segment of the left lower lobe	
Congenital lobar emphysema **(Fig. 17C)**	• Soon after birth, it may show opacification of the affected lobe • Later, the affected lung is overexpanded and hyperlucent, and the adjacent lung appears dense and compressed	

Contd...

Contd…

Disease conditions	*X-ray findings*	*USG findings*
Congenital diaphragmatic hernia **(Fig. 17B)**	• Herniated bowel contents • Shift of mediastinum toward the opposite side • Compressive atelectasis of the opposite lung	• On the affected side, absence of a pleural line with no lung sliding and visible loops of the bowel (may show peristalsis) • Heart may appear displaced
Eventration **(Fig. 17D)**	The affected side may be seen as smooth hump or elevation	
TEF **(Fig. 17E)**	• Coiling of the tube in the upper esophagus • Lateral X-ray to delineate the extent of gap between upper and lower pouch • Absent stomach bubble signifies esophageal atresia	

(BPD: bronchopulmonary dysplasia; CPAM: congenital pulmonary airway malformation; RDS: respiratory distress syndrome; TEF: tracheoesophageal fistula; USG: ultrasonography)

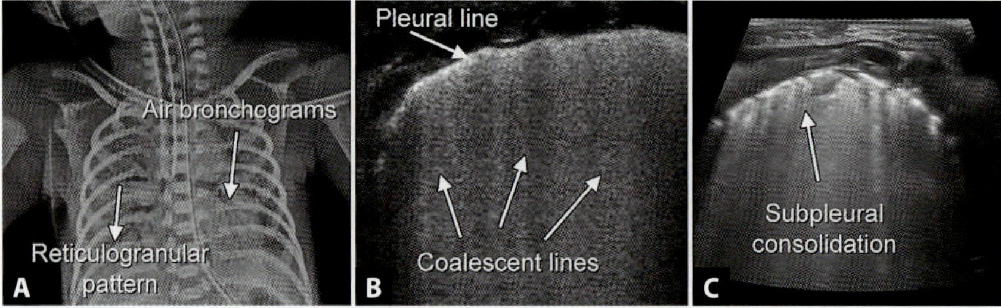

Figs. 6A to C: Neonatal respiratory distress syndrome imaging—chest X-ray and ultrasonography (USG).

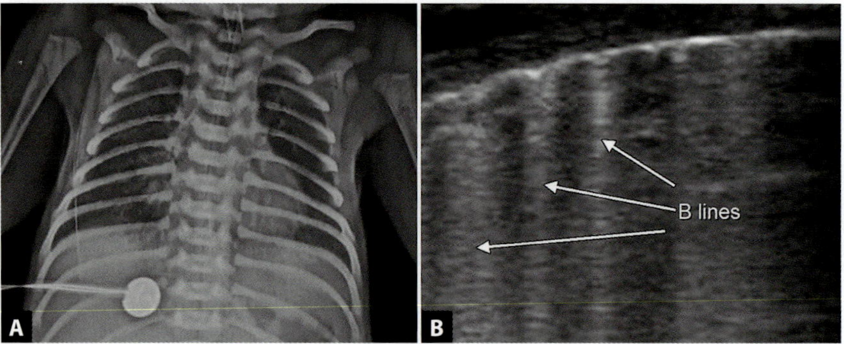

Figs. 7A and B: Transient tachypnea of newborn.

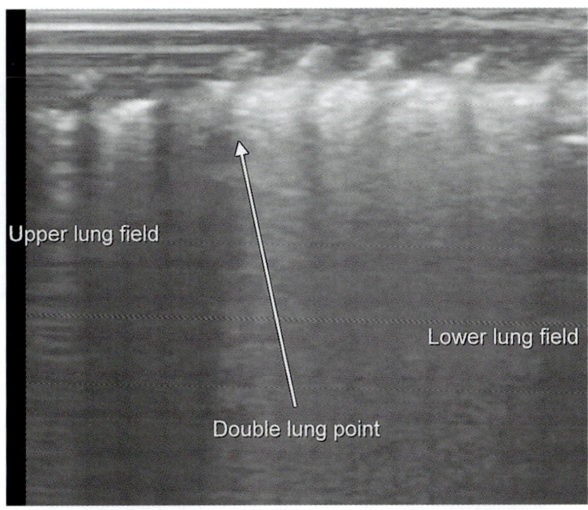

Fig. 8: Double lung point—note the difference between the severity of B lines of upper and lower lung fields in lung ultrasonography (USG).

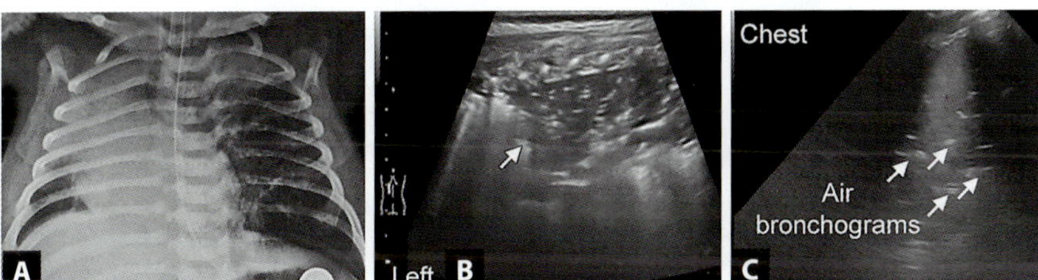

Figs. 9A to C: (A) Neonatal chest X-ray showing collapse consolidation of the left upper and middle zone; (B) Shred sign; (C) Speckled snowflake-like appearance of air bronchograms.

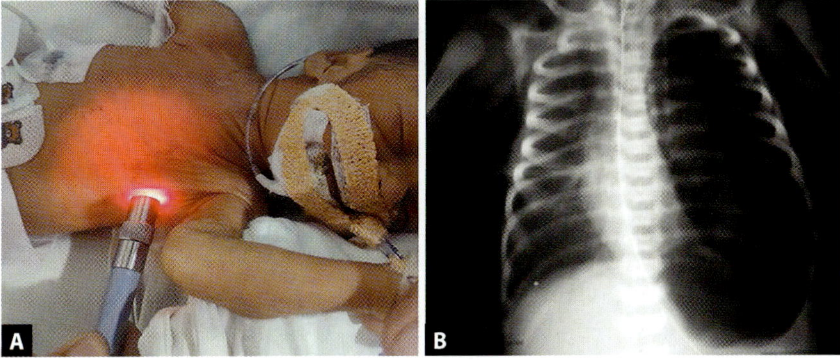

Figs. 10A and B

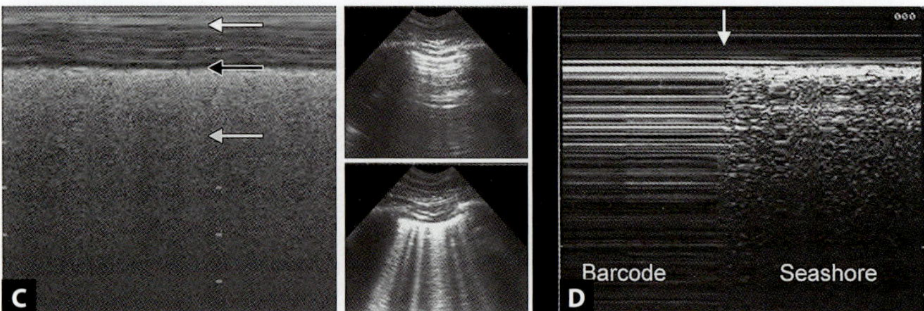

Figs. 10C and D

Figs. 10A to D: (A) Fiber-optic source light showing transillumination in a left-sided pneumothorax; (B) Chest X-ray showing large left-sided pneumothorax with shift of mediastinum toward the opposite side; (C) Sandy beach appearance/seashore sign—normal lung; (D) Barcode sign—pneumothorax.

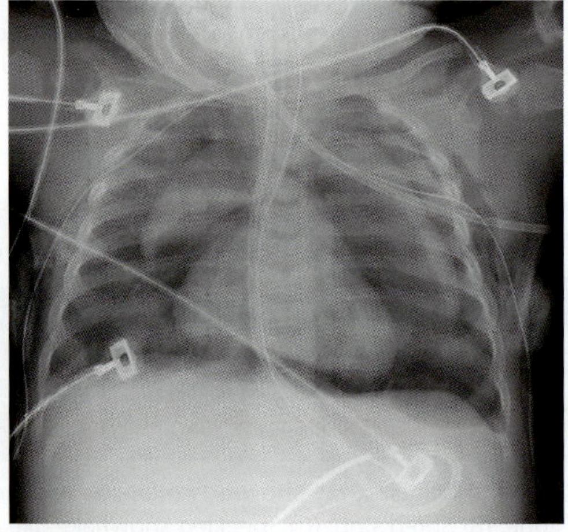

Fig. 11: Spinnaker sign (pneumomediastinum).

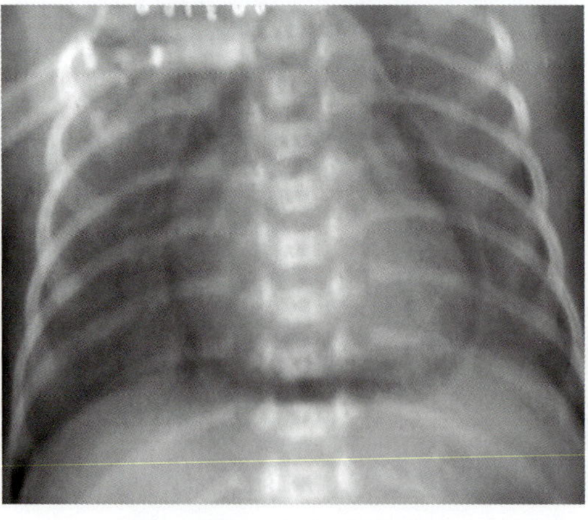

Fig. 12: Pneumopericardium.

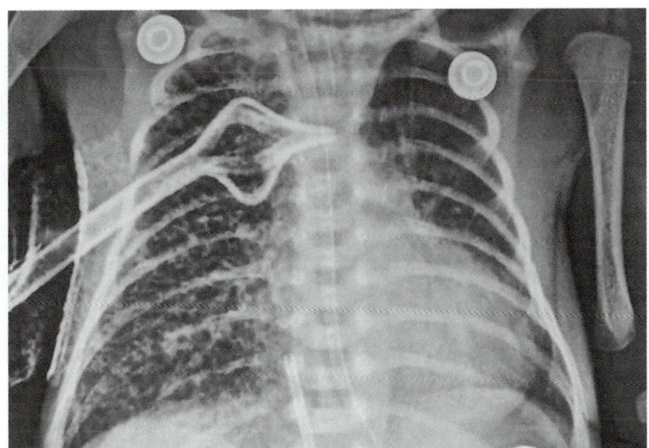

Fig. 13: Pulmonary interstitial emphysema—note the streaky radiolucencies in bilateral lung fields.

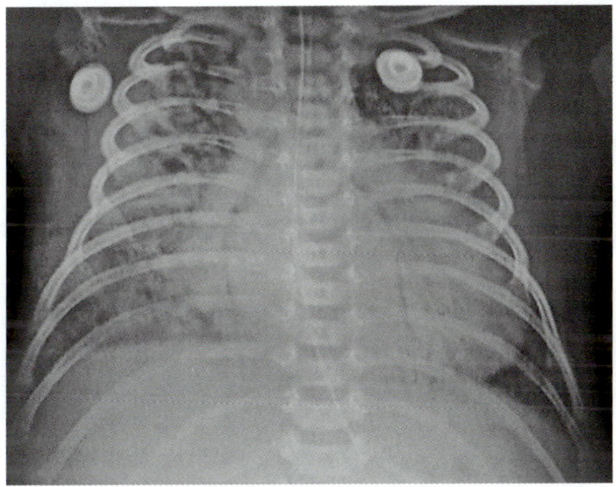

Fig. 14: Neonatal pulmonary hemorrhage secondary to hemodynamically significant patent ductus arteriosus (hsPDA). Note the cardiomegaly secondary to patent ductus arteriosus (PDA) in 26 weeks extremely low birth weight neonate.

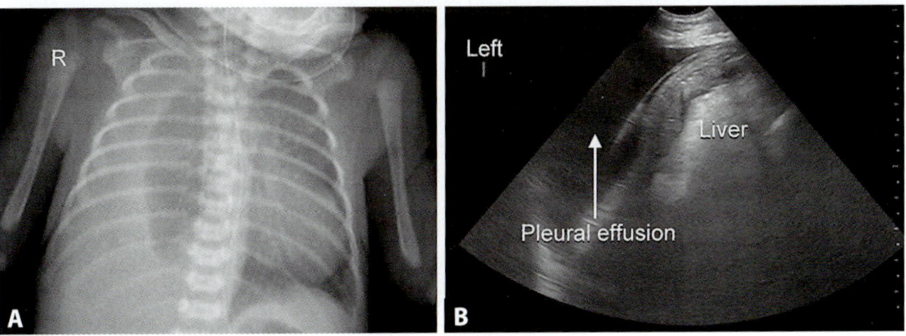

Figs. 15A and B

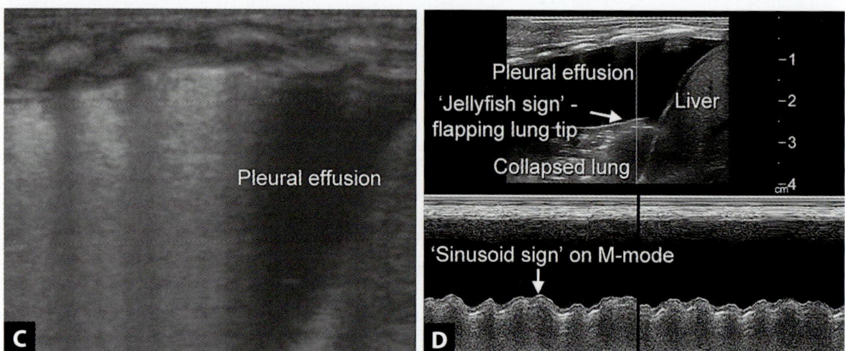

Figs. 15C and D

Figs. 15A to D: (A) Chest X-ray and (B to D) lung ultrasonography (USG) images and different signs of pleural effusion.

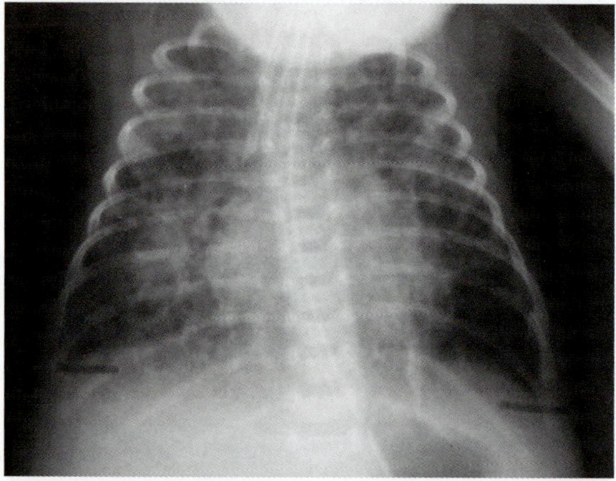

Fig. 16: Stage 3 bronchopulmonary dysplasia (BPD) (Northway classification).

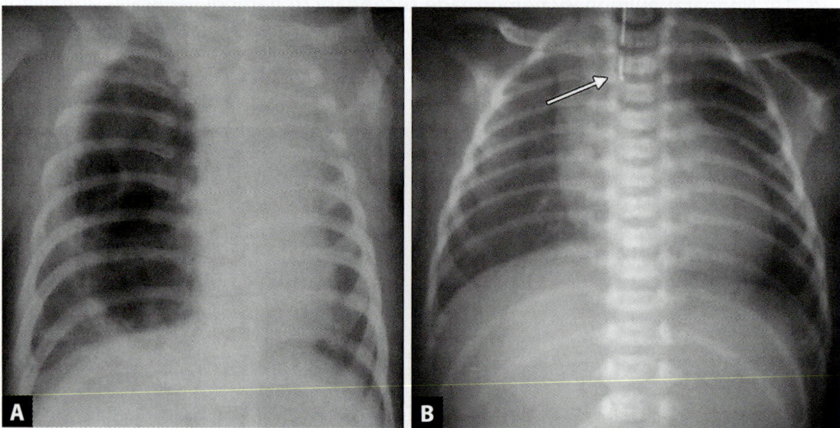

Figs. 17A and B

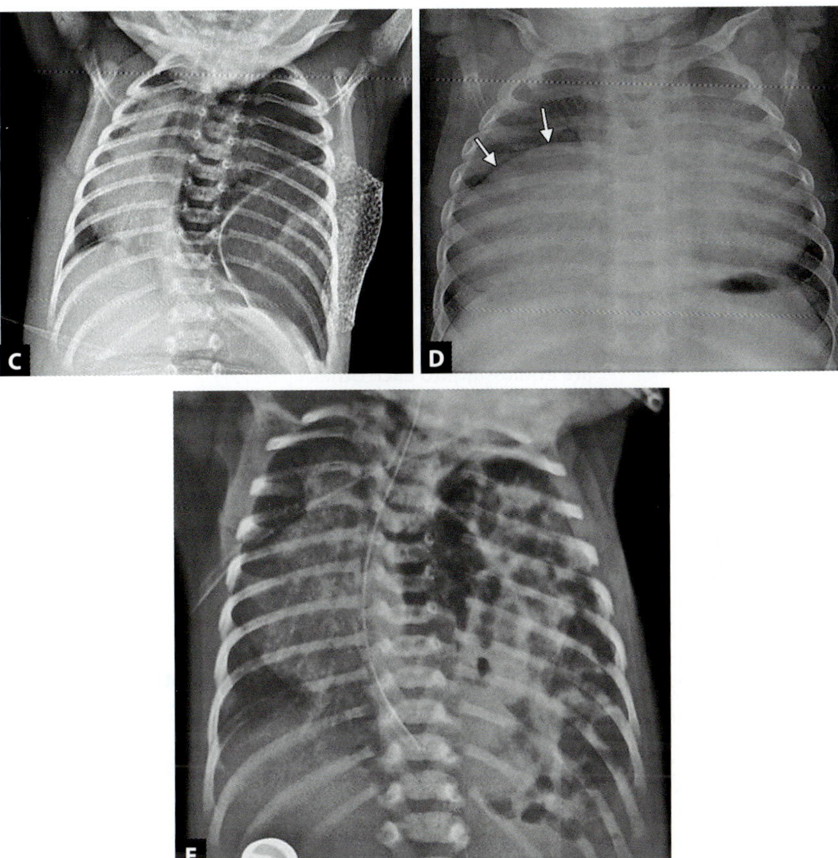

Figs. 17C to E

Figs. 17A to E: Congenital anomalies of the lung in a neonate: (A) Right congenital pulmonary airway malformation (CPAM); (B) Left-sided congenital diaphragmatic hernia; (C) Congenital lobar emphysema; (D) Right-sided eventration of the diaphragm; (E) Esophageal atresia [nasogastric (NG) tube coiling in the upper esophagus].

Table 2 enumerates the different signs that can be appreciated on X-ray and USG in neonatal conditions.

PITFALLS AND PRACTICAL TIPS

- *Asepsis:* Handwashing should be done before doing chest X-ray by the X-ray technician and before lung USG by doctor/resident. Ultrasound probe should be cleaned with alcohol each time before and after use.
- Do not place baby directly in contact with X-ray plate—cover with sterile plastic sheet.
- Left and right markings should be placed carefully.
- Shield yourself and patient's gonads.

TABLE 2: Different signs of chest X-ray and lung ultrasonography (USG).

Signs seen in neonatal chest X-ray	
Sail sign	A sail-like, triangular projection from the mediastinum, which is a shadow of thymus. It is not pathological
Spinnaker sign	It refers to thymus being outlined by air and the lobes of the thymus are displaced off the mediastinal structures by air in the mediastinum. It is pathological and seen in pneumomediastinum
Signs seen in neonatal lung USG	
A lines	Horizontal, reverberation artifacts of the pleural line. A lines are equidistant to each other
B lines	Vertical, laser-like, hyperechoic lines arise from pleural line and extend to the edge of the screen without fading. Erases A lines. The occurrence of three or more B lines in one intercostal space indicates interstitial or alveolar fluid
Comet tail sign	Less echoic than the pleural line, vanishes after 2–4 cm, does not erase A lines
Sliding sign	The parietal pleura and visceral pleura appear sliding over each other. Absent in pneumothorax
Double lung point	Areas within a lung with a sharp cutoff point between two lung fields of different severity of B lines, e.g., transient tachypnea of the newborn (TTNB)
Lung point	B-mode USG, transition area between an area of absence of lung sliding and the adjacent area with normal sliding, e.g., mild to moderate pneumothorax
Sandy beach sign/ seashore sign	*M-mode USG:* Above the pleural line, the tissues are generally not moving, and they appear as sand on a beach. Below the pleural line, the lung moves with breathing movements and appears as uniform dot echoes like sand on beach. Absent in pneumothorax
Stratosphere sign/ barcode sign	*M-mode USG:* When lung movement is impaired, granular dot is replaced by a series of horizontal parallel lines, e.g., air leak
Shred sign/fractal sign	The boundary between consolidated lung tissue and adjacent aerated tissue that appears shredded
Air bronchograms	Dense, speckled, and snowflake-like, e.g. consolidation and atelectasis

- Exposure settings should be noted to determine optimal exposure for the baby.
- Expose only the area that is required.
- Baby's back should be in full contact with the plate to avoid any air pocket in between.
- Try to avoid rotation in the neck and spine.

- While reading the X-ray, use ABCDEF approach to avoid missing on important findings.
- Use ultrasound gel that has been prewarmed to body temperature (can be done by placing it under warmer).
- Avoid air bubbles between the transducer and the skin surface.

CONCLUSION

Chest X-ray and USG chest are the primary imaging modalities, with computed tomography (CT) and magnetic resonance imaging (MRI) reserved for complex cases. Early, accurate, and systematic interpretation of neonatal chest imaging is critical for diagnosing respiratory illnesses. Lung USG is increasingly being recognized as a valuable tool for point-of-care assessment, but it is operator-dependent. A multimodal approach combining clinical findings and imaging results is necessary.

To assess the E-videos on lung USG, scan below:

SUGGESTED READING

1. Ammirabile A, Buonsenso D, Di Mauro A. Lung Ultrasound in Pediatrics and Neonatology: An Update. Healthcare (Basel). 2021;9(8):1015.
2. Jain SN, Modi T, Varma RU. Decoding the neonatal chest radiograph: An insight into neonatal respiratory distress. Indian J Radiol Imaging. 2020;30(4):482-92.
3. Keszler M, Suresh GK, Goldsmith JP, (Eds). Goldsmith's Assisted Ventilation of the Neonate: An Evidence-based Approach to Newborn Respiratory Care. 7th ed. Philadelphia: Elsevier; 2021.
4. Northway WH Jr., Rosan RC, Porter DY. Pulmonary disease following respirator therapy of hyaline-membrane disease. Bronchopulmonary dysplasia. N Engl J Med. 1967;276(7):357-68.
5. Rath C, Suryawanshi P. Point of care lung USG in neonatology. J Neonatol. 2018;32(1):27-37.

CHAPTER

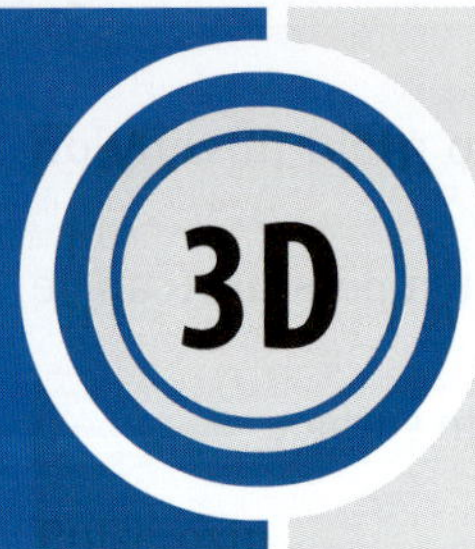

Noninvasive Monitoring of Gas Exchange

Murugesan A, Chaitra Angadi

INTRODUCTION

Monitoring of gas exchange involves monitoring of both oxygenation and CO_2 removal. Although the reference standard to assess gas exchange is arterial blood gas analysis, it is invasive and not always necessary. Both indirect measures and surrogate markers of assessment of gas exchange are preferred whenever possible. The various methods of assessment of gas exchange at different levels of microcirculation is shown in **Figure 1**. We will discuss some commonly used monitoring devices/techniques in this chapter.

CLINICAL MONITORING

Respiratory Distress Scoring

Downes and Silverman Anderson scores (SAS) are commonly used respiratory distress severity scores in neonates. While Downes score can be used in both term and preterm infants, SAS is used in preterm infants only as shown in **Tables 1 and 2**. A score of 4–6 usually indicates moderate respiratory distress

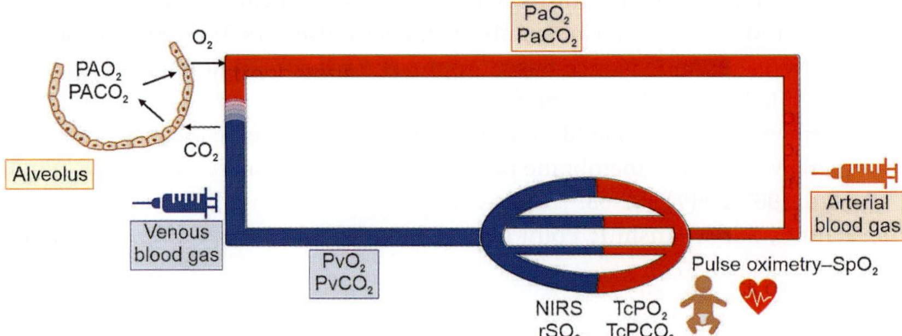

Fig. 1: Alveolocapillary interface and gas exchange at different levels of microcirculation. Various methods of assessment of gas exchange at different levels are also depicted. (PaO_2: partial pressure of arterial oxygen; $PaCO_2$: partial pressure of arterial CO_2; $TcPO_2$: transcutaneous PO_2 at capillary level; $TcPCO_2$: transcutaneous PCO_2 at capillary level; NIRS: near infrared spectroscopy; rSO_2: regional oxygen saturation; PvO_2: partial pressure of venous oxygen; $PvCO_2$: partial pressure of venous CO_2; PAO_2: partial pressure of alveolar oxygen; $PACO_2$: partial pressure of alveolar CO_2)

TABLE 1: Downes score.

Score	*0*	*1*	*2*
Respiratory rate/min	<60	60–80	>80
Cyanosis[#]	Absent	In room air	In 40% O_2
Retractions	Absent	Mild	Moderate to severe
Grunting	Absent	Audible with stethoscope	Audible without stethoscope
Air entry*	Clear	Delayed or decreased	Barely audible

*Air entry as measured in mid axillary line.
[#]For infants on respiratory support, this can be taken as fraction of inspired oxygen (FiO_2) required to maintain target oxygen saturation (SpO_2) (0: 21%; 1: 22–39%; 2: 40% or more).
Interpretation:
- *Score 1–3:* Mild respiratory distress
- *Score 4–6:* Moderate respiratory distress
- *Score >6:* Impending respiratory failure

TABLE 2: Silverman Anderson score.

Score	*0*	*1*	*2*
Upper chest retractions	Synchrony between upper chest and lower chest during breathing	Upper chest lags during inspiration	See-saw respiration
Lower chest retractions*	Absent	Just visible	Marked
Xiphoid retractions	Absent	Just visible	Marked
Nasal flaring	Absent	Minimal	Marked
Grunting	Clear	With stethoscope only	Audible without stethoscope

*To be examined tangentially from the side below the level of mid-axillary line.
Interpretation:
- *Score 1–6:* Respiratory distress
- *Score >6:* Impending respiratory failure

which can be managed with noninvasive support. A score of >6 is associated with respiratory failure and death and may require invasive ventilation. Though the respiratory distress severity scores do not provide quantitative assessment of partial pressure of carbon dioxide (pCO_2) and partial pressure of oxygen (pO_2), they have been shown to be useful in deciding escalation/de-escalation of respiratory support and/or surfactant administration and are easy to assess bedside. Additionally, they may be the only guide for clinicians in resource-constrained settings.

MONITORING USING POINT-OF-CARE EQUIPMENT

The various point-of-care equipment, their working principle, utility, and limitations are shown in **Table 3**.

Pulse Oximetry

Pulse oximetry is a noninvasive measure of oxygenation, and it has been in use in neonates since mid-1980s. It measures the percentage of hemoglobin that is saturated with oxygen (measured as SpO_2 values). It is based on the Beer–Lambert law, which states that the absorption of light of a given wavelength is directly proportional to the concentration of the substance that absorbs light (Hb in case of pulse oximetry) and the path length, which the light beam has to traverse. Working principles behind pulse oximetry are:

- Spectrophotometry (oxygenated Hb absorbs light in infrared spectrum, while deoxygenated blood absorbs light in the red spectrum)
- Photoplethysmography (amount of light absorbed by tissues varies according to arterial pulse)

TABLE 3: Commonly available point-of-care equipment for noninvasive monitoring of gas exchange.

Measurement	*What is measured and how?*	*Utility*	*Limitations*
SpO_2	Ratio of oxygenated to reduced Hb by spectrophotometry	Routinely used in delivery points, NICU for oxygen targeting and for CCHD screening	Less reliable in lower saturation limits (<80%); cannot measure CO_2
$TcPO_2$, $TcPCO_2$	Transcutaneous measurement of both PO_2 and PCO_2 by electrophoresis	Can measure both O_2 and CO_2	Skin burns. Need frequent change of site
Capnography	Measured at the level of endotracheal tube, by infrared absorption spectroscopy	Bedside assessment of CO_2	• Detector adds to dead space • Leaks around ET may affect measurement
NIRS	Similar to SpO_2; but measures tissue oxygenation rather than arterial saturation	Gives idea about regional oxygenation and oxygen extraction	• Lack of normative values • Use of NIRS has not improved clinical outcomes

(CCHD: critical congenital heart disease; SpO_2: oxygen saturation; NICU: neonatal intensive care unit; NIRS: near infrared spectroscopy; PCO_2: partial pressure of carbon dioxide; PO_2: partial pressure of oxygen; $TcPCO_2$ transcutaneous partial pressure of carbon dioxide; $TcPO_2$: transcutaneous oxygen pressure)

The use of signal extraction technology (SET) has improved accuracy of pulse oximetry to ±2% in neonates whose SpO_2 >80%. Recently introduced blue sensors with SET have shown good accuracy (±5%) in infants with SpO_2 between 60 and 80%. There is enough evidence to suggest that targeting SpO_2 of 91–95% protects against the harmful effects of both hypoxemia and hyperoxia. Targeting a lower SpO_2 of 85–89% is associated with a 16% higher incidence of death and 33% higher incidence of necrotizing enterocolitis (NEC).

Measurement of oxygenation by pulse oximetry is relevant in:

- *SpO_2 targeting:* Target SpO_2 for preterm infants is 91–95%. Alarm limits are set at 89 and 96%.
- For screening of critical congenital heart disease.

Important practical points:

- Attach the pulse oximetry probe correctly **(Fig. 1)** in such a way that the light source is exactly opposite to the sensor. Inaccurate attachment may lead to air interference and incorrect values. It is useful to cover the sensor to protect it from the ambient light in the room, which again may interfere with the readings.
- Use right hand/wrist for preductal SpO_2, and either of the feet for postductal SpO_2.
- Target SpO_2 at 1, 2, 3, 4, 5, and 10 minutes of life are: 60–65%, 65–70%, 70–75%, 75–80%, 80–85%, and 85–95%, respectively.
- Motion artefacts, low heart rate, and poor peripheral perfusion will affect SpO_2 values.
- To get a stable reading quickly, particularly in the delivery room settings, the steps are to be followed in order: (1) Connect pulse oximetry cable to monitor, (2) switch on the monitor, (3) connect probe to infant, (4) then connect the probe to the pulse oximeter cable.
- It is important to remember the effect of oxygen dissociation curve (ODC) on SpO_2 readings. As we know, increase in temperature, H^+, 2,3 DPG, and adult Hb will shift the ODC to right (PaO_2 will be higher for the same SpO_2). A preterm infant born at 30 weeks has almost 90% of Hb as HbF. Liberal transfusions in preterm infants with adult Hb increase the risk of retinopathy of prematurity (ROP) and bronchopulmonary dysplasia (BPD), because of this reason.
- Pulse oximeters used for neonatal use should have clinically proven technology to detect saturation in low perfusion states and to avoid motion artefacts. Signal extraction technology is one of the techniques which incorporates adaptive filtering, thereby limiting the effect of noise and motion artefacts.

Limitations of pulse oximetry:

- Pulse oximetry can give an idea about oxygenation but not gas exchange/ CO_2 removal.

- Conditions which shift the ODC to right/left (temperature, pH, fetal Hb, 2.3-DPG) affect the interpretation of measured values.
- Due to sigmoidal nature of ODC, larger changes in pO_2 will have only smaller increments/decrements in SpO_2 at the higher and lower plateaus of the curve **(Fig. 1)**; hence, pulse oximetry is slow to detect hypoxemia and hyperoxia.
- There is often a lag between measured SpO_2 and fall/rise in pO_2, with pulse oximetry lagging by 5–15 seconds. Actual changes in oxygenation usually precede changes visualized in pulse oximetry.
- Other forms of Hb (Met Hb and carboxy Hb) are usually found in lower concentrations in the blood and may not affect SpO_2 measurement in normal individuals, but SpO_2 values may be unreliable with significant levels of these forms of Hb in blood.
- Pulse oximetry values are reliable in the SpO_2 range between 80 and 95%.
- Affected by skin pigmentation.

Newer pulse oximeters have ORI (oxygen reserve index) measurement, which gives an approximate measure of pO_2. It is based on Fick's principle which takes into account the change in light absorption with increasing pO_2 (whereas Beer–Lambert law uses the principle of differential light absorption based on concentration of substance that absorbs light, i.e., Hb). ORI is a value between 0 and 1, where if all ORIs were above 0.24, the pO_2 values were also above 100 mm Hg, and almost 96% of all ORIs were above 0.55 if the pO_2 value was above 150 mm Hg. However, it needs additional validation in neonates.

Transcutaneous Oxygen ($TcPO_2$) and CO_2 ($TcPCO_2$) Measurement

Transcutaneous oxygen ($TcPO_2$) and CO_2 ($TcPCO_2$) measurement helps to circumvent one major limitation of pulse oximetry, which is the inability to measure pO_2 and pCO_2. Both of them have similar principles in that, they use a round sensor of about 1.5 cm diameter, which is usually placed over the anterior abdominal wall or thigh. The sensor has an adhesive, a polyethylene film separating a thin film of electrolyte solution and a cathode and anode. Based on the electrical signal detected, the value of pO_2 or pCO_2 is calculated. Though originally sensors were different for pO_2 and pCO_2, newer machines have made it possible to measure pO_2 or pCO_2 and SpO_2, with the same sensor.

The major limitation of these sensors is that the calibration takes some time (about 20 minutes, especially for $TcPO_2$) and the skin is heated up to 41–43°C (to arterialize the capillaries), which may cause erythema and injury to the skin.

Capnography

Cerebral blood flow is primarily influenced by arterial CO_2 ($PaCO_2$) levels. Therefore, an elevation in $PaCO_2$ levels leads to an augmentation in the cerebral blood flow and vice versa. In mechanically ventilated extremely preterm babies, variations in $PaCO_2$ levels increase the risk of intraventricular hemorrhage (associated with hypercapnia) and periventricular leukomalacia and BPD (linked to hypocapnia). Capnography offers breath-by-breath assessment of exhaled CO_2, represented graphically to illustrate carbon dioxide levels in the conducting airways throughout a respiratory cycle. Due to its high diffusibility in blood, CO_2 from the pulmonary capillary diffuses into the alveolus and rapidly equilibrates with the alveolar pCO_2 ($PACO_2$). Therefore, $PaCO_2$ is considered as proxy marker of $PACO_2$. The capnogram in each respiratory cycle encompasses four phases and represents the end tidal CO_2 ($EtCO_2$) **(Fig. 2)**.

Clinical Applications in NICU

Capnography facilitates the evaluation of effectiveness of ventilation and directs ventilatory management in mechanically ventilated infants, for minimizing fluctuations in CO_2, detecting accidental extubation, monitoring

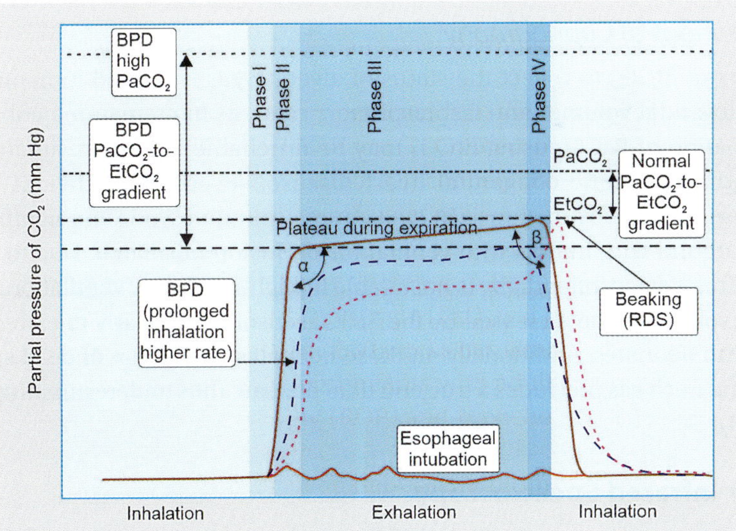

Fig. 2: Phase 1 depicts the gas from apparatus and anatomical dead space with minimal CO_2. Phase II exhibits a swift S-shaped ascent, due to mixture of alveolar gas with dead space gas. Phase III denotes exhaled gas from the alveoli, abundant in CO_2. Phase IV, or beaking, is observed in respiratory distress syndrome (RDS) resulting from the collapse and emission of alveolar gas. The alterations in the waveform concerning RDS, bronchopulmonary dysplasia (BPD), and esophageal intubation are also depicted.
Source: Rajiv PK, Lakshminrusimha S, Vidyasagar D, (Eds). Essentials of Neonatal Ventilation, 1st edition. New Delhi: Elsevier India; 2019.

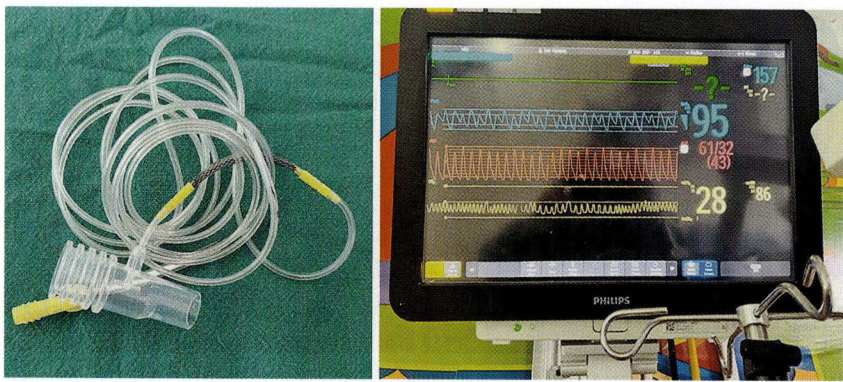

Fig. 3: $EtCO_2$ detector (with sampling line and airway adapter) on the left and monitor showing CO_2 on the right.

during transport. $EtCO_2$ monitoring is the conventional care for assessing neonates during anesthesia, as it facilitates real time evaluation of airway adequacy in intubated neonates. Additionally, it can be used to monitor hyperventilation in neonates with hypoxic ischemic encephalopathy (HIE), and to evaluate the effectiveness of cardiopulmonary resuscitation. The $EtCO_2$ detector and the monitor are shown in **Figure 3**.

Limitations of Capnography

Ability of $EtCO_2$ to reflect the status of alveolar gas is limited in neonates with low tidal volumes and fast respiratory rates, as in premature neonates. Estimation of $PaCO_2$ using $EtCO_2$ may be unreliable in certain situations, including cyanotic congenital heart disease, severe parenchymal lung disease, airway obstruction as in meconium aspiration syndrome significant leak around ETT, infants with ventilation-perfusion mismatch. Due to very rapid rates set, capnography is unsuitable in high-frequency ventilation. The dead space may be increased by the $EtCO_2$ sensor, particularly in extremely preterm neonates. Additionally, in these neonates, admixture of dead space gas and fresh gas precludes a true end tidal plateau, thus underestimating the $PaCO_2$.

Near Infrared Spectroscopy

Near infrared spectroscopy (NIRS) is an indirect assessment of tissue oxygen utilization. Tissue oxygenation relies on the oxygen supply which is fundamentally affected by cardiac output, hemoglobin saturation, and hemoglobin content. A state of oxygen deficit arises when the tissue's demand for oxygen surpasses its supply, potentially resulting in adverse consequences. NIRS provides a reliable and continuous noninvasive monitoring of regional oxygen saturation (rSO_2) in several organs.

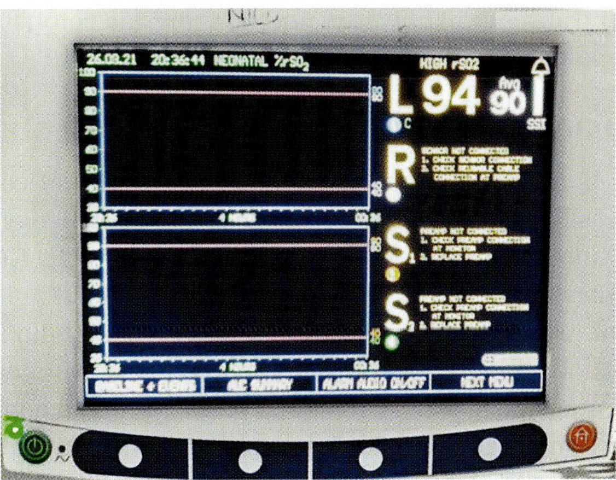

Fig. 4: Near infrared spectroscopy (NIRS) monitor showing regional oxygen saturation ($CrSO_2$).

The regions most monitored are cerebral ($CrSO_2$) **(Fig. 4)** renal ($RrSO_2$) and splanchnic ($SrSO_2$) oxygenation.

Its operational principle is based on the modified Beer–Lambert law. Light of specific wavelengths (700–1,000 nm) produced by light emitting diodes, traverses various tissues in arc-like configuration, depending on the transparency of biological tissue to near infrared spectrum of light and its differential absorption by various chromophores, such as hemoglobin, myoglobin, and cytochrome aa3. The penetration depth of the transmitted light is directly proportional to the distance between the transmitting and receiving optode. The receiving optode detects the reflected light, which is quantified and processed to estimate the concentrations of oxygenated hemoglobin and deoxyhemoglobin in the intervening tissue. NIR oximetry assesses a weighted average of arterial, capillary, and venous compartments and assumes a fixed ratio of venous to arterial blood volume, typically 70:30.

Clinical Applications

Cerebral oximetry has been extensively used to monitor cerebral oxygenation in neonates with hypoxic-ischemic injury, hypotension, patent ductus arteriosus, during cardiac surgery and those requiring invasive ventilation. There is available literature on utilization NIRS in monitoring splanchnic perfusion in monitoring of necrotizing enterocolitis. $CrSO_2$, $SrSO_2$, and $RrSO_2$ have been evaluated to assess the need for red blood cell transfusion and the response to transfusion.

Limitations

Though it is a promising tool, there is a lack of normative data for rSO_2 across two organs. Wide intravariability in the readings from different areas of the same organ and absence of universal normal value and cutoff that mandates action are some significant limitations of NIRS.

CONCLUSION

Noninvasive monitoring of gas exchange is an essential component of neonatal care, allowing continuous, bedside assessment of oxygenation, and ventilation without the risks of repeated invasive sampling. Clinical scores such as Downes and Silverman Anderson remain useful guides for early recognition of respiratory distress, especially in resource-limited settings. Advances in pulse oximetry, transcutaneous monitoring, capnography, and near-infrared spectroscopy have significantly enhanced our ability to detect and respond to hypoxemia, hyperoxia, and fluctuations in CO_2. Each modality, however, carries inherent limitations that must be understood to avoid misinterpretation and inappropriate interventions. Optimal neonatal monitoring thus requires a judicious combination of clinical assessment, noninvasive technologies, and selective use of arterial blood gases. Integrating these tools in a complementary manner improves precision in respiratory management and ultimately contributes to safer, more effective neonatal outcomes.

SUGGESTED READING

1. Askie LM, Darlow BA, Finer N, Schmidt B, Stenson B, Tarnow-Mordi W, et al; Neonatal Oxygenation Prospective Meta-analysis (NeOProM) Collaboration. Association Between Oxygen Saturation Targeting and Death or Disability in Extremely Preterm Infants in the Neonatal Oxygenation Prospective Meta-analysis Collaboration. JAMA. 2018;319(21):2190-201.
2. Chotas W, Edwards EM, Horn D, Soll R, Ehret DEY. Using a simplified Downes score to predict the receipt of surfactant in a highly resourced setting. J Perinatol. 2025;45(1):30-5.
3. Hedstrom AB, Gove NE, Mayock DE, Batra M. Performance of the Silverman Andersen Respiratory Severity Score in predicting PCO_2 and respiratory support in newborns: a prospective cohort study. J Perinatol. 2018;38(5):505-11.
4. Kim EH, Lee JH, Song IK, Kim HS, Jang YE, Yoo S, et al. Accuracy of pulse oximeters at low oxygen saturations in children with congenital cyanotic heart disease: an observational study. Paediatr Anaesth. 2019;29(6):597-603.
5. Sankaran D, Zeinali L, Iqbal S, Chandrasekharan P, Lakshminrusimha S. Non-invasive carbon dioxide monitoring in neonates: methods, benefits, and pitfalls. J Perinatol. 2021;41(11):2580-9.
6. Sood BG, McLaughlin K, Cortez J. Near-infrared spectroscopy: applications in neonates. Semin Fetal Neonatal Med. 2015;20(3):164-72.
7. van Weteringen W, van Essen T, Gangaram-Panday NH, Goos TG, de Jonge RCJ, Reiss IKM. Validation of a New Transcutaneous $tcPO_2/tcPCO_2$ Sensor with an Optical Oxygen Measurement in Preterm Neonates. Neonatology. 2020;117(5):628-36.

SECTION

Basics of Mechanical Ventilation-modes and Knobology

CHAPTER

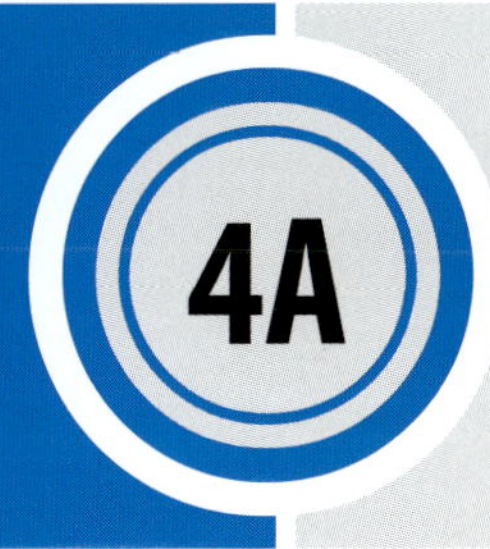

Basic Modes of Ventilation Including Patient-triggered Ventilation

Tejo Pratap Oleti

INTRODUCTION

Overview of Mechanical Ventilation in Neonatology

The mechanical ventilation for neonates has evolved lately by leaps and bounds. The year 1963 reminds us of the death of President Kennedy's son due to lack of adequate respiratory supports. However, with advances in technology and research, we are having very advanced ventilators currently.

Neonates are unique and have significantly different pathophysiology compared to children and adults. The shorter inspiratory time (Ti) due to low compliant lungs leading to higher respiratory rates poses unique challenge in designing the ventilator. The rapid respiratory rates (RRs) do pose a challenge to make adequate flow reaching the terminal alveoli for delivering desired pressure and volume. The uncuffed tubes used also can give rise to a significant leak during inspiration and also makes the measurement of tiny tidal volumes difficult.

VENTILATION MODES: TERMINOLOGY

All the new ventilators will work on the principle of delivering either set pressure or volume. Before learning the modes of ventilation, everyone should have an idea on these basic concepts which will determine the way the breath is delivered to the neonate in every mode. During each breath, the ventilator delivers a positive flow during inspiration and creates a negative flow during expiration. To avoid confusion between a breath and inspiration, we can use the word "inflation". The mechanism to initiate an inflation (trigger) and terminating it to go into expiration (cycling) apart from intended parameter (limit/control) to get achieved by gas flow regulation will determine the mode of the ventilator **(Fig. 1; Table 1)**.

- *Limit:* It is the maximum limit of the variable set in the ventilator which may or may not be able to reach in each breath. The ventilator would start decreasing the flow if it is achieved early during the inspiration. The neonatal ventilators will have either pressure or volume as their limit parameters.
- *Control:* The parameter at which the gas flow will get ceased during inflation. The ventilator uses either pressure [pressure control (PC)] or

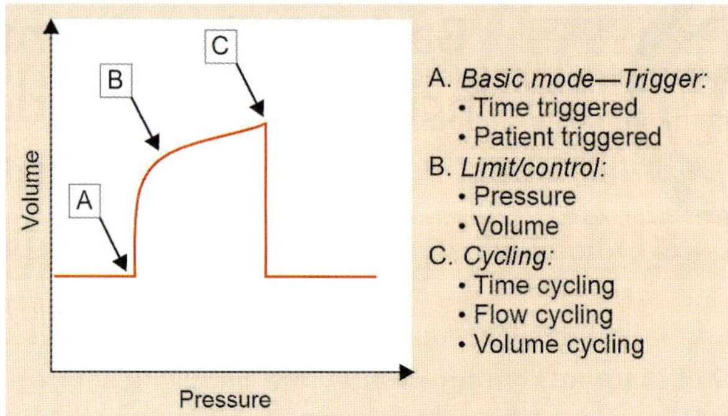

Fig. 1: Determinants of mode.

TABLE 1: Terminologies involved in the modes.

Limit/control	*Trigger*	*Cycling*
Pressure control (PC)	Time	Time (SIMV-TCPLV)
Volume control (VC)	*Baby:* • Pressure • Flow • Volume	*Flow*: Pressure support ventilation (PSV)
		Volume control ventilation (VCV)

(SIMV: synchronized intermittent mandatory ventilation; TCPLV: time-cycled, pressure-limited ventilation)

volume [volume control (VC)] as their control parameters. In neonates, we usually use pressure as the control parameter.

- *Trigger:* The parameter which initiates the inflation in a ventilator is called a trigger. The trigger can be independent of patient effort (time triggered) or dependent on patient efforts (pressure, flow, or volume). The patient-triggered inflation will get initiated when the patient creates a negative flow (requires a flow sensor) or pressure (pressure transducer) measured with the sensors. Few old ventilators are used to initiate the inflation by looking at the thoracic impendence and abdominal movements.
- *Cycling:* The cycling parameter will determine the switching of phase of respiration. This parameter will guide the ventilator to switch from inspiration to expiration. The parameters used in neonatal ventilators include time (time cycled), flow (flow cycled), and volume (volume cycled).

Pressure versus Volume Control Ventilation (Table 2)

The basic difference between the two modes is the set limit or control that terminates the airflow. In neonates, most used mode is PC while in adults it

TABLE 2: Differences between pressure versus volume control modes.

Pressure control ventilation	*Volume control ventilation*
Advantages: • Initial higher-pressure peak assisted by higher flow will improve the alveolar opening • Duration of recruited alveolar phase is more • Delivered mean airway pressure is more • Work of breathing and comfort is better due to higher MAP • The variation in the pressure delivered in each breath is less which might protect against VILI	*Advantages:* • Guaranteed tidal volumes produces a more consistent minute volume • The minute volume might remain stable even with changing pulmonary characteristics • The initial flow rate is lower than in pressure-controlled modes and avoid a high resistance-related pressure peak
Disadvantages: • The volume delivered in each breath (tidal volume) is variable as it is dependent on changing respiratory compliance • Variations and uncontrolled volume may result in more volutrauma especially due to overdistension • Initial high inspiratory flow may exceed the pressure limit if the airway resistance is too high	*Disadvantages:* • The mean airway pressure delivered is lower • Recruitment may be poorer in lung conditions with poor compliance • If there are higher leaks, the mean airway pressure may be variable • Inadequate flow may aggravate patient-ventilator dyssynchrony

(MAP: mean arterial pressure; VILI: ventilator-induced lung injury)

is VC. With improvements in technology, new sensors have the capability to detect very low volumes which is helping the neonatologists to combine the modes. The topic will be discussed in the subsequent chapters.

In PC mode, the inspiratory pressure, the targeted control variable, and ventilator adjust the air flow accordingly to maintain a stable inspiratory pressure. The increase in flow from baseline [maintaining positive end-expiratory pressure (PEEP)] will help to achieve the desired peak inspiratory pressures (PIPs). The pressure waveform appears like a square as shown in the figure below. Once the PIP is reached, the flow rates will decrease and comes to "zero" and remains the same till the inspiratory phase concludes. The plateau PIP **(Fig. 2)** is maintained throughout the inspiratory phase.

In volume control ventilation (VCV), the control variable is the volume. The set inspiratory flow will remain constant and will remain the same till we achieve the set tidal volume. The pressure is not controlled and can be variable in VCV. The pressure graph will appear like a parabola as the lungs start distending. The pressure waveform graph **(Fig. 2)** is highly variable

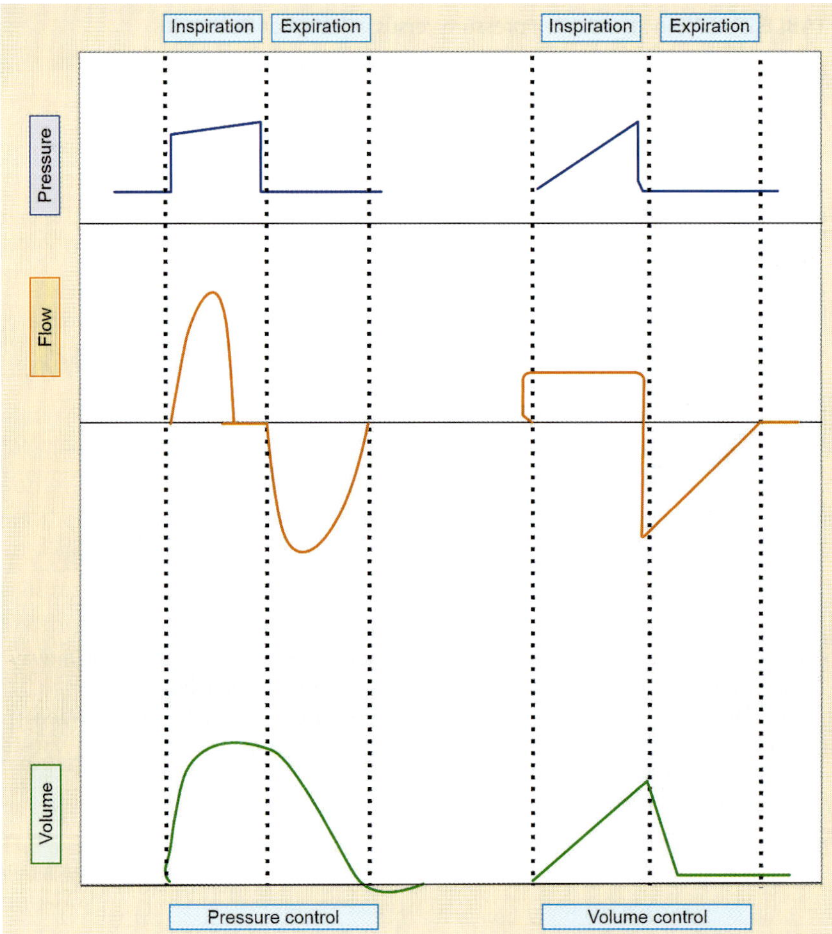

Fig. 2: Pressure versus volume control modes.

during VCV as the waveform pattern depends on the lung characteristics like compliance and resistance.

CONCEPT OF SYNCHRONY AND TRIGGERING

Earlier, the common mode used was intermittent mandatory ventilation. In this mode, the ventilator will deliver set number of breaths. These breaths can get initiated irrespective of the state of the efforts of the neonate. It can lead to improper delivery of the pressure and volume. This asynchrony **(Fig. 3)** can lead to air-trapping, air-leak syndromes, poor gas-exchange, fluctuations in the intracranial pressure leading to intraventricular hemorrhage, respiratory muscle fatigue, and adverse effects on hemodynamics. This "asynchrony" can lead to both increase in the complications related to ventilation and also effect on the duration of the ventilation. Prior to the innovation of good

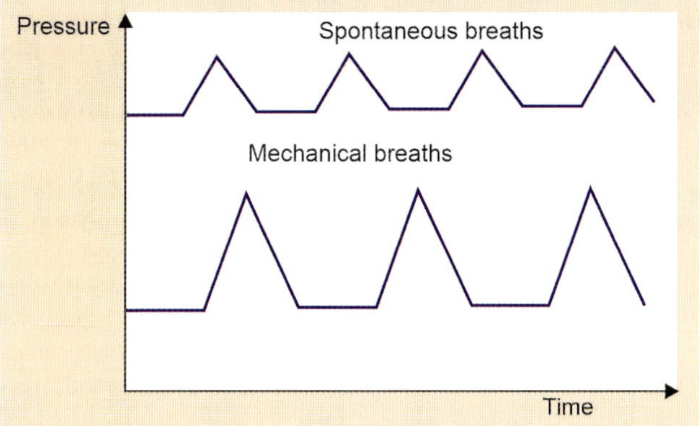

Fig. 3: Patient-ventilator asynchrony in intermittent mandatory ventilation.

triggering technology, the clinicians use medications for sedation and muscle paralysis which can lead to the prolonged duration of the ventilation.

The triggering mechanism for the patients efforts as mentioned above can utilize movements of thorax/abdomen and flow or pressure or volume changes across the flow sensors which are placed above the ET adapter. Few machines use the sensors available inside the machine itself instead of the distal sensors. Different mechanisms of triggering are described in **Table 3**.

An ideal trigger sensor should:

- Have good sensitivity to sense weakest of breathing effort by patient
- Lesser response time
- Should have leak compensation from the side of the tube
- Can able to counter routine artifacts of motion not related to breathing movements.

How to set trigger sensitivity?

- Start with best sensitivity (where all patient's efforts are sensed by the sensor and mimics of the movements are reasonable not detected).
- Reduce and monitor for autotriggering. Autotriggering is false triggering of the breath due to flow of gas across the flow sensor due to nonbreathing efforts like water in the tube.
- This can be achieved by looking at the breathing efforts for effective triggering. One should adjust and see that we are not missing breaths of the baby because of ineffective breaths or double triggering.

Inspiratory synchrony can be improved by improving the trigger mechanism. This can be achieved by flow triggering as it is very sensitive. One should also choose correct ET size to prevent air leaks.

If neural adjusted ventilatory assist (NAVA) is available in the machine and the clinical team has sufficient expertise, it can become the better triggering mechanism. The neonate's respiratory muscle activity is assessed

TABLE 3: Different triggering sensor devices available.

Sensor	*Mechanism*	*Remarks*
Pressure transducer	Negative pressure created by the breathing efforts	• Simple device • Lesser sensitivity • Longer trigger delay
Hotwire anemometer	Air flow changes across the sensor create difference in the temperature due to heat changes	• Can measure tidal volume • Sensitivity is better • Dead space is more • Air leaks can cause the erroneous measurement
Pneumotachograph	Measures the airflow by comparing the pressure drop across a resistive field to the flow	• Good sensitivity • Rapid measurement • More dead space • As it is flow dependent, air leaks can cause erroneous measurements
Thoracic impedance by ECG leads	Electrical activity of the muscles	• Adhesion issues • No dead space
Abdominal motion by Graseby capsule	Detect the abdominal movement	• No dead space • False triggering is an issue
Electrical activity of the diaphragm (EAdi)/ transesophageal electromyography	Electrical changes happening in the diaphragm	• Costly • Semi-invasive • More accurate • Less trigger delay

by continuous recording of diaphragmatic electric activity (EAdi) via a multiple-array esophageal electrode on a nasogastric catheter.

Patient-triggered Modes (Table 4)

The three commonly used patient-triggered modes are:
1. Synchronized intermittent mandatory ventilation (SIMV)
2. Assist control ventilation (ACV)
3. Pressure support ventilation (PSV)

Synchronized Intermittent Mandatory Ventilation

In this mode, breaths are mechanically delivered at a pre-set rate which are synchronized to the onset of spontaneous infant's breaths. If the neonate breaths faster than the set rate, these additional spontaneous breaths are allowed. However, the excess breaths are not supported by the ventilator.

If neonate does not initiate a breath or fails to trigger ventilator sensors with ineffective breath, then ventilator will deliver breath at the set rate.

TABLE 4: Parameters to be set by a clinician, cycling method and synchrony status in different patient-triggered ventilation modes.

Parameter	*SIMV*	*ACV*	*PSV*
PIP and PEEP	Clinician	Clinician	Clinician
Respiratory rate (RR)	Clinician	Neonate	Neonate
Inspiratory time (Ti)	Clinician	Clinician	Neonate
Cycling	Time	Time	Flow
Inspiratory synchrony	Partial	Complete	Complete
Expiratory synchrony	Nil	Nil	Complete

(ACV: assist control ventilation; PEEP: positive end-expiratory pressure; PIP: peak inspiratory pressure; PSV: pressure support ventilation; SIMV: synchronized intermittent mandatory ventilation)

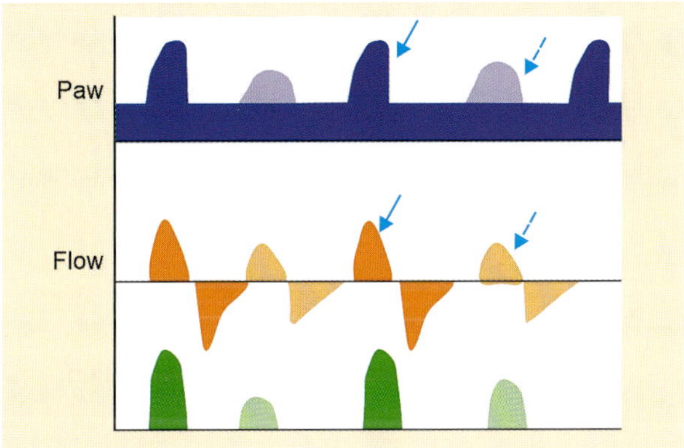

Fig. 4: Synchronized intermittent mandatory ventilation (*solid arrows indicated supported mandatory breaths; dotted arrows indicate spontaneous breaths which are not supported*).

The ventilator "waits" for the neonate to initiate the breath for a period known as "assist window". With SIMV mode, we can understand that few breaths triggered by the neonates are synchronized with the ventilator well **(Fig. 4)**. It will reduce the inspiratory asynchrony. However, the Ti is fixed as SIMV is a time-cycled ventilation. There is possibility that the expiration is not initiated according to the neonate's efforts which can lead to expiratory asynchrony.

Assist Control Ventilation

In this mode, the breaths are delivered in a synchronized manner. Every spontaneous breath is detected (assist) and assisted **(Fig. 5)**. If the neonate fails to initiate a breath, the ventilator will deliver a mechanical breath at a preset rate (control). This will create complete inspiratory synchronization. However, still expiratory synchrony will continue.

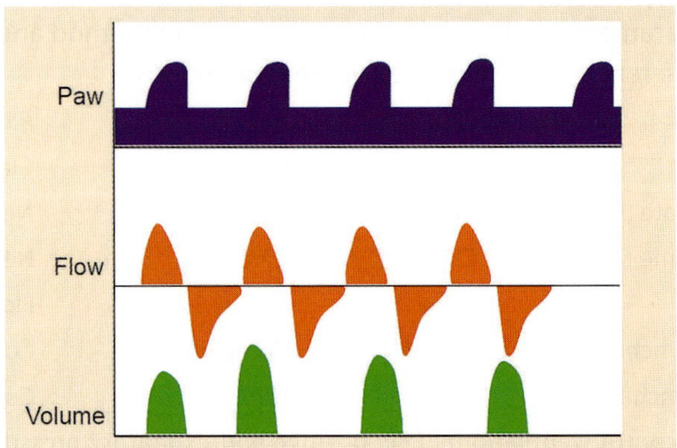

Fig. 5: Assist control ventilation mode (*all breaths are supported*).

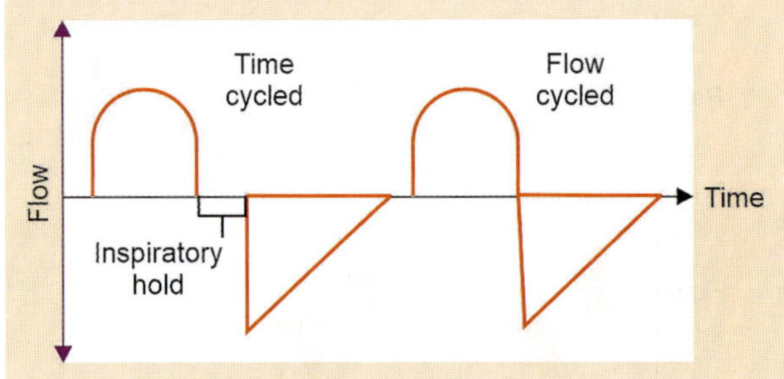

Fig. 6: Time-cycled versus flow-cycled ventilation.

The unique feature of ACV mode is that the respiratory rate will be decided by the neonate. The backup ventilatory rate set ensures and helps the neonate to breath during the apneas and counters the ineffectively triggered breaths. In rare cases, if the respiratory rates are too high due to nonlung-related condition, then it can lead to either hyperventilation or air trapping.

Pressure Support Ventilation

Pressure support ventilation is a patient-triggered, pressure-limited, and flow-cycled mode of ventilation. It is designed to assist all the spontaneous breathing efforts with a pressure boost. Many of the ventilators will not have a backup rate in this mode. We should ensure that neonate has good breathing efforts before initiation of this mode. It is more physiological and suited as even weaning mode.

Understanding the flow cycling is very important as it is the differentiating factor between other modes. In this, the neonate initiates inspiration, controls flow and the inspiratory time **(Fig. 6)**. The set PIP will be delivered during the inspiration with adjustments in the flow. Once the set pressure is achieved, the neonate will go into expiration with the switch in the flow. The flow cycling helps to reduce the mean arterial pressure (MAP) exposed as it limits Ti as shown in **Figure 6**. The pressure is chosen to deliver a full tidal volume breath; it is referred to as PS_{max}. The initiated positive pressure breath will be terminated according to redecided termination sensitivity.

Termination of inspiratory flow happens in this mode due to an embedded feature called "termination sensitivity". Flow sensor measures air flow which is delivered by ventilator to achieve desired pressure/volume. As ventilator breath progresses till the set targets of pressure/volume are achieved. After achieving the same, the flow will start decreasing. Once the flow decreases to a point, expiration is initiated and thereby helping to achieve expiratory synchronization. The clinician can adjust this termination sensitivity level to end a ventilator breath when flow declines to 0–25% of peak flow **(Fig. 7)**. Many of the ventilators have preset termination sensitivity. When we are manually setting the same, we should keep the lung mechanics determining the Ti and Te in the neonates.

Pressure support ventilation can be used as standalone mode and also can be combined with SIMV to support additional breaths. As PSV mode **(Fig. 8)** is more physiological, the ventilation-induced lung injury is lesser. The synchrony is good in both the inspiration and expiration. The clinician need to set only PIP, PEEP, and fraction of inspired oxygen (FiO_2) in this mode. The Ti and the respiratory rate will be decided by the neonates themselves.

Understanding the patient-triggered modes is very important. Evidence shows that patient-triggered ventilation (PTV) modes will reduce the duration of ventilation and incidence of air-leak syndromes.

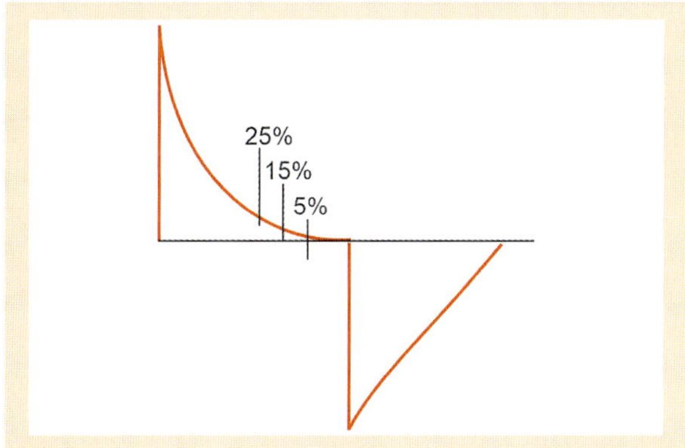

Fig. 7: Termination sensitivity.

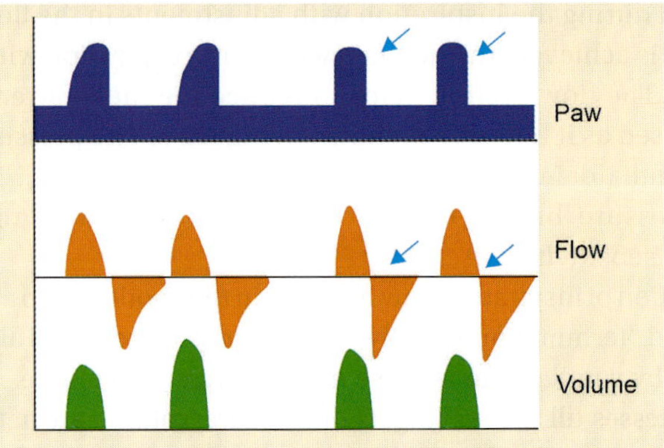

Fig. 8: Pressure support ventilation (*note the first 2 breaths are SIMV and other 2 are PSV mode; no inspiratory hold*). (PSV: pressure support ventilation; SIMV: synchronized intermittent mandatory ventilation)

CONCLUSION

Mechanical ventilation in neonates requires careful selection of modes based on their unique physiology. Patient-triggered strategies such as SIMV, ACV, and PSV improve synchrony, reduce complications, and support timely weaning, helping achieve effective ventilation with minimal risk of lung injury.

SUGGESTED READING

1. Greenough A. Update on patient-triggered ventilation. Clin Perinatol. 2001;28(3):533-46.
2. Keszler M, Gautham KS. Goldsmith's Assisted Ventilation of the Neonate, 7th edition. Amsterdam: Elsevier Inc.; 2022.
3. Keszler M. Update on mechanical ventilatory strategies. Neoreviews. 2013;14(5):e237-51.
4. Sarkar S, Donn SM. In support of pressure support. Clin Perinatol. 2007;34(1): 117-28, vii.

CHAPTER

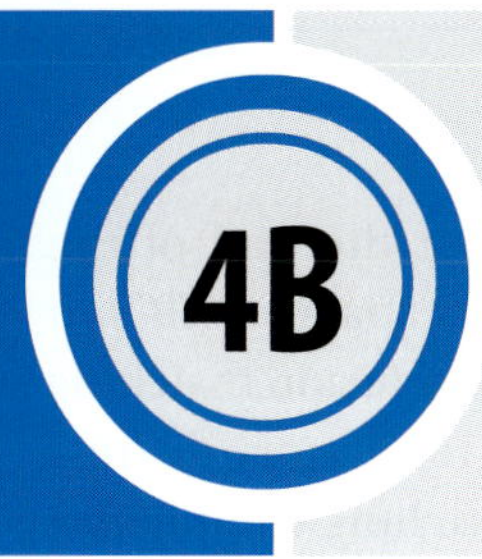

Knobology in Neonatal Ventilators

Sushil Choudhary

INTRODUCTION

Knobs: Hardware buttons or digital touch screen that allows the treating physician to adjust the ventilator setting and also helps in monitor the status of machine and patient. Modern ventilators have combination of digital displays and hardware knobs.

COMMONLY USED VENTILATOR PARAMETERS AND KNOBS

Peak Inspiratory Pressure

Peak inspiratory pressure (PIP): Peak inspiratory pressure is relative to atmospheric pressure. Some ventilators show pressure gradient between onset and end of inspiration [ΔP = PIP – positive end-expiratory pressure (PEEP)].

Tidal volume and minute ventilation are mainly affected by the PIP. Clinically, appropriate PIP can be decided by observation of the chest wall movement. Just visible chest rise is acceptable for start of ventilation. Further changes in PIP can be made depending on the disease and condition of the neonate.

Flow sensor at patient end also measures tidal volume. This can also use to decide adequate PIP. Small tidal volume (4–6 mL/kg) is recommended in initiation of ventilation in neonates.

An increase in PIP will increase tidal volume and minute ventilation thus increases CO_2 elimination. It also increases in mean airway pressure and thus improves oxygenation.

High PIP increases the risk of ventilator-induced lung injury (barotrauma/volutrauma) and thereby increases the risk of bronchopulmonary dysplasia, pneumothorax, pneumomediastinum, and pulmonary interstitial emphysema.

It is important to adjust PIP based on primary pathology and lung compliance. Excessive chest rise should be avoided in neonates. Adjustment of PIP is particularly important in preterm neonates after surfactant therapy.

Positive End-expiratory Pressure

Positive end-expiratory pressure keeps alveoli open at the end of the expiration and helps in maintaining functional residual capacity (FRC). It also prevents alveolar collapse and improves ventilation/perfusion matching in neonates with reduced expiratory lung volume [e.g., respiratory distress syndrome (RDS)]. Adequate PEEP is required to improve lung compliance and reduce the risk of atelectotrauma.

Optimal PEEP maximizes lung compliance and may allow the use of lower peak pressures to achieve the same tidal volume. Optimal PEEP maximizes oxygenation for a given mean airway pressure. Adjusting PEEP to maintain an open lung is judged by finding a point where fraction of inspired oxygen (FiO_2) is at its lowest with hemodynamic stability and acceptable blood gases. Pulmonary vascular resistance is minimum when the lung is neither under- nor overinflated.

For a healthy lung, starting PEEP should be 3–4 cmH_2O. In a case of poor lung compliance (e.g., RDS), PEEP should be 5–8 cmH_2O.

Adverse effects of high PEEP:
- Overdistended lung, increased risk of pneumothorax
- Impaired CO_2 elimination
- Elevated pulmonary vascular resistance
- Decrease cardiac output and worsening of shock.

Frequency (or Rate)

The ventilator frequency (f) determines minute ventilation ($MV = f \times VT$). Very high frequencies are used in high-frequency ventilation to deliver adequate minute ventilation while using lower peak inspiratory pressures and tidal volumes.

CO_2 removal and ventilator frequency relationship is not linear. It depends on primary disease and baseline rates. Neonates with smaller noncompliant lungs (RDS) tend to breathe faster to minimize work. In these neonates, further increase in ventilators rate will not have much effect on CO_2 removal. Increasing ventilator rates in neonates with lower baseline respiratory rates will help in elimination of CO_2. Very high rates lead to insufficient expiratory time and gas trapping and also insufficient inspiratory time (TI) leads to decreased tidal volume.

Inspiratory Time, Inspiratory to Expiratory Ratio

A sufficient TI is necessary for adequate tidal volume delivery and CO_2 elimination. 3–5 times constant is required for complete inspiration. TI of 0.2–0.4 seconds is usually adequate for newborns with RDS. Neonates with established bronchopulmonary dysplasia require longer TI (0.6–0.8 seconds). Longer TI (>0.5 ses) generally does not improve ventilation or gas exchange and may lead to asynchrony and hyperinflation. A very short TI will lead to incomplete inspiration and decreased tidal volume. A very short TE or high inspiratory to expiratory ratio (I:E) ratio can lead to incomplete expiration and increased gas trapping which leads to decreased tidal volume. Incomplete inspiration and expiration can be detected on the pulmonary graphics and TI and TE can be adjusted accordingly.

Inspired Oxygen Concentration (FiO_2)

Oxygenation depends on mean airway pressure and FiO_2. High FiO_2 generates more free radicals and damages the lung tissue. Optimization of FiO_2 is necessary to minimize lung injury. When FiO_2 is above 0.6–0.7, increases in mean airway pressure are generally required. When FiO_2 is below 0.3–0.4, decreases in mean airway pressure are generally preferred.

Flow

Preset flow rate has effects on airway pressure rise time. Higher flow rates lead to faster pressure rise and higher peak inspiratory flow. Effect of these flow rates on gas exchange is minimal in neonatal ventilation if sufficient flow is used. Inadequate flow (i.e., long pressure rise time and low peak inspiratory flow) may contribute to air hunger, asynchrony, and increased work of breathing. Higher flow rates and steeper inspiratory pressure slopes may be needed at high ventilator rates with short TI to maintain adequate flow for complete inspiration. Excessive flow may contribute to turbulence, inefficient gas exchange, and inadvertent PEEP.

In summary, depending upon the condition of neonates, clinical assessment, chest X-ray, and blood gases, the following ventilator parameters can be optimized **(Table 1)**.

VENTILATION MODES

Basic classification of different ventilation modes is described in **Flowchart 1**.

Choice of Ventilator Mode

In neonatal population, synchronized intermittent mandatory ventilation (SIMV) and assist control (A/C) modes are mostly used as primary mode. Recent evidence does not indicate any superiority of one mode or the other. Choice of mode depends on the personal experience. Any mode which requires minimum number of knob adjustments is preferred over a complex mode where multiple parameters are adjusted. A/C mode is preferred for small preterm babies due to more uniform tidal volumes and less work of breathing.

Different modes of neonatal ventilation, their basic characteristic, and advantage are compared in **Table 2**.

TABLE 1: Commonly used ventilator parameters for neonatal ventilation.

Parameters	*Initial setting*	*How to decide optimize setting*	*Remarks*
PIP	12–20 cmH_2O	Adequate oxygenation, acceptable blood gases	Avoid hyperinflation
PEEP	5–7 cmH_2O	FiO_2 is at its lowest with hemodynamic stability and acceptable lung expansion	Excessive PEEP can decrease lung compliance and decrease cardiac output
Tidal volume	4–6 mL/kg	Just visible chest rise	Avoid excessive chest rise. Proximal flow sensor can detect reliable tidal volumes
Inspiratory time	• *Term:* 0.4–0.5 seconds • *Preterm:* 0.2–0.4 seconds	Incomplete inspiration and expiration can be detected on the pulmonary graphics	Bronchopulmonary dysplasia requires longer inspiratory time (0.6–0.8 seconds)
FiO_2	0.21–0.4	Target saturation 90–94%	When FiO_2 requirements is more than 0.6–0.7, optimize the inflation pressures
Rate	40–60/minute	Decided by primary disease (e.g., RDS—high rates, CNS depression and established BPD—low rates)	Minute ventilation is more important for CO_2 elimination. Excessive rates can decrease alveolar minute ventilation

(CNS: central nervous system; FiO_2: fraction of inspired oxygen; PEEP: positive end-expiratory pressure; PIP: peak inspiratory pressure; RDS: respiratory distress syndrome)

Flowchart 1: Basic classification of ventilation modes.

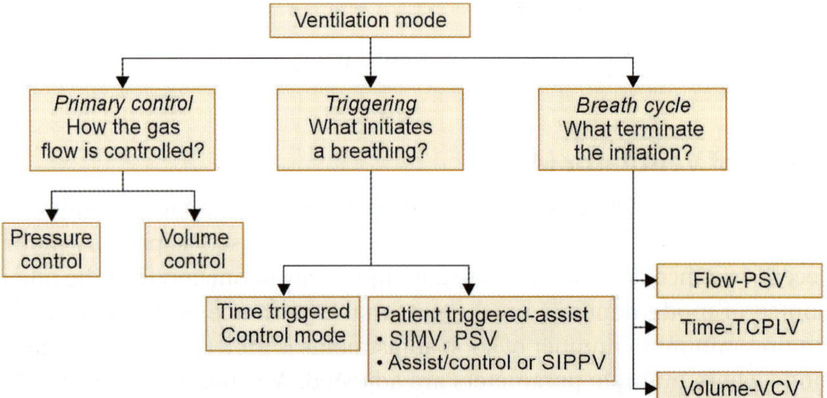

(PSV: pressure support ventilation; SIMV: synchronized intermittent mandatory ventilation; TCPLV: time-cycled, pressure-limited ventilation; VCV: volume control ventilation)

TABLE 2: Basics characteristics of different mode of ventilation.

	Intermittent mandatory ventilation (IMV)	*Synchronized intermittent mandatory ventilation (SIMV)*	*Assist control (A/C)/SIPPV/PTV*	*Pressure support ventilation (PSV)*	*SIMV + PSV*
Control	Pressure/volume	Pressure/volume	Pressure/volume	Pressure	Pressure/volume
Triggering	None	Patient triggered but set no of breaths	Every spontaneous breath	Every spontaneous breath	Every spontaneous breath with different support
Cycling	Time	Time	Time	Flow	Time and flow
Rate	Decided by operator	Decided by operator	Decided by neonate	Decided by neonate	
Backup rate in apnea	Same rates	Fixed no of breaths	Set rates are actually backup rates	No backup rates. Apnea mode is used in modern ventilators	Fixed number of breaths
Advantage	Rate and triggering is decided by machine. Can be useful in complete apnea or muscle paralysis	• Synchrony with the neonates • Greater patient comfort • Decrease need of sedation	• More uniform tidal volume • Less work of breathing • Rates are decided by neonates, so only one parameter (pressure) is adjusted in case of weaning	• Less inspiratory hold • More synchrony	More uniform tidal volume. Less work of breathing
Disadvantage	Complete asynchrony	Only fixed number of breaths are supported. Increased work of breathing in neonates with high respiratory rates	• Risk of hyperventilation • Risk of CO_2 washout	• No backup rate in case of apnea • Risk of CO_2 washout	Multiple parameters need to be adjusted during weaning. PSV pressures, SIMV pressure, and SIMV rates

CONCLUSION

Knobology in neonatal ventilation emphasizes precise adjustment of parameters to balance effective gas exchange with minimal lung injury. Individualized settings, guided by clinical condition and monitoring, ensure safe, synchronized, and outcome-oriented respiratory support in neonates.

SUGGESTED READING

1. Klingenberg C, Wheeler KI, McCallion N, Morley CJ, Davis PG. Volume-targeted versus pressure-limited ventilation in neonates. Cochrane Database Syst Rev. 2017;(10):CD003666.
2. Patel DS, Rafferty GF, Lee S, Hannam S, Greenough A. Work of breathing during SIMV with and without pressure support. Arch Dis Child. 2009;94(6):434-6.
3. Peng W, Zhu H, Shi H, Liu E. Volume-targeted ventilation is more suitable than pressure-limited ventilation for preterm infants: a systematic review and meta-analysis. Arch Dis Child Fetal Neonatal Ed. 2014;99(2):F158-65.
4. Perlman JM, Goodman S, Kreusser KL, Volpe JJ. Reduction in Intraventricular Hemorrhage by Elimination of Fluctuating Cerebral Blood-Flow Velocity in Preterm Infants with Respiratory Distress Syndrome. N Engl J Med. 1985;312(21):1353-7.
5. Reyes ZC, Claure N, Tauscher MK, D'Ugard C, Vanbuskirk S, Bancalari E. Randomized, Controlled Trial Comparing Synchronized Intermittent Mandatory Ventilation and Synchronized Intermittent Mandatory Ventilation Plus Pressure Support in Preterm Infants. Pediatrics. 2006;118(4):1409-17.
6. Sweet DG, Carnielli VP, Greisen G, Hallman M, Klebermass-Schrehof K, Ozek E, et al. European Consensus Guidelines on the Management of Respiratory Distress Syndrome: 2022 Update. Neonatology. 2023;120(1):3-23.

SECTION

Disease Specific Ventilation, Weaning, Extubation, and Postextubation Care of Neonates

CHAPTER

Indications for Invasive Mechanical Ventilation: Choosing Appropriate Ventilation Mode

Viraraghavan Vadakkencherry Ramaswamy

INTRODUCTION

The primary goal of mechanical ventilation is to maintain acceptable gas exchange avoiding serious side effects and to wean from invasive support at the earliest opportunity. The secondary goals include comfort, reducing the work of breathing, and minimizing oxygen consumption.

INDICATIONS FOR CONVENTIONAL MECHANICAL VENTILATION IN NEONATES

The threshold for initiating invasive mechanical ventilation (IMV) is multifactorial in the neonatal population. It depends upon a myriad of factors such as gestational age, postnatal age, coexisting morbidities, and, most importantly, the availability of resources to not only initiate IMV, but also to continuously monitor and provide auxiliary care for the newly born infant on IMV.

The common general indications for IMV in preterm or term neonates [who are most often initially managed on noninvasive respiratory support (NRS) modalities] are:

- Severe apnea (not responding to methylxanthines/NRS modalities); defined as >4 episodes/hour requiring stimulation or any episode requiring positive pressure ventilation (PPV)
- Hypoxemia [requirement of fraction of inspired oxygen (FiO_2)] >0.60 on NRS to maintain oxygen saturation (SpO_2) in the range 90–94%
- Respiratory acidosis [pH <7.20 with partial pressure of carbon dioxide ($PaCO_2$) of >60 mm Hg; in <28 weeks' gestational age (GA): $PaCO_2$ >50 mm Hg (day 0–3), >55 mm Hg (day 4–6), >60 mm Hg (>day 7)]
- Shock requiring inotrope/vasopressor therapy
- Impending respiratory failure defined as Silverman Anderson score (SAS) or Downes score >6.

Other clinical indications include:

- Neonates born at threshold of viability (22–24 weeks' GA) with respiratory distress syndrome (RDS) who have severe respiratory distress requiring surfactant administration. Usually, these neonates are continued on IMV for hours to days based on unit protocol. There may be a subgroup of more mature preterm neonates with RDS who may require continuing IMV which could be based on many factors such as requirement of high FiO_2 even after surfactant administration, presence of cardiovascular instability, and poor respiratory efforts.

- *Moderate to severe respiratory distress with contraindications to provide NRS:* Congenital diaphragmatic hernia (CDH), choanal atresia, cleft palate who cannot be managed with NRS, necrotizing enterocolitis (NEC) stage 2 or more, pre- and postsurgical repair of tracheoesophageal fistula, intestinal obstruction, perforation, and ileus.

INDICATIONS FOR HIGH-FREQUENCY OSCILLATION VENTILATION

High-frequency oscillation ventilation (HFOV) is usually used as a rescue modality in scenarios where conventional IMV fails. In certain scenarios, it may be used as the first line choice. The common indications for HFOV are:

- *Failure of conventional IMV to maintain adequate oxygenation and ventilation:* The IMV settings at which its failure is to be considered vary based on unit/regional protocol. In preterm neonates, a requirement of peak inspiratory pressure (PIP) ≥25 cmH_2O and in term infants, a PIP requirement of ≥28 cmH_2O on conventional IMV are a common indication to initiate HFOV.
- In neonates with severe persistent pulmonary hypertension of newborn (PPHN) due to any etiology, with an oxygenation index (OI) of >15 which mandates inhaled nitric oxide (iNO) therapy is another indication for HFOV. The synergistic effect of HFOV along with iNO has been demonstrated in many preclinical and clinical studies.
- In preterm neonates with severe NEC requiring high mean airway pressure (MAP) on conventional IMV, HFOV is used in some units as a lung-protective strategy as the primary pathophysiology is the distended abdomen with the lungs being normal.

CHOOSING APPROPRIATE VENTILATION MODE

There are severe modes of conventional IMV, and the routinely used mode in neonatology is synchronized intermittent positive pressure ventilation (SIPPV) which is also termed as patient-triggered ventilation (PTV) and assist control ventilation (ACV) based on the ventilator being used. Volume targeting or volume guarantee is a standard of care while using any of the modes of IMV. Synchronized intermittent mandatory ventilation with pressure support ventilation (SIMV-PSV) is also a routinely used modality in the neonatal population. The initial settings for conventional IMV and HFOV based on the disease pathophysiology are provided in **Tables 1 and 2**, respectively.

TABLE 1: Initial ventilator settings in conventional IMV for the various diseases in neonates.

Disease	*Pathophysiology*	*Tidal volume (mL/kg)*	*PEEP (cmH_2O)*	*Rate (breaths/ minute)*	*Ti (seconds)*
Pulmonary condition:					
RDS/congenital pneumonia in preterm neonate	Low lung compliance, compliant chest wall, diffuse micro atelectasis, ventilation:perfusion mismatch, fragile lungs	4–6	6–8	40–60	0.30–0.35
Pulmonary hemorrhage	Poor lung compliance, surfactant inactivation, pulmonary edema	4–6	6–8	40–50	0.40–0.50
MAS (obstructive pathology)	High airway resistance, low compliance, heterogeneous inflation, prolonged time constants	5–6	5–6	25–35	0.45–0.50
MAS (homogenous low volume lungs)	Surfactant inactivation and diffuse alveolar disease same as RDS	5–6	6–7	30–45	0.45–0.50
BPD	*Different lung mechanics in various segments of lungs:* Low compliance and increased resistance, poorly supported airways prone to collapse, decreased alveolarization with less gas-exchanging surface and fewer pulmonary capillaries and increased pulmonary artery pressure	6–10	8–10	25–35	0.40–0.50
PPHN	Reduced pulmonary blood flow secondary to increased pulmonary artery pressures superimposed on underlying lung disease	4–6	6–8	40–45	0.40–0.45
CDH	Low lung compliance due to decreased lung volume. Increased risk of lung injury, and pulmonary hypertension	4–5	4–6	40–50	0.45–0.55

Contd...

Contd…

Disease	*Pathophysiology*	*Tidal volume (mL/kg)*	*PEEP (cmH_2O)*	*Rate (breaths/minute)*	*Ti (seconds)*
Apnea	• Preterm infant with apnea of prematurity • RDS with impending respiratory failure	4–5	4–5	15–20	0.40–0.50
Air leak	Compression of airspaces by interstitial gas resulting in poor compliance, and high airway resistance	4–5	4–6	50–60	0.30–0.35
Cardiac conditions:					
Left to right shunts	Pulmonary overcirculation with decreased lung compliance	5–7	5–8	40–50	0.40–0.50
Airway problems:					
Large airway obstruction	Increased respiratory effort because of airway collapse	4–6	6–10	15–30	0.45–0.50
Small airway obstruction	• Inflammation, airway secretions, smooth muscle hypertrophy leading to fixed airway obstruction • There may be a variable bronchospasm component • The above factors lead to the prolongation of Te and gas trapping. Expiratory flow limitation at low lung volumes	4–6	6–8	15–30	0.50–0.60
Pre-/postoperative support:					
Sedation/paralysis	Suppression of respiratory drive because of sedation. Limitation of respiratory excursion because of pain	4–5	4–6	15–20	0.40–0.50
Abdominal surgery	Raised intra-abdominal pressure leading to diaphragmatic splinting	4–5	6–8	15–20	0.40–0.50

(BPD: bronchopulmonary dysplasia; CDH: congenital diaphragmatic hernia; IMV: invasive mechanical ventilation; PEEP: positive end-expiratory pressure; PPHN: persistent pulmonary hypertension of newborn; RDS: respiratory distress syndrome; Ti: inspiratory time)

TABLE 2: Initial HFOV settings for the various diseases in neonates.

Disease	*Mean airway pressure (cmH_2O)*	*Frequency (Hz)*	*Amplitude/ $Amplitude_{max}$*
RDS/congenital pneumonia	2 above the requirement in conventional IMV	8–12	• *If volume guarantee is used:* Refer to foot notes* • *If volume guarantee not used:* Twice the MAP set
MAS (hyperinflated chest/obstructive pathology)	3–5 above the requirement in conventional IMV	6–8	Same as above
MAS (chemical pneumonitis/low volume lungs and homogenous)	Same as for RDS	Same as for RDS	Same as above
BPD	3–5 above the requirement in conventional IMV	6–8	Same as above
PPHN	Same settings as in conventional IMV to avoid hyperinflation, purpose of HFOV is to synergize the effect of iNO	8–10	Same as above
CDH and lung hypoplasia	Same as that used in conventional IMV	8–10	Same as above

Note:

**HFOV aspects common to all disease pathologies:*

- I:E ratio is usually 1:2. If all measures to improve oxygenation fail, then I:E ratio of 1:1 could be used
- HFOV with volume guarantee is now routinely utilized. The volume used is 1–3 mL/kg. Start with 2 mL/kg. Evaluate the blood gas after half an hour. Based on the $PaCO_2$, increase or decrease the volume by 0.5 mL/kg. Once a stable $PaCO_2$ is obtained, never change the volume
- In HFOV with volume guarantee, the amplitude max is set. It is usually set 5 above the required amplitude to deliver a particular tidal volume
- Never alter the frequency in HFOV with or without volume guarantee as it results in huge fluctuations in $PaCO_2$. You may alter the amplitude max to achieve the desired tidal volume
- Raining out is a frequent issue in HFOV, make sure the ventilator tubing is placed below the level of the endotracheal tube to prevent VAP
- Recruitment maneuvers are the most important aspect of HFOV
- Do not frequently interrupt the closed loop ventilator circuit as it can result in decruitment
- Repeated chest radiography may be warranted to see for adequate chest expansion and lung recruitment

Contd...

Contd...

Recruitment maneuver:

With HFOV, the key aspect is recruitment of the alveoli, maintain optimal lung inflation obtained by the recruitment maneuver thereby using the lowest acceptable mean airway pressure to obtain adequate gas exchange. The process is as follows:

- Step-wise increase (by 2 cmH_2O) in MAP to recruit atelectatic alveoli, which would be indicated by lowering of required FiO_2 (opening pressure)
- Step-wise reduction in MAP to a point at which FiO_2 requirement starts increasing again (closing pressure)
- Repeating the step 1 to recruit the alveoli again and then bring down the MAP to 2–3 cm H_2O above the closing pressure
- Recruitment maneuver should be done with utmost care in heterogeneous lung diseases such as MAS, pneumonia, etc., where hyperinflation of the normal alveoli may result in air leak syndrome
- The mean arterial blood pressure needs to be monitored while increasing the MAP during the recruiting process

(BPD: bronchopulmonary dysplasia; CDH: congenital diaphragmatic hernia; HFOV: high-frequency oscillation ventilation; IMV: invasive mechanical ventilation; iNO: inhaled nitric oxide; MAP: mean airway pressure; PPHN: persistent pulmonary hypertension of newborn; RDS: respiratory distress syndrome)

CONCLUSION

The decision to initiate invasive mechanical ventilation in neonates requires careful clinical judgment, balancing the need for adequate gas exchange with the risks of ventilator-associated complications. Indications for ventilation are multifactorial and include severe apnea, hypoxemia, respiratory acidosis, shock, and impending respiratory failure, with disease-specific considerations such as congenital anomalies or postsurgical states. High-frequency oscillation ventilation serves as a valuable rescue or adjunctive strategy, particularly in refractory hypoxemia and conditions like PPHN or severe air-leak syndromes. Selecting the appropriate ventilation mode—whether conventional IMV with volume targeting or HFOV—should be guided by the underlying pathophysiology, unit protocols, and resource availability. Ultimately, a structured, individualized approach ensures optimal outcomes while minimizing lung injury and long-term morbidity.

SUGGESTED READING

1. Keszler M. Mechanical ventilation strategies. Semin Fetal Neonatal Med. 2017;22(4):267-74.
2. Ramaswamy VV, More K, Roehr CC, Bandiya P, Nangia S. Efficacy of noninvasive respiratory support modes for primary respiratory support in preterm neonates with respiratory distress syndrome: Systematic review and network meta-analysis. Pediatr Pulmonol. 2020;55(11):2940-63.
3. Rocha G, Soares P, Gonçalves A, Silva AI, Almeida D, Figueiredo S, et al. Respiratory care for the ventilated neonate. Can Respir J. 2018;2018:7472964.

4. Sant'Anna GM, Keszler M. Developing a neonatal unit ventilation protocol for the preterm baby. Early Hum Dev. 2012;88(12):925-9.
5. Shalish W, Sant'Anna G, Keszler M. Weaning and extubation from mechanical ventilation. In: Keszler M, Gautham KS (Eds). Goldsmith's Assisted Ventilation of the Neonate. Philadelphia: Elsevier; 2022. pp. 303-14.
6. Snoek KG, Reiss IK, Greenough A, Capolupo I, Urlesberger B, Wessel L, et al. CDH EURO Consortium. Standardized Postnatal Management of Infants with Congenital Diaphragmatic Hernia in Europe: The CDH EURO Consortium Consensus - 2015 Update. Neonatology. 2016;110(1):66-74.
7. Yoder BA, Grubb PH. Mechanical ventilation: Disease-specific strategies. In: Keszler M, Gautham KS (Eds). Goldsmith's Assisted Ventilation of the Neonate. Philadelphia: Elsevier; 2022. pp. 288-302.

CHAPTER

5B Lung-protective Ventilation

Pankaj Kumar Mohanty

INTRODUCTION

The preterm lung is susceptible to various forms of ventilation-induced lung injuries (VILIs). Even a few large breaths in the delivery room can initiate a lung injury cascade. The preterm is born at various stages of lung development, mainly at the canalicular or saccular stage. The alveoli of these micro premises are surfactant deficient; septations are prematurely formed and functionally so immature. Ventilating the surfactant-deficient lung with high pressure, which is complicated by antenatal inflammation (chorioamnionitis), chronic maternal condition (diabetes, preeclampsia/eclampsia, and placental vascular disease), and postnatal inflammation (sepsis and pneumonia), opens the gateway to VILI.

The various forms of VILI are due to alveolar/saccular overdistension (avoiding volutrauma), alveolar collapse (atelectotrauma), alveolar overdistension due to high positive pressure (barotrauma), inflammatory process mediated injury (biotrauma), and oxygen toxicity (free radical injury due to 100% oxygen).

Mitigating VILI is a daunting task, as injuries occur despite all precautions and protective strategies being followed. The foundation of lung-protective strategies is avoiding/preventing lung injury cascade by providing evidence-based respiratory care mimicking physiology (lung-protective strategies), practicing noninvasive respiratory support, supporting adequate nutrition (enteral and parenteral), avoiding oxygen toxicity, practicing asepsis, and trying to extubate the neonate early.

The standard principle of neonatologists is ventilating the lung after the recruitment of alveoli, stabilizing the alveoli, otherwise called the open lung strategy. So, the open lung strategy, together with permissive hypercapnia with targeted saturations, is termed lung-protective ventilation, supported by many preclinical studies.

The principles of lung-protective ventilation:
- The neonates should be ventilated in the middle of the pressure–volume loop (P-V) to avoid atelectasis and overdistension
- Opening the alveoli with sufficient positive end-expiratory pressure (PEEP) to avoid microatelectasis will prevent repeated alveolar opening and collapse (RACE) and maintain alveolar-capillary integrity

- Low tidal volume ventilation should be followed, stabilizing already recruited alveoli with adequate peak inspiratory pressure (PIP) and PEEP
- Avoid administering high FiO_2, which may generate oxygen-free radicals and cause lung injury
- Open lung ventilation strategies, volume target/volume guarantee, and permissive hypercapnia.

OPEN LUNG VENTILATION STRATEGY

The aim is to optimize lung volume by recruiting alveoli and stabilizing the lung at the outset. The "*open the lung and keep it open*" concept is emulated here. Open lung ventilation, which uses high PIP and PEEP to recruit and stabilize alveoli, has been proven to decrease VILI irrespective of type/mode of ventilation. It holds good for high-frequency oscillation ventilation (HFOV) ventilation as well **(Fig. 1)**.

Volume Target Ventilation

The primary target is to deliver a set tidal volume (TV) of 5–6 mL/kg. This decreases the chance of hypo-/hypercapnia and volutrauma, reducing VILI. During volume control ventilation (VCV), the ventilator delivers target VT by real-time microprocessor adjusting inflation pressure. This is regulated TV delivery based on flow measurement in both phases of respiration.

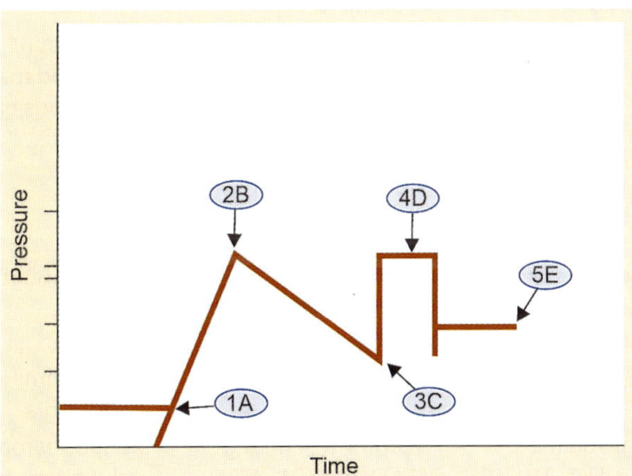

Fig. 1: At the *1A* position, the mean airway pressure (MAP) is low, FiO_2 is high, and the alveoli are closed; pressure is gradually increased, facilitating recruitment, improving oxygenation, and decreasing shunt fraction; by the time, there will be a gradual reduction in FiO_2. The mean airway pressure (MAP) is increased until FiO_2, 30% or oxygenation reaches the summit. At *2B*, the pressure is called opening pressure, where most alveoli are open. Then, the MAP decreased gradually till oxygenation deteriorated (SpO_2 fell drastically) till point *3C*, which is called closing pressure. This happens after the opening pressure is already known *(4D)*. The MAP is set to 2 cmH_2O above the closing pressure *(3C)*, ensuring alveolar full recruitment and stabilization *(5E)*. (FiO_2: fraction of inspired oxygen; SpO_2: oxygen saturation)

Volume Guarantee Mode

This mode can be used with synchronized intermittent mandatory ventilation (SIMV), patient-triggered ventilation (PTV), or pressure support ventilation (PSV) mode. The ventilator delivers a PIP targeted to deliver set TV, and the measures depend on the expired VT. If this delivered TV deviates from the set VT, the PIP is automatically adjusted to match the set VT as much as possible.

Understanding lung pathophysiology and mechanics before applying disease-specific ventilation strategies is vital. The person managing the baby on a ventilator is more crucial than the ventilator itself, so it is not all about changing the knob on the ventilator. Still, one should understand disease progression and its impact on other systems.

RESPIRATORY DISTRESS SYNDROME (TABLE 1)

The respiratory distress syndrome (RDS) is a homogenous, diffuse alveolar disease due to surfactant deficiency. The surfactant pool varies according

TABLE 1: Initial ventilatory support (conventional ventilation) parameters for RDS.

Conventional invasive ventilation with VG mode/PS mode (initial setting)		*Weaning*	*Remark*
1.	PIP (16–20 cmH$_2$O) to adjust tidal volume 5–6 mL/kg	Auto wean in VG mode; if not, keep PIP $<$16 cmH$_2$O	To deliver TV, PIP will adjust and auto-wean
2.	PEEP (5–8 cmH$_2$O)	PEEP wean up to 5 if FiO$_2$ $\leq$25%	To maintain FRC, decrease RACE, and maintain continuous gas exchange
3.	Set pressure support (PS) to achieve 65–75% of set tidal volume (TV)	Wean as indicated above for PIP	
4.	Inspiratory time 0.30–0.35	Keep same	Allow enough expiratory time
5.	Ventilatory rate 30–60 breaths/minute	Rate wean to 15–20 if PCO$_2$ $<$50	Keep PCO$_2$ at target range (40–55 mm Hg), avoid hypocarbia
6.	VG, tidal volume 5–6 mL/kg, FiO$_2$ 21–30% to start with, relative humidity 100%	Wean TV to 4 mL/kg if PCO$_2$ $<$50, 21–25% keeping SPO$_2$ target	Reduce barotrauma and volutrauma, keep target SPO$_2$, 90–95%, avoid hypoxia/hyperoxia
7.	FiO$_2$ 21–30% to start with, relative humidity 100%	21–25% keeping SpO$_2$ target	Keep target SpO$_2$, 90–95%, avoid hypoxia/hyperoxia

(FRC: functional residual capacity; PEEP: positive end-expiratory pressure; PIP: peak inspiratory pressure; RACE: repetitive alveolar collapse and expansion; VG: volume guarantee; FiO$_2$: fraction of inspired oxygen; SpO$_2$: oxygen saturation)

to gestational age and premature status. It is essential to understand lung biology. Among the five stages of lung development, canalicular and early saccular stages (26–36 weeks) are essential because most babies are managed in this lung growth stage. The aim of the neonatologist should be to treat RDS and simultaneously prevent the development of long-term adverse effects like bronchopulmonary dysplasia (BPD).

Principles

The primary objective is to apply lung-protective strategies while ventilating the baby.

- A volume guarantee should be applied in conventional ventilation mode, and surfactant replacement should be considered.
- Reduce the duration of invasive ventilation and promote early weaning.
- Managing factors that may contribute to failure of extubation [early onset sepsis, hemodynamic significant patent ductus arteriosus (PDA)].

Principles and Indication If the Initial Setting is High-frequency Oscillation Ventilation (Table 2)

- Recruitment of alveoli, maintaining optimum lung volume and gas exchange
- Keep mean airway pressure (MAP) lowest acceptable range
- Initial stepwise MAP increment to recruit alveoli to a point when FiO_2 will be needed to increase to maintain target saturation—open lung strategy.

TABLE 2: Initial ventilatory support (high-frequency ventilation) parameters for RDS.

HFOV initial setting		*Weaning and extubation*	*Remark*
1.	Frequency 8–12 Hz	Frequency 8–10 Hz	Keep PCO_2 ≤55 mm Hg after amplitude is adjusted
2.	MAP 10–12	8–9, keeping FiO_2 ≤30%, posterior rib space <8 rib	Keep 2–3 more MAP than con. ventilator
3.	Amplitude (delta P), twice MAP 25–30	Keep the same or 16–18; wean to keep PCO_2 at an acceptable range	Keep PCO_2 ≤55 mm Hg
4.	% Inspiratory time 33% (sensor medics ventilator), I:E 1:2 (SLE ventilator)	Remain unchanged	
5.	FiO_2, 21–100%	Keep FiO_2 <40%	

(FiO_2: fraction of inspired oxygen; HFOV: high-frequency oscillation ventilation; MAP: mean airway pressure; RDS: respiratory distress syndrome)

MECONIUM ASPIRATION SYNDROME LUNG-PROTECTIVE STRATEGY PRINCIPLE (FLOWCHART 1; TABLE 3)

- Gentle ventilation strategy, accepting permissive hypercarbia, lower pH, and lower PaO_2 to prevent lung injury.
- Ventilate the baby with moderate PIP, not exceeding 25 cmH_2O, a relatively rapid ventilator rate (40–60/min), a moderate positive end-expiratory pressure (4–6 cmH_2O), and an adequate expiratory time (0.5–0.7 seconds) to prevent gas trapping and air leaks.

LUNG-PROTECTIVE STRATEGY PRINCIPLE IN BRONCHOPULMONARY DYSPLASIA (TABLE 4)

- Moderate/severe BPD is a heterogeneous lung disease with variable lung compliance and resistance. Two classical parenchymal abnormalities, i.e.,

Flowchart 1: Lung-protective strategies and weaning and extubation protocol.

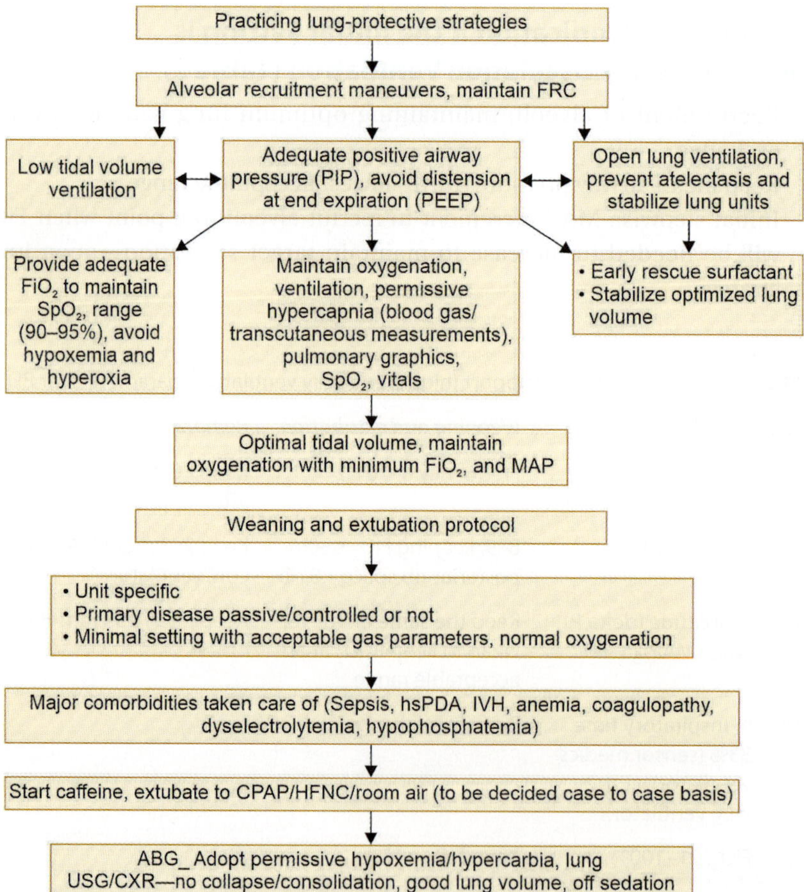

(ABG: arterial blood gas; CPAP: continuous positive airway pressure; CXR: chest X-ray; FRC: functional residual capacity; HFNC: high-flow nasal cannula; PEEP: positive end-expiratory pressure; PIP: peak inspiratory pressure; USG: ultrasound)

TABLE 3: Initial ventilatory support, weaning (conventional and HFOV) parameters for MAS.

Conventional invasive ventilation with VG mode/PS mode (initial setting)		*Weaning and extubation*	*HFOV setting*	*Weaning*
MAS	PIP 16–20, PEEP 4–7 cmH_2O, keep TV 5–6 mL/kg, rate <30 breath/min, I:E ratio 0.35–0.50 seconds, with VG mode—keep TV 5–6 mL/kg, PIP adjust to deliver set TV, with PS mode, needs to achieve 65–75% of set TV, Surfactant ± iNO	Wean FiO_2 <40%, PIP then ventilatory rate, and PEEP at last, PIP <16, PEEP <5–6, FiO_2 <40%, PS 6–8 rate 16–20 breath/min, acceptable blood gas	HFOV rate 10–12 Hz, amplitude (delta P) to just be able to see wiggles over the chest, MAP 13–14, twice >conventional ventilation, rib space 8–9 expansion, I:E 1:2, surfactant ± iNO	Wean amplitude then wean MAP, minimum MAP 10–12, amplitude 15–20, frequency 8, FiO_2 <40%

(FiO_2: fraction of inspired oxygen; HFOV: high-frequency oscillation ventilation; MAP: mean airway pressure; MAS: meconium aspiration syndrome; iNO: inhaled nitric oxide; PEEP: positive end-expiratory pressure; PIP: peak inspiratory pressure; PS: pressure support; TV: tidal volume; VG: volume guarantee)

TABLE 4: Initial ventilatory support, weaning (conventional and HFOV) parameters BPD.

Conventional invasive ventilation with VG mode/PS mode (initial setting)		*Weaning and extubation*	*HFOV setting*	*Weaning*
BPD	Use volume target (VG) 6–8 mL/kg, PIP can be adjusted to deliver set TV, PEEP 5–8 cmH_2O, ventilator rate 20–40 breath/min; inspiratory time 0.35–0.45 seconds, PS mode, needs to achieve 65–75% of set TV, with established BPD, keep PS 6–12 cmH_2O	PIP <16, PEEP <5–6, FiO_2 <35%, PS 6–8 rate 15–25 breath/min, acceptable blood gas (permissive hypercapnia)	Similar to MAS	Similar to MAS

(BPD: bronchopulmonary dysplasia; FiO_2: fraction of inspired oxygen; HFOV: high-frequency oscillation ventilation; MAS: meconium aspiration syndrome; PEEP: positive end-expiratory pressure; PIP: peak inspiratory pressure; PS: pressure support; TV: tidal volume; VG: volume guarantee)

atelectatic (require high PEEP)/overexpanded lung (require low PEEP), need to be ascertained by doing a chest X-ray.

- The strategy applied is high TV 6–8 mL/kg, low ventilatory rate (20–25/min), and prolonged Ti (0.5–0.8 seconds), PEEP kept relatively high (6–8 cmH_2O), SpO_2 target (92–98%)

TABLE 5: Initial ventilatory support, weaning (conventional and HFOV) parameters for CDH/lung hypoplasia.

Conventional invasive ventilation with VG mode/PS mode (initial setting)		*Weaning*	*HFOV setting*	*Weaning*
Lung hypoplasia/ congenital diaphragmatic hernia (CDH)	Keep TV 4–6 mL/kg, PIP <26 cmH_2O, rate 40–60/min Inspiratory time 0.30–0.40 seconds, PEEP 3–5 cmH_2O, FiO_2 40%, rib space, target saturations 92–98%	Wean TV and PIP, the wean rate and PEEP see follow permissive hypercarbia/ hypoxemia, perform ECHO	MAP 10–12, frequency 8–10 Hz, delta P—2× MAP, I:E 1:2, FiO_2 40%, adjust to see wiggle on chest	Wean FiO_2, 60%, wean iNO, follow preductal saturation targets

(FiO_2: fraction of inspired oxygen; HFOV: high-frequency oscillation ventilation; iNO: inhaled nitric oxide; MAP: mean airway pressure; PEEP: positive end-expiratory pressure; PIP: peak inspiratory pressure; PS: pressure support; TV: tidal volume; VG: volume guarantee)

- Permissive hypercapnia (PCO_2 55–65 mm Hg) is followed, keeping pH >7.25.

GENTLE VENTILATION STRATEGIES ADOPTED FOR CONGENITAL DIAPHRAGMATIC HERNIA/LUNG HYPOPLASIA (TABLE 5)

- Optimize lung inflation; ventilate the lung with low TV and a high rate, which seems physiological to lung hypoplasia. Physiologic TV (5 mL/kg) may produce volutrauma, which should be avoided. Keep ABG limits (PCO_2 45–55 mm Hg). Chest X-ray—contralateral chest expansion up to 8–9 rib space.
- HFOV may be used as the preferred mode; use of lower MAP and low frequency. The *VICI trial* revealed that starting with low MAP in HFO is associated with a lower requirement of inhaled nitric oxide (iNO), inotropes, and, subsequently, extracorporeal membrane oxygenation (ECMO) in managing the baby.

LUNG-PROTECTIVE STRATEGY PRINCIPLE IN PERSISTENT PULMONARY HYPERTENSION OF NEWBORN (TABLE 6)

- Gentle ventilation with permissive hypercapnia, avoiding hypoxemia, should be practiced.

TABLE 6: Initial ventilatory support, weaning (conventional and HFOV) parameters for PPHN.

Conventional invasive ventilation with VG mode/PS mode (initial setting)		*Weaning*	*HFOV setting*	*Weaning*
PPHN	Gentle ventilation with permissive hypercapnia and avoids hypoxemia, optimal MAP, relatively low PIP and PEEP, TV 4–6 mL/kg targeted, set PIP to deliver TV in VG mode, acceptable blood gas, (pH >7.25, PCO_2 <50 use iNO as indicated, ECHO parameters)	Wean FiO_2 to 60%, wean PIP <16–18, and rate, wean PEEP to 4–5 cmH_2O,	Minimize lung hyperinflation and acceptable blood gas, and use inhaled nitric oxide (iNO) as indicated	Same like MAS

(FiO_2: fraction of inspired oxygen; HFOV: high-frequency oscillation ventilation; MAP: mean airway pressure; MAS: meconium aspiration syndrome; PPHN: persistent pulmonary hypertension of newborn; PEEP: positive end-expiratory pressure; PIP: peak inspiratory pressure; PS: pressure support; TV: tidal volume; VG: volume guarantee)

- Use exogenous surfactant as per guidelines to improve compliance. The HFOV is beneficial in persistent pulmonary hypertension of newborn (PPHN) secondary to congenital diaphragmatic hernia (CDH)/lung hypoplasia.
- Selective pulmonary vasodilator should be used in severe disease in late preterm and term neonates (oxygenation index >15–20, ECHO—S/O severe PPHN).

POSTEXTUBATION MANAGEMENT

The success of extubation and preventing reintubations depends upon many predictors, which should be taken care of before weaning from a ventilator. Understanding the primary pathology for which the baby was intubated and the comorbidities that the baby develops during management are essential. Anticipating extubation failure and possible invasive support that the baby may require should be discussed beforehand.

The three most important factors which are crucial to successful extubation and care are:

1. *Anticipated respiratory support/no support:* Continuous positive airway pressure (CPAP)/noninvasive mechanical ventilation (NIMV)/heated humidified high flow nasal cannula (HHHFNC) or room air
2. *Therapies proved beneficial at periextubation/postextubation period:* Caffeine, nebulized epinephrine/dexamethasone, short course post-extubation steroid for stridor/glottic edema, chest physiotherapy

3. Intensive monitoring, prepare for any catastrophe/any reintubation indications.

Noninvasive respiratory support helps to prevent extubation failure in extremely low birth weight (ELBW) babies. Maintaining functional residual capacity (FRC) in such babies is prudent to prevent postextubation collapse, given the compliant chest wall and premature alveoli. Meta-analysis on caffeine at periextubation/postextubation revealed that the loading dose (20 mg/g) and maintenance dose (10 mg/kg) reduce the risk of reintubation (RR 0.51, CI 0.36–0.71), given that the side effects of caffeine (tachycardia, reflux, diuresis, weight loss, feeding intolerance, and seizure), it should be used judiciously.

Chest wall percussion with vibrator and oropharyngeal suction subsequently every 2 hours helps reduce reintubation.

Postextubation monitoring is vital; every intensive care unit should have a clearly defined protocol for extubation preparedness and postextubation care.

CONCLUSION

Lung-protective ventilation in neonates is central to minimizing ventilator-induced lung injury while ensuring adequate gas exchange across diverse pulmonary pathologies. Strategies such as open-lung recruitment, volume-targeted ventilation, permissive hypercapnia, and careful titration of FiO_2 form the foundation of safe respiratory management. Disease-specific modifications—whether for RDS, MAS, BPD, CDH, or PPHN—require a nuanced understanding of lung physiology and progression of illness. Successful outcomes depend not only on technology but also on the clinician's expertise in tailoring support, anticipating extubation readiness, and implementing vigilant postextubation care. Ultimately, a balanced approach that integrates physiology-driven ventilation, early noninvasive support, and structured extubation protocols offers the best opportunity to reduce both short-term morbidity and long-term pulmonary sequelae in vulnerable neonates.

SUGGESTED READING

1. Al-Mandari H, Shalish W, Dempsey E, Keszler M, Davis PG, Sant'Anna G. International survey on periextubation practices in extremely preterm infants. Arch Dis Child Fetal Neonatal Ed. 2015;100(5):F428-31.
2. Kalikkot Thekkeveedu R, El-Saie A, Prakash V, Katakam L, Shivanna B. Ventilation-induced lung injury (VILI) in neonates: Evidence-based concepts and lung-protective strategies. J Clin Med. 2022;11(3):557.

3. Keszler M, Gautham KS. Goldsmith's Assisted Ventilation of the Neonate, 7th edition. Amsterdam: Elsevier; 2022. pp. 241-314.
4. Keszler M, Sant'Anna G. Mechanical ventilation and bronchopulmonary dysplasia. Clin Perinatol. 2015;42:781-96.
5. Reiterer F, Schwaberger B, Freidl T, Schmölzer G, Pichler G, Urlesberger B. Lung-protective ventilatory strategies in intubated preterm neonates with RDS. Paediatr Respir Rev. 2017;23:89-96.
6. Snoek KG, Capolupo I, van Rosmalen J, Hout Lde J, Vijfhuize S, Greenough A, et al. Conventional mechanical ventilation versus high-frequency oscillatory ventilation for congenital diaphragmatic hernia: A randomized clinical trial (The VICI-trial). Ann Surg. 2016;263(5):867-74.
7. Van Kaam AH, De Luca D, Hentschel R, Hutten J, Sindelar R, Thome U, et al. Modes and strategies for providing conventional mechanical ventilation in neonates. Pediatr Res. 2021;90(5):957-62.

CHAPTER

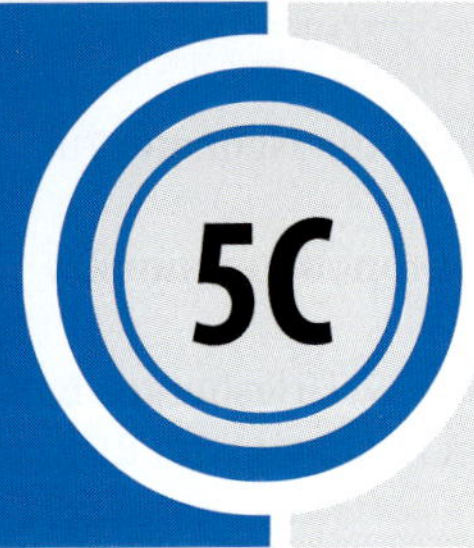

Initial Setting for Common Disease Conditions in Pressure Controlled Ventilation

Pratima Anand

INTRODUCTION

The success of invasive ventilation depends on understanding the rationale of ventilating any neonate. The knowledge of the normal physiology and physiology of diseased lungs helps us titrate the ventilator setting at initiation as well as adjusting the settings subsequently.

The commonly used ventilatory parameters which have been discussed in the previous chapters are peak inspiratory pressure (PIP), peak end-expiratory pressure (PEEP), fraction of inspired oxygen (FiO_2), inspiratory time (Ti), inspiratory to expiratory ratio (I:E), and respiratory rate (RR). As we have learnt, mean airway pressure (MAP) is determined by combination of these parameters.

The initial settings of these parameters largely depend on the cause of respiratory failure. For example, the pathophysiology respiratory distress of a preterm neonate with respiratory distress syndrome (RDS) is very different from that of distress in a term neonate with meconium aspiration syndrome (MAS).

The broad categories of lung diseases in neonates are diffuse alveolar pathology (preterm neonate with RDS, term neonate with pulmonary hemorrhage, and term neonate with pulmonary edema), heterogeneous or localized pathology (MAS and pneumonia), normal lung parenchyma with a central cause (birth asphyxia and apnea of prematurity). The other underlying lung pathologies in neonates are depicted in **Flowchart 1**.

The context specific pathophysiology helps decide the initial settings, since the parameters to be set on ventilator depends on the underlying compliance and resistance of the diseased lung.

Table 1 shows the underlying change in lung physiology and subsequent consequences on the initial settings.

It should be remembered that these settings are a broad guide for initiation of invasive ventilation as soon as the baby is intubated and connected to the ventilator. Continuous bedside monitoring is critical for precise titration of the settings subsequently **(Box 1)**.

Flowchart 1: Categories of diseases that may warrant invasive ventilation in neonates.

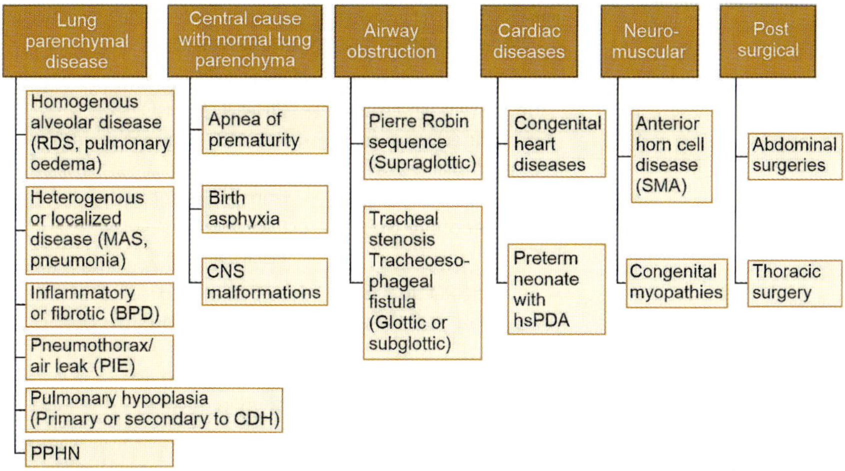

- Lung parenchymal disease
  - Homogenous alveolar disease (RDS, pulmonary oedema)
  - Heterogenous or localized disease (MAS, pneumonia)
  - Inflammatory or fibrotic (BPD)
  - Pneumothorax/ air leak (PIE)
  - Pulmonary hypoplasia (Primary or secondary to CDH)
  - PPHN
- Central cause with normal lung parenchyma
  - Apnea of prematurity
  - Birth asphyxia
  - CNS malformations
- Airway obstruction
  - Pierre Robin sequence (Supraglottic)
  - Tracheal stenosis Tracheoeso- phageal fistula (Glottic or subglottic)
- Cardiac diseases
  - Congenital heart diseases
  - Preterm neonate with hsPDA
- Neuro- muscular
  - Anterior horn cell disease (SMA)
  - Congenital myopathies
- Post surgical
  - Abdominal surgeries
  - Thoracic surgery

(BPD: bronchopulmonary dysplasia; CDH: congenital diaphragmatic hernia; CNS: central nervous system; hsPDA: hemodynamically significant patent ductus arteriosus; MAS: meconium aspiration syndrome; PIE: pulmonary interstitial emphysema; PPHN: persistent pulmonary hypertension of the newborn; RDS: respiratory distress syndrome; SMA: spinal muscular atrophy)

TABLE 1: Disease specific initial settings for neonatal ventilation.

Disease	*Underlying pathophysiology*	*Initial settings*
Lung parenchymal diseases		
Respiratory distress syndrome **(Table 2** shows settings as per birth weight in RDS)	• Compliance is reduced • Resistance unchanged so shorter time constants are needed	• Initial settings • PIP 14–16 cmH_2O or Vt of 5–6 mL/kg • Rate 40–60/min • Ti 0.35 seconds
Meconium aspiration syndrome (MAS) (**Table 3** shows initial settings based on underlying pathophysiology of different MAS presentations)	• Compliance may be normal • Resistance is increased	• Use lower PEEP 3.5–4 if risk of air leak is high • Vt 5–6 mL/kg on PIP adjusted to achieve Vt of 5–6 mL/kg • Rate < 30 • Ti 0.35–0.50 seconds • PEEP 4–7 cmH_2O if atelectatic picture and lower if air trapping
Air leak	Compliance reduced, resistance may be increased, time constants needed are longer	Goal is to reduce positive pressure and provide oxygenation with increased FiO_2

Contd...

Contd…

Disease	*Underlying pathophysiology*	*Initial settings*
Lung hypoplasia	• Context of preterm neonate born after prolonged rupture of membranes or oligohydramnios • Term neonate with CDH	• Vt 4–5 mL/kg • PIP <26 cmH_2O • Rate 40–60 breaths per minute • I-time 0.25 seconds to 0.40 seconds • PEEP 3–5 cmH_2O
• BPD • Early/mild moderate • Chronic severe	• Severe BPD goal is to wean off as early as possible • Longer Ti (0.5 to 1.0 seconds) lower SIMV rates, longer expiratory times • Higher PEEP is needed when airway malacia is severe • Higher PIPs may be needed since lungs are stiff • BPD spells (oxygenation and airway resistance worsen rapidly due to larger airway collapse and respond to increase in PEEP (>7–8 cm)	• Vt 6–8 mL/kg • Rate 20–40 breaths per minute • I-time 0.35–0.45 seconds • PEEP 5–8 cmH_2O • PS to achieve 2/3 or ¾ set Vt • Chronic may need higher Vt 7–12 mL/kg or higher • Second increased dead space • I-time: 0.50–1.00 seconds; longer to overcome airway resistance • Rate: 15–30 breaths per minute; slower to allow adequate lung emptying • PEEP: Quite variable; may need 8–12 cmH_2O to "stent" airway open
PPHN	• Primary PPHN or PPHN with parenchymal lung disease • PPHN with parenchymal lung disease	• PEEP 4 cmH_2O • Vt 4–5 mL/kg • PEEP 5–6 cmH_2O • Vt 4–6 mL/kg • Minimize hyperinflation • Adjunct therapies
TTNB	• Compliance reduced variably depending on fluid in the lung	• PIP 12–16 cmH_2O • Vt of 4–5 mL/kg • PEEP 4–5 cmH_2O • Rate 40–60/min • Ti 0.35–0.45 seconds
Pulmonary hemorrhage and pulmonary edema	Compliance variably affected due to alveoli filled with fluid/blood	• High PEEP of 7–8 cmH_2O • PIP 12–16 cmH_2O • Vt of 4–5 mL/kg • PEEP 4–5 cmH_2O • Rate 40–60/min • Ti 0.35–0.45 seconds

Contd…

Contd…

Disease	*Underlying pathophysiology*	*Initial settings*
Central cause with normal lung parenchyma		
Apnea of prematurity	• Lungs essentially normal • Compliance may be reduced due to prematurity • Resistance is unaffected, time constant is shorter	• PIP 12–14 cmH_2O • Vt 4–5 mL/kg • PEEP 4 cmH_2O • Rate 20–30/min • Ti 0.40 seconds
Birth asphyxia CNS malformations	Normal lung and normal resistance and compliance	• PIP 12–14 cmH_2O • Vt 4–5 mL/kg • PEEP 4 cmH_2O • Rate 20–30/min • Ti 0.40 seconds
Airway malformations		
Supraglottic	• Lung compliance normal • Alveolar hypoventilation	• PIP 12–14 cmH_2O • Vt 4–6 mL/kg • PEEP 4–6 cmH_2O • Rate 20–30/min • Ti 0.40 seconds
Subglottic or glottic	• Air trapping • Prolongation of expiration leading to alveolar hypoventilation	• PIP 12–14 cmH_2O • Vt 4–6 mL/kg • PEEP 4–6 cmH_2O • Rate 20–30/min • Ti 0.40 seconds
Cardiac diseases		
• Mixing lesions with pulmonary overload such as TGA and TAPVC • Preterm neonate with PDA • Term neonates with large VSD, endocardial cushion defects	Lung compliance is reduced because of pulmonary congestion and edema	• High PEEP of 7–8 cmH_2O • PIP 12–16 cmH_2O • Vt of 4–5 mL/kg • PEEP 4–5 cmH_2O • Rate 40–60/min • Ti 0.35–0.45 seconds
Neuromuscular diseases		
Congenital myopathies, SMA	Low tidal volume and functional residual capacity due to respiratory muscle weakness	• PEEP between 5 and 6 cmH_2O • PIP 12–14 cmH_2O • Vt 4–6 mL/kg • Rates 30–40/minute

Contd…

Contd...

Disease	*Underlying pathophysiology*	*Initial settings*
Postsurgical		
Thoracic and abdominal surgeries	• PEEP necessary to maintain the recruitment of alveoli • Low tidal volumes can predispose to atelectasis • Respiratory drive may be compromised due to intraoperative sedation and medications • Pain relief measures to be ensured postoperatively • Thoracic surgeries such as TEF and CDH are predisposed to air leaks, so pressures need to be used cautiously	• Tidal volumes >5 mL/kg • PEEP between 5–7 cmH_2O • PIP 12–14 cmH_2O • Rates 30–40 minute

(BPD: bronchopulmonary dysplasia; CDH: congenital diaphragmatic hernia; CNS: central nervous system; FiO_2: fraction of inspired oxygen; PEEP: positive end-expiratory pressure; PIP: peak inspiratory pressure; PPHN: persistent pulmonary hypertension of the newborn; PS: pressure support; RDS: respiratory distress syndrome; SIMV: synchronized intermittent mandatory ventilation; SMA: spinal muscular atrophy; TAPVC: total anomalous pulmonary venous connection; TEF: tracheoesophageal fistula; TGA: transposition of great arteries; Ti: inspiratory time; VSD: ventricular septal defect; Vt: tidal volume)

TABLE 2: Initial settings in RDS based on birth weight.

	Weight (g)		
Ventilator mode	<1,000	1,000–2,500	>2,500
Conventional SIMV			
Rate	30–60	30–60	20–40
Vt (mL/kg)	5–6	5	4–5
PEEP (cmH_2O)	5–8	5–8	6–9
I-time (sec)	Start 0.3–0.4 seconds		
PS (cmH_2O)	Start at 8–12 adjust as needed to two-thirds of PIP for Vt		

(PEEP: positive end-expiratory pressure; PIP: peak inspiratory pressure; PS: pressure support; RDS: respiratory distress syndrome; SIMV: synchronized intermittent mandatory ventilation; Vt: tidal volume)

TABLE 3: Initial settings in MAS based on presentation.

Ventilator mode	*Airway obstruction with evidence of gas trapping*	*Alveolar disease with evidence of low lung volume*	*Pulmonary hypertension*
Pathophysiology	• Increased resistance • Increased time constant • Lung hyperexpansion	• Reduced surfactant function • Reduced lung compliance • Increased ventilation perfusion mismatch	• Reduced nitric oxide synthase • Hypoxemia • Acidosis
Conventional SIMV PC	• PIP for adequate chest rise • Lower Ti • Adjust PIP to desired Vt • PEEP 4–6 cmH_2O • PS three-fourths set PIP	• Surfactant therapy • Monitor lung volume higher PEEP as needed	• Consider inodilators • Inhaled NO

(MAS: meconium aspiration syndrome; NO: nitric oxide; PC: pressure-controlled; PEEP: positive end-expiratory pressure; PIP: peak inspiratory pressure; PS: pressure support; SIMV: synchronized intermittent mandatory ventilation; Ti: inspiratory time; Vt: tidal volume)

BOX 1: Continuous clinical monitoring after initial settings on ventilator.

Clinical monitoring
- Chest excursion
- Work of breathing retractions
- Perfusion
- Synchrony between the baby and ventilator
- Auscultation: Breath sounds

Noninvasive monitoring
- Pulse oximetry
- Chest X-ray if indicated

Pulmonary graphics
- Flow and volume scalars
- Loops
- Tidal volume delivered

CONCLUSION

The selection of initial ventilator settings in neonates must be tailored to the underlying disease pathophysiology. Understanding lung compliance, resistance, and time constants provides the foundation for setting appropriate parameters in pressure-controlled ventilation. Conditions such as RDS, MAS, BPD, PPHN, TTNB, and central or structural causes each demand specific adjustments to optimize gas exchange while minimizing ventilator-induced lung injury. Importantly, these initial settings are only a starting point; meticulous clinical assessment and continuous bedside monitoring remain essential for dynamic titration and achieving safe, effective respiratory support.

SUGGESTED READING

1. Dargaville PA, Keszler M. Setting the ventilator in the NICU. In: Rimensberge PC (Ed). Paediatric and Neonatal Mechanical Ventilation. London: Springer Nature; 2013. pp. 1101-25.
2. Eichenwald EC, Hansen AR, Martin CR, Stark AR. Cloherty and Stark's Manual of Neonatal Care, 8th edition. Philadelphia: Lippincott Williams & Wilkins; 2017.
3. Keszler M, Gautham K, Goldsmith JP. Goldsmith's Assisted Ventilation of the Neonate: An Evidence-Based Approach to Newborn Respiratory Care, 7th edition. Amsterdam: Elsevier; 2022. p. 500.
4. Rajiv PK, Lakshminrusimha S, Vidyasagar D. Essentials of Neonatal Ventilation, 1st edition. Amsterdam: Elsevier; 2018.

CHAPTER

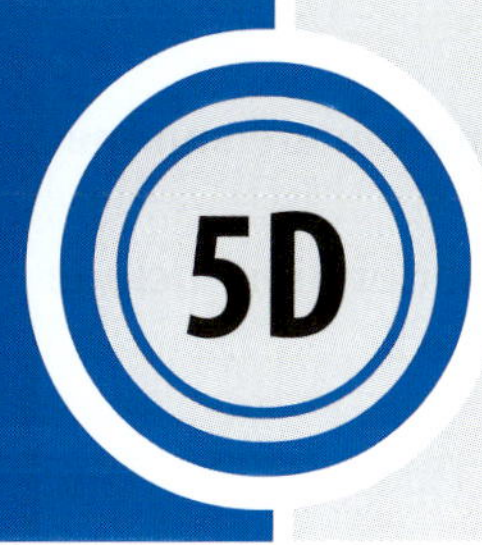

Acute Deterioration of a Neonate on Ventilator

Prathik Bandiya

INTRODUCTION

Neonatal mechanical ventilation has improved the survival of sick neonates over the years. Despite advances in mechanical ventilation, complications and adverse events due to ventilation still exist. One of the dreaded event for a neonate on ventilator is acute deterioration. These events are nightmare not only for clinician but also for parents. Early and prompt recognition of such events will not only prevent complications but also improve outcome in long term. In this chapter, we will go through about the algorithmic approach in recognition and management of acute deterioration of neonate on ventilator.

In the majority of cases, acute deterioration is not actually acute but a gradual deterioration leading to acute terminal event. Most of the catastrophic events which occur in neonatal intensive care unit (NICU) are usually due to failure by the treating team to recognize the clinical symptoms and signs preceding the event. The usual course of events leading to acute deterioration is shown in **Figure 1**.

Acute deterioration is manifested as *collapse* of a neonate on respiratory support (either *noninvasive or invasive*) with one or more of the following clinical symptoms:

- Desaturation
- Cyanosis
- Bradycardia
- Hypotension
- Cardiorespiratory arrest

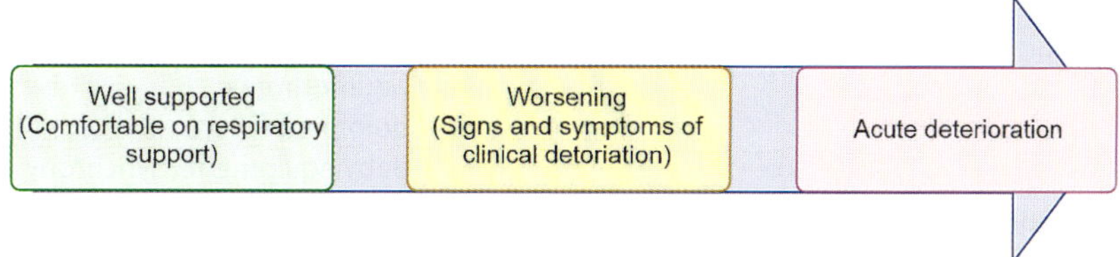

Fig. 1: Course of events preceding acute deterioration.

The causes and possibilities leading to acute deterioration are summarized in **Table 1**.

The other commonly used mnemonics for acute deterioration include the following and the causes have been mentioned in **Table 2**.

- *DOPE*
- *DOPE + SIP*
- *BOLD PEEP*

Let us see each important cause which leads to deterioration on ventilator:

- *Displacement of endotracheal (ET) tube:*
    - *History and examination:* Sequence of events prior to desaturation like loose ET tape, secretions pooling in oral cavity, etc. There might be a history of recent handling as well.

On examination, no response to manual ventilation, no chest rise, no air entry over axilla and audible leak and or gurgling sound over stomach.

- *Ventilator alarms and graphics:* Ventilator may give alarms such as "leak", "low tidal volume", and "low minute ventilation".

TABLE 1: Acute deterioration causes.

Machine	*Interface*	*Pulmonary/systemic*
Ventilator malfunction	Accidental extubation	Pneumothorax
Leak in circuit	Interface blocked with secretion/blood	Worsening lung disease
Blender/compressor failure	Kinked/compressed ET tube	PPHN/opening of PDA
Inappropriate settings	Interface displacement	Shock/acute blood loss
Improper alarm settings	Nasal block (in noninvasive ventilation)	Arrhythmias

(ET: endotracheal; PDA: patent ductus arteriosus; PPHN: persistent pulmonary hypertension of newborn)

TABLE 2: Commonly used mnemonic for acute deterioration on ventilator.

DOPE	*DOPE + SIP*	*BOLD PEEP*
D—Displacement O—Obstruction P—Pneumothorax E—Equipment failure	S—Shock I—Intraventricular hemorrhage P—PDA/PPHN	B—Bad or worsening lung disease O—Obstructed ET/interface L—Long ET D—Displaced interface P—Pneumothorax E—Equipment failure EP—Baby equipment asynchrony

(ET: endotracheal; PDA: patent ductus arteriosus; PPHN: persistent pulmonary hypertension of newborn)

In graphics: No expiratory flow in flow time and flow volume loops. In PV loop, the expiratory loop will not be touching the baseline.

- *Action:* Remove the ET tube—start bag and mask ventilation and then reintubate.

- *Obstruction:*
  - *History and examination:* History of frequent suctioning, thick secretions, previous history of tube change due to block, progressive increase in FiO_2 requirement in last few hours.
    On examination: There will be presence worsening respiratory distress, especially retractions. The baby will be breathing independent of ventilator (especially in case of complete block).
  - *Ventilator alarms and graphics:* Tube block alarm or tube obstruction alarm depending on the ventilator, low VT alarm. Graphics may show serrated pattern in flow time curve and flow volume loops.
  - *Action:* Suction first, if there is no improvement then reintubate.
- *Pneumothorax:*
  - *History and examination:* There will be sudden deterioration in clinical condition with bradycardia, desaturation and hypotension with sudden increase in FiO_2. On examination, there will be asymmetry in chest wall, decreased air entry and positive transillumination test.
  - *Ventilator alarms and graphics:* Air trapping trend before and air leak pattern after the event. There will be presence of auto-PEEP.
  - *Action:* Needle drainage for emergency evacuation and intercostal chest drain (ICD) tube insertion.
- *Equipment failure:*
  - *History and examination:* Failure of pressure in gas supply lines, alarm failure, with failure of staff to realize ventilator is disconnected, expiratory port occlusion producing inadvertent overdistention of lungs.
  - *Ventilator alarms and graphics:* Blunting of loops in case of leaks, system failure alarm in case of major malfunction.
  - *Action:* Disconnect the baby from the ventilator and start manual ventilation. Improvement on bag and tube/T Piece is an indicator of equipment malfunction.
- *Bad/worsening lung disease:*
  - *History and examination:* Progressively increasing FiO_2 and pressure requirement in ventilator (PIP)
  - *Ventilator parameters:* Graphics may show flattening of PV loops or increased expiratory airway resistance in PV loop and flow volume curves

    - *Action:* Increasing the pressure and FiO_2 requirement on ventilator. Neonates with worsening respiratory distress syndrome (RDS) might require treatment with surfactant and those with pneumonia require antibiotic treatment. Bronchodilators in neonates with bronchospasm.
- *Long ET tube:*
    - *History and examination:* Desaturations on ventilator and no improvement. Increased air entry on right side with absent or decreased air entry on left side.
    - *Ventilator parameters:* X-ray may show hyperinflated right lung field with ET tube beyond T2 vertebra
    - *Action:* Pull out ET tube
- *Other conditions:* Pulmonary hemorrhage, large intraventricular hemorrhage (IVH), and persistent pulmonary hypertension of newborn (PPHN).

STEPWISE APPROACH

Whenever we encounter a neonate who deteriorates acutely on ventilator, it is very important to maintain calm and not to panic as there are few causes which lead to acute deterioration and stepwise approach leads to successful outcome. The first step is usually to disconnect the baby from the ventilator and start positive pressure ventilation with a self-inflating bag **(Flowcharts 1 to 4)**.

Flowchart 1: Approach to acute deterioration.

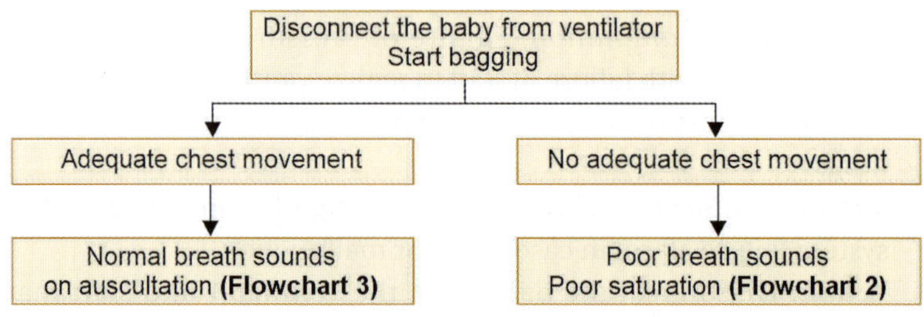

Flowchart 2: Assessment in a neonate with inadequate chest movement and poor breath sounds and saturation.

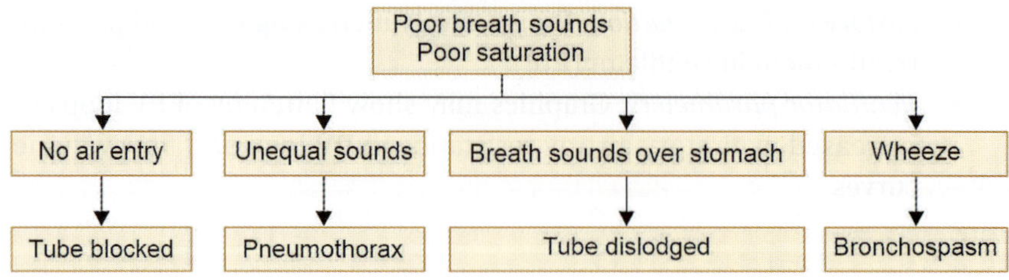

Flowchart 3: Action for a neonate with inadequate chest movement and poor breath sounds and saturation.

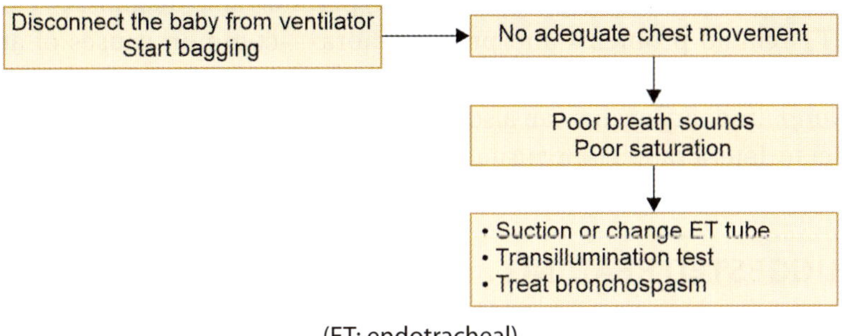

(ET: endotracheal)

Flowchart 4: Assessment in a neonate with adequate chest movement and good breath sounds and poor saturation.

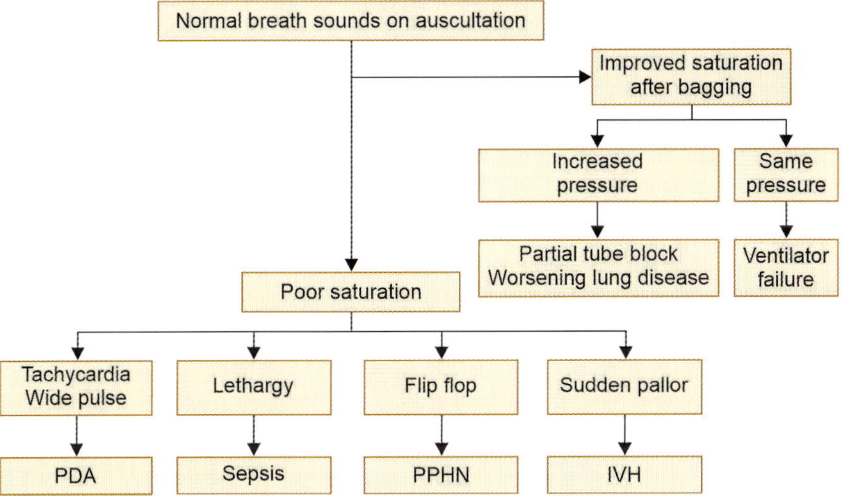

(IVH: intraventricular hemorrhage; PDA: patent ductus arteriosus; PPHN: persistent pulmonary hypertension of newborn)

PREVENTION OF ACUTE DETERIORATION

- *Endotracheal tube (ETT):* Fixation, care, timely suction when required
- Regular monitoring of baby
- Be aware of what are you dealing with
- Training of nurses and physicians with simulation and debriefing
- Upkeep of equipment with periodic maintenance is essential.

In any neonate with acute deterioration, algorithmic approach based on quick clinical examination and diagnosis can help in crisis aversion. One should anticipate that such issue can occur and should be able to take appropriate action before a major deterioration.

CONCLUSION

- Stepwise algorithmic approach (DOPE) permits rapid diagnosis.
- ETT-related problems and pneumothorax—common causes of acute deterioration.
- Nonpulmonary events can also cause deterioration.
- Acute deterioration is not usually acute, most of the time it is due to failure of timely detection.

SUGGESTED READING

1. Keszler M, Gautham KS. Goldsmith's Assisted Ventilation of the Neonate, 7th edition. Amsterdam: Elsevier; 2022.
2. Rajiv PK, Vidyasagar D, Lakshminrusimha S. Essentials of Neonatal Ventilation. Amsterdam: Elsevier; 2018.

CHAPTER

Weaning of a Neonate from Ventilator: Extubation and Postextubation Management

Pradeep Sharma

INTRODUCTION

Mechanical ventilation is lifesaving but invasive and associated with complications such as pneumonia, sepsis, bronchopulmonary dysplasia (BPD), periventricular leukomalacia, and adverse long-term neurological outcomes. Therefore, clinicians should make every effort to wean the baby as soon as possible.

The basic weaning strategy for a neonate on pressure, volume-controlled, and high-frequency ventilation is shown in **Table 1**.

- *Pressure-targeted ventilation (PTV):* The basic principle is to create enough pressure to open the airway, overcome the respiratory tract and parenchymal resistance and result in the gas flow to the alveoli which depends on the lung compliance, inspiratory pressure, time, flow, and synchronization of the breaths of the ventilator and the baby. Start weaning with reducing peak inspiratory pressure and rate. The extubation can be done at >20 breaths per minute. If the respiratory drive is good, the tidal volume should not be allowed to fall below 4–5 mL/kg unless spontaneous ventilation supplements the minute volume.
- *Synchronized intermittent mandatory ventilation (SIMV):* In SIMV, the lack of support beyond the SIMV rate may result in increased work of breathing during weaning in extremely low birthweight babies with

TABLE 1: Weaning strategy for various modes of mechanical ventilation.

Change in blood gas parameter	*Action:* SIMV	*Action:* AC or PSV	*Action:* Volume-targeted ventilation	*Action:* HFV
Increase PCO_2	Reduce PIP, rate	Reduce PIP	Reduce rate, tidal volume to 4 mL/kg	Reduce amplitude
Decrease PO_2	Reduce FiO_2, PEEP	Reduce FiO_2, PEEP	Reduce FiO_2, PEEP	Reduce FiO_2, MAP

(AC: assist control; HFV: high-frequency ventilation; MAP: mean airway pressure; PEEP: positive end expiratory pressure; PIP: peak inspiratory pressure; PSV: pressure support ventilation; SIMV: synchronized intermittent mandatory ventilation)

narrow endotracheal tubes leading to high airway resistance. Poor muscle power and excessive chest wall compliance results in small ineffective tidal volumes, increased dead space, and decreased alveolar ventilation. It is better to add pressure support to SIMV when the rate falls below 30 per minute. This will reduce the work of breathing and make weaning faster.

- In difficult weaning, neurally adjusted ventilatory assist (NAVA) mode may help as the electrical signals from the diaphragm are detected in the NAVA system triggering respiratory assistance which is applied simultaneously with the diaphragmatic movement and this synchronized respiratory support with the neonate's spontaneous efforts may facilitate weaning.
- *Pressure support ventilation (PSV):* PSV mode ensures better inspiratory and expiratory synchronization and auto-weaning happens when targeted tidal volume (TTV) is put on.
- *Volume-targeted ventilation (VTV):* Pressure reduction occurs automatically in VTV as the lung compliance improves. The decrease in respiratory support occurs in real time and may accelerate weaning. The ventilation support is reduced automatically to achieve the desired tidal volume but the target tidal volume if reduced below average physiologic values will lead to increased work of breathing. Long-term ventilator-dependent babies require higher tidal volumes over time due to increased anatomic and physiologic dead space due to acquired tracheomegaly and segmental atelectasis. The tidal volume should not fall below 4–5 mL/kg during weaning to prevent increased work of breathing as there is heterogeneous aeration of the lungs. Ventilation with higher tidal volumes may cause alveolar injury and volume trauma. Delaying extubation until a very low tidal volume may cause atelectasis and alveolar collapse and increases the chances of extubation failure. Therefore, a tidal volume of 5–7 mL/kg is recommended during weaning.
- *High-frequency ventilation (HFV):* The neonates can be directly extubated from HFV and may need not go through the process of conventional ventilation during weaning. Some studies have shown a lower incidence of BPD and a shorter number of ventilation days with this approach.

ASSESSMENT OF EXTUBATION READINESS

Extubation failure is defined as the need for reintubation in the first 2–7 days after extubation. The ventilation settings for extubation of neonates <14 days of postnatal age are given in **Box 1**. Prediction of the extubation success depends on adequate neural signals and neuromuscular synapsis, the functional capacity of the respiratory muscles, and the primary lung pathology. The improvement in the lung pathology and its complications is one of the most important determinants of successful weaning and extubation.

BOX 1: Ventilation settings for extubation of neonates <2 weeks of postnatal age.

Conventional ventilation:
- *SIMV:* PIP ≤16 cmH_2O, PEEP ≤6 cmH_2O, rate ≤20, FiO_2 ≤0.30
- *AC/PSV, BW, <1000 g:* MAP ≤7 cmH_2O and FiO_2 ≤0.30
- *AC/PSV, BW ≥1,000 g:* MAP ≤8 cmH_2O and FiO_2 ≤0.30

Volume-targeted ventilation (tidal volume measured at the endotracheal tube):
Tidal volume ≤4.0–4.5 mL/kg (5–6 mL/kg if, <700 g or >2 weeks of age) and FiO_2 ≤0.30

High-frequency oscillatory ventilation:
- *BW <1,000 g:* MAP ≤7 cmH_2O and FiO_2 ≤0.30
- *BW ≥1,000 g:* MAP ≤9 cmH_2O and FiO_2 ≤0.30

(AC: assist control; MAP: mean airway pressure; PEEP: positive end expiratory pressure; PIP: peak inspiratory pressure; PSV: pressure support ventilation; SIMV: synchronized intermittent mandatory ventilation)

BOX 2: Tools to assess readiness for extubation.

- Minute ventilation
- Minimal ventilatory settings
- Spontaneous breath test
- Tension time index
- Heart rate variability
- Respiratory variability index

Clinical Assessment

Different methods and techniques have been used for the clinical assessment of neonates before and following extubation some of which are summarized in **Box 2**.

Minute Ventilation

Measuring minute ventilation on continuous positive airway pressure (CPAP) for 10 minutes and comparing it to that on mechanical ventilation has also been reported to increase extubation success.

Minimal Ventilatory Settings

Another parameter to assess the readiness for extubation is the *minimal ventilatory settings* before extubation but there is no consensus on these settings.

Spontaneous Breath Test

Spontaneous breath test of 3–10 minutes has high sensitivity and positive predictive value but low specificity and negative predictive value in evaluating the neonate's readiness for extubation. This may be due to increased resistance and dead space of the endotracheal tubes in very preterm neonates on CPAP leading to increased work of breathing. Those who can tolerate this added work have a higher chance of successful extubation.

Tension Time Index

Tension time index (TTI) evaluates respiratory muscle strength as a tool to determine readiness for extubation.

Autonomic Nervous System Function

A lack of heart rate variability (HRV) in preterm neonates has high specificity and positive predictive value for extubation failure.

Respiratory Variability Index

A lower respiratory variability index (RVI) has a higher chance of extubation failure, the combination of RVI and spontaneous breathing trial (SBT) had high sensitivity and specificity in predicting successful extubation. An automated tool analyzed by MATLAB compiler with the use of machine learning and automated RVI and HRV assessment methods can reduce the extubation failure from 20% to <5% **(Table 1)**.

EXTUBATION CHECKLIST

The extubation checklists criteria that a neonate should meet 24 hours before extubation are as given in **Box 3**.

The CPAP devices should be kept ready one hour before extubation, nursing care and observation of the neonate for signs of increased work of breathing are performed half an hour before extubation.

Quality Improvement Studies

A plan-do-check-act (PDCA) cycle tool was implemented by Prasad et al., and the rate of reintubation following extubation decreased from 41.7% preprotocol period to 23.8%. Unplanned extubations with the need for reintubation should be tracked. Severe and dangerous postextubation

BOX 3: Extubation checklist.

- Stable vitals including HR, SpO_2 on ventilation during the previous 24 hour
- The underlying disease is resolving
- CDP machine is ready
- Nebulizer device preferably inline should be kept ready
- Sedation should be off for at least the duration of the half-life of the drug
- There should be adequate monitoring and intubation backup facility for the next couple of hours

(CDP: continuous distending pressure)

complications should be closely monitored and documented during the first 24 hours including hemodynamic instability, severe or prolonged hypoxia, intraventricular hemorrhage (IVH), and death.

EXTUBATION FAILURE

Risk factors for extubation failure are lower gestational age, prolonged mechanical ventilation for >2 weeks, blood gas abnormalities before extubation, high ventilatory settings, glottic and subglottic edema, respiratory muscle weakness, hemodynamically significant patent duct arteriosus (HSPDA), etc., as given in **Box 4**.

The other factors leading to extubation failure may be related to neonatal intensive care unit (NICU) policies like inadequate training, lack of protocols for initiation and termination of mechanical ventilation, use of sedatives and muscle relaxant, and lack of proper postextubation continuous distending pressure (CDP) after extubation.

POSTEXTUBATION MANAGEMENT

Preterm neonates may have inadequate respiratory drive and muscle strength to maintain functional residual capacity (FRC). The evidence-based treatment modalities for preventing extubation failure are as given in **Box 5**.

After extubation, the vocal cords may be edematous preventing effective grunting depriving the neonate of endogenous distending pressure to

BOX 4: Risk factors for extubation failure.

- Lower gestational age and birth weight
- Prolonged mechanical ventilation for >2 weeks
- Low pH and higher PCO_2 before extubation
- High ventilatory settings like high MAP and FiO_2
- Glottic and subglottic edema
- Poor respiratory control
- Respiratory muscle weakness
- Airway abnormalities
- Hemodynamically significant patent duct arteriosus (HSPDA)
- Nosocomial infections such as ventilator-associated pneumonia and lung injury

(MAP: mean airway pressure)

BOX 5: Therapies for preventing extubation failure.

- Continuous distending pressure support
- Caffeine
- Postnatal steroids
- Diuretics
- Chest physiotherapy
- Nutritional support
- Developmentally supportive care

augment end expiratory volume. Therefore, it is necessary to provide CDP to all preterm neonates after extubation. The various modalities available are noninvasive positive pressure ventilation (NIPPV), synchronized noninvasive positive pressure ventilation (SNIPPV), nasal continuous positive airway pressure (nasal CPAP), and heated humidified high-flow nasal cannula (HHHFNC). Noninvasive neurally adjusted ventilatory assist (NAVA) and noninvasive high-frequency oscillatory ventilation (NHFOV) may be more effective than NCPAP. Synchronized NIPPV was more effective than nonsynchronized NIPPV.

Caffeine

Caffeine administration before extubation increases the chance of successful extubation and improves the neurological outcome of very preterm neonates. A systematic review showed that a higher maintenance dose of caffeine was associated with lower mortality and BPD rates.

Postnatal Steroids

Postnatal steroids can be considered for late administration in babies who cannot be weaned from mechanical ventilation. National Institute of Child Health and Human Development (NICHD) has developed a software tool which includes the gestation, gender, need for respiratory support to decide for the administration of postnatal steroids. A low-dose dexamethasone <0.2 mg/kg per day facilitates extubation. Corticosteroids can also be used during the weaning process and after extubation to treat stridor. The risk factors for stridor include prolonged ventilation, multiple intubations, and previous extubation failure. Steroid therapy should be prescribed for a short time, and the risk benefits should be discussed with parents. Inhaled, intratracheal, or intranasal steroids are also acceptable but more evidence is required.

Diuretics

Diuretics improve lung mechanics in respiratory distress syndrome (RDS) and BPD. These babies often suffer from pulmonary interstitial edema leading to increased accumulation of fluid in the alveoli. In these babies, fluid restriction is also helpful.

Chest Physiotherapy

Chest physiotherapy with percussion and vibration may prevent atelectasis and facilitate the removal of secretions and improve pulmonary function before extubation.

Nutritional Support

All neonates should be provided with aggressive nutritional support which also helps in better long-term neurological outcome.

Developmentally Supportive Care

Mechanically ventilated neonates placed in a sideline position and wrapped with a mother scented cloth had significantly lower distress, pain, and higher SpO_2 values. These techniques might help in early extubation by improving oxygenation, but more studies are required.

The commonly followed protocol for extubation is to initially decrease the FiO_2 to 30% while maintaining the saturation between 91 and 95%. Based on the PCO_2, reduce the tidal volume and rate. With improving oxygenation, positive end expiratory pressure (PEEP) is decreased and caffeine is loaded 20 mg/kg salt especially in very low birth weight preterm neonates and all sedatives are discontinued before weaning. The neonate may be placed on CPAP for 3–10 minutes and if there is no increased work of breathing, desaturation, or bradycardia, the neonate is extubated to NIPPV or nasal CPAP.

CONCLUSION

Weaning and extubation in neonates require a careful balance between minimizing ventilator-associated complications and ensuring adequate respiratory support. Successful extubation depends on appropriate selection of weaning strategies tailored to the ventilation mode, vigilant assessment of extubation readiness using clinical and physiological tools, and adherence to structured checklists. Preventive strategies—including continuous distending pressure, caffeine therapy, cautious use of steroids, optimized nutrition, physiotherapy, and developmentally supportive care—play a pivotal role in reducing extubation failure. Ultimately, individualized, evidence-based approaches supported by quality improvement initiatives are essential to enhance extubation success, reduce morbidity, and improve both short- and long-term outcomes in critically ill neonates.

SUGGESTED READING

1. Fu M, Hu Z, Yu G, Luo Y, Xiong X, Yang Q, et al. Predictors of extubation failure in newborns: a systematic review and meta-analysis. Ital J Pediatr. 2023;49(1): 133.
2. Gizzi C, Moretti C, Agostino R. Weaning from mechanical ventilation. J Matern Fetal Neonatal Med. 2011;24(Suppl)1:61-3.
3. Sangsari R, Saeedi M, Maddah M, Mirnia K, Goldsmith JP. Weaning and extubation from neonatal mechanical ventilation: an evidenced-based review. BMC Pulm Med. 2022;22(1):421.
4. Shalish W, Sant'Anna GM. Optimal timing of extubation in preterm infants. Semin Fetal Neonatal Med. 2023;28(5):101489.

SECTION

Volume-targeted Ventilation

CHAPTER

Volume-targeted Ventilation

Sindhu Sivanandan

INTRODUCTION

Pressure-controlled ventilation (PCV) was the most commonly used mode of ventilation in the past era due to the ease of use, lack of ventilators with microprocessor technology, and ability to cope with leaks around uncuffed endotracheal tubes (ETT). In PCV mode, pressure is the primary control variable, and tidal volume (VT) is the dependent variable, which changes depending on lung mechanics and the patient's spontaneous efforts. In volume-controlled ventilation (VCV), VT is the primary control variable, and the pressure varies depending on the resistive and elastic forces of the lungs.

LIMITATIONS OF PRESSURE-CONTROLLED VENTILATION MODE OF VENTILATION

The disadvantage of PCV is the risk of volutrauma as VT delivery may be excessive when lung compliance improves, resulting in hypocapnia, bronchopulmonary dysplasia (BPD), and air leaks.

LIMITATIONS OF VOLUME-CONTROLLED VENTILATION MODE OF VENTILATION

The disadvantage with VCV in neonates is that a set VT is delivered into the ventilator end of the circuit, and loss of this volume due to compression of gas within the circuit and humidifier, distention of the compliant circuit, and leak around the ETT is not accounted. So, the actual VT that gets into the neonate's lungs may be half of the set VT, necessitating the user to monitor the exhaled VT to adjust the set VT frequently.

HYBRID MODES

Volume-targeted ventilation (VTV) is a hybrid mode that combines the advantages of PCV and VCV modalities by automatically adjusting inflation pressure to maintain a target VT. It is also called the volume guarantee (VG) or volume-targeted pressure-limited ventilation. In this mode, the microprocessor compares the exhaled VT of the previous breath to the desired target and adjusts the working pressure up or down to achieve the target VT. As lung compliance improves, the inflation pressure autoweans in real-time compared to manual reduction in response to blood gas measurement. A systematic review of 20 randomized controlled trials showed that VTV mode had the advantage of reduced rates of death or BPD, pneumothorax, hypocarbia, severe forms of brain injury such as severe intraventricular hemorrhage and periventricular leukomalacia and reduced duration of mechanical ventilation compared to PCV mode.

ALGORITHM OF VOLUME-TARGETED VENTILATION

The clinician chooses a target VT and a pressure limit (Pmax) up to which the device can adjust the peak inspiratory pressure (PIP). The pressure required to deliver the VT is the working pressure or measured PIP. The microprocessor then compares the exhaled VT of the previous inflation and adjusts the working pressure up or down to try to achieve the set VT. A functioning flow sensor is essential in this mode, and exhaled VT is used, because it is a better estimate of the actual VT that entered the lungs. However, when the ETT leak exceeds 40%, VTV mode does not work well. There are several safety features, as noted further. The pressure increment from one cycle to the next is limited to avoid dramatic fluctuations, and several cycles are needed to reach the target VT. The pressure adjustment is made from one inflation to the next and is not based on averaging several cycles. The device also has a separate control algorithm for patient- and machine-triggered breaths. If the inspired VT exceeds 130% of the target (for example, 6.5 mL for a set target of 5 mL), the microprocessor terminates the inflation. The measured VT fluctuates around the target VT due to the variable contribution of the patient's spontaneous breathing. If a complete ETT obstruction is noted (due to secretions or kinking), the working pressure drops to about half its original value. This is a precaution against the risk of overshooting if the obstruction is temporary and gets relieved rapidly.

INDICATIONS AND CONTRAINDICATIONS

Volume-targeted ventilation, being a lung-friendly mode, should be employed as soon as possible. Situations include respiratory distress syndrome, evolving and established BPD, meconium aspiration syndrome, pneumonia, congenital diaphragmatic hernia, and ventilation for other reasons with a normal lung. There are no contraindications except when the ETT leak is >40% unless the ventilator has an adequate leak compensation. A better option would be to reintubate with an ETT of an appropriate size to reduce the leak. Similarly, care should be taken when using VTV during surfactant administration as a complete ETT block by surfactant may result in a dramatic drop in working pressure. However, postinstillation, VTV mode helps the pressure to autowean as lung compliance improves.

SETTING THE VOLUME-TARGETED VENTILATION MODE

The initial setting and further adjustment when using VTV mode are illustrated in **Flowchart 1**. Choosing the appropriate VT is the first step, and similar to the saying, one size does not fit all; the choice depends on the infant's size, postnatal age, and underlying lung disease. Generally, extremely small infants (<1,000 grams birth weight) require a slightly larger VT/kg (5 mL/kg) due to the proportionally larger fixed dead space of the flow sensor in addition to the ETT compared to late preterm and term infants (4 mL/kg). Those with lung disease characterized by increased alveolar dead space [e.g., meconium aspiration syndrome (MAS; 5–5.5 mL/g) and BPD (5–7 mL/kg or more)] also require relatively larger VT.

ALARMS AND TROUBLESHOOTING

Volume-targeted ventilation mode generates more alarms than PCV mode. These alarms indicate changes in the ventilation, such as worsening lung compliance, decreased spontaneous respiratory effort, impending

Flowchart 1: Initiation, adjustment, and weaning of volume-targeted ventilation.

Initial settings

Mode: Assist control or pressure support ventilation + volume target
Select VT (4–5 mL/kg) based on neonate's age, size, and disease process
Pmax: 3–5 cm H_2O above expected PIP need
Set other parameters: Rate, inspiratory time, PEEP, and FiO_2
- Ensure that flow sensor is calibrated and functioning properly
- Check ET position and leak percentage

Adjustments

- Monitor chest rise, air entry, SpO_2, and obtain blood gas
- Adjust VT in steps of 0.5 mL/kg to ensure chest rise and acceptable blood gas. Do not wean <4 mL/kg
- Consider both pH and $PaCO_2$; accept higher PCO_2 if pH is OK
- Record both working PIP and Pmax
- Pmax should be kept 3–5 cm above upper end of working PIP
- Assess patient's respiratory rate, comfort, oxygen requirement and working pressure, not just blood gas. Increase VT if necessary to achieve adequate support

Weaning

- Maintain pH < 7.35 to ensure respiratory drive and automatic weaning
- Do not lower target VT below 4 mL/kg
- As PIP decreases, increase PEEP to maintain distending pressure
- Avoid using SIMV without PS during weaning
- Do not wean backup rate on PC-AC or PC PSV

Consider extubation when the disease process improves, baby has good spontaneous drive, working pressure is reasonable (12–16) to deliver the target VT and FiO_2 requirement is less than 30%

(AC: assist control; FiO_2: fraction of inspired oxygen; $PaCO_2$: partial pressure of arterial carbon dioxide; PC: pressure-controlled; PCO_2: partial pressure of carbon dioxide; PIP: peak inspiratory pressure; PEEP: positive end-expiratory pressure; PSV: pressure support ventilation; SIMV: synchronized intermittent mandatory ventilation; VT: tidal volume) accidental extubation, ETT obstruction, and forced exhalation episodes. However, unnecessary alarms can be avoided by optimizing settings and alarm limits, such as the use of longer alarm delay settings, appropriate pressure limit settings, correction of ET leak, appropriate ET position, and adequate physical comfort measures.

A common alarm encountered is "low VT," which indicates that the device cannot reach the VT target at the set PIP limit. The actions include the following:

- The PIP limit may need to be increased.
- Check if ETT is impinging on the carina or selectively at the right main bronchus.
- Check for ET block and kink
- Worsening lung compliance
- Check if the ET leak exceeds 40%
- Rule out pneumothorax.

CONCLUSION

Volume-targeted ventilation (VTV) represents a significant advancement in neonatal respiratory support, combining the benefits of both pressure- and volume-controlled modes. By automatically adjusting inspiratory pressure to achieve consistent tidal volumes, VTV minimizes risks of volutrauma, hypocarbia, and severe brain injury while reducing the duration of ventilation. Its application across a wide range of neonatal respiratory conditions underscores its versatility and lung-protective potential. Careful attention to initial settings, monitoring of exhaled volumes, and appropriate troubleshooting of alarms are essential to maximize its effectiveness and safety. Thus, VTV should be considered the preferred mode of ventilation in neonates whenever feasible.

SUGGESTED READING

1. Keszler M, Abubakar MK. Volume-targeted ventilation. Semin Perinatol. 2024;48(2):151886.
2. Keszler M. Volume-targeted ventilation. Early Hum Dev. 2006;82(12):811-8.
3. Klingenberg C, Wheeler KI, McCallion N, Morley CJ, Davis PG. Volume-targeted versus pressure-limited ventilation in neonates. Cochrane Database Syst Rev. 2017;10(10):CD003666.
4. Sant'Anna GM, Keszler M. Developing a neonatal unit ventilation protocol for the preterm baby. Early Hum Dev. 2012;88(12):925-9.
5. van Kaam AH. Optimal Strategies of Mechanical Ventilation: Can We Avoid or Reduce Lung Injury? Neonatology. 2024;121(5):570-5.

SECTION

High-frequency Ventilation

CHAPTER

High-frequency Ventilation

Tapas Bandyopadhyay

INTRODUCTION

Despite significant technological advancement in ventilation devices as well as neonatal respiratory care management, bronchopulmonary dysplasia (BPD) remains the most prevalent chronic respiratory morbidity among very preterm neonates. The main pathophysiological mechanism behind BPD is ventilator-induced lung injury (VILI).

High-frequency ventilation (HFV) is a form of assisted ventilation that uses small tidal volumes (less than anatomic dead space) and very rapid ventilator rates (2.5–25 Hz or 150–1,500 cycles per minute).

As compared to conventional mechanical ventilation (CMV), HFV uses lower peak airway pressures; oxygenation and ventilation are independently handled in the recruited lung, and the preservation of normal lung architecture even when using high mean airway pressures (MAPs).

PHYSIOLOGY

The physiology responsible for gas transport during involves several contributing mechanisms, which are briefly reviewed as shown in **Figure 1**.

- *Bulk convection:* Even with small tidal volumes, gas flow may reach proximal alveoli and participate in direct alveolar ventilation.
- *Pendelluft:* At high frequencies, gas distribution is influenced by inequalities in time-constant, and there is redistribution from units with lower to units with higher time constant.
- *Asymmetric velocity profiles:* Inspiratory gas tends to pass along the center of the airway, while expiratory gas escapes along the outer wall.
- *Taylor dispersion:* Superimposition of convective gas flow into diffusive process leads to an increased diffusion of the high-velocity central gases to the margins of the airway.
- *Molecular diffusion:* As in physiological mechanism, there is movement of molecules from higher concentration to lower concentration.

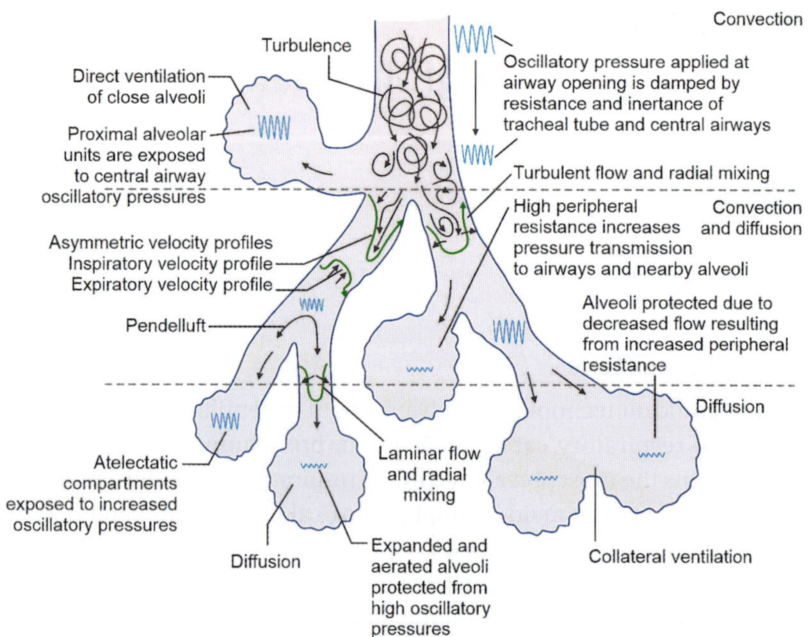

Fig. 1: Gas exchange mechanism in high-frequency ventilation.

Source: Adapted from Slutsky S, Drazen JM. Ventilation with small tidal volumes. N Engl J Med. 2002;347:630-1.

BASIC CONCEPTS

Factors Influencing Oxygenation and Ventilation

Oxygenation

The two most important players of oxygenation are MAP and fraction of inspired oxygen (FiO_2). Since, the lack of alveolar recruitment is the major pathophysiology behind neonatal lung disease. Hence, providing a higher MAP improves the recruitment and reduces ventilation-perfusion mismatching.

Achieving an optimal MAP is important as higher MAP can cause hyperinflation, which restricts venous return, and compromises cardiac output. Additionally, a higher airway pressures exert compressive forces against the capillaries within the alveolar wall and may also increase pulmonary vascular resistance and impede pulmonary blood flow and consequently impairs oxygenation. On the other hand, a low MAP leads to hypoventilation, worsening ventilation/perfusion mismatch and impairs oxygenation.

As compared to the CMV, in high-frequency oscillatory ventilation (HFOV) the pressure at the proximal airway opening is considerably higher

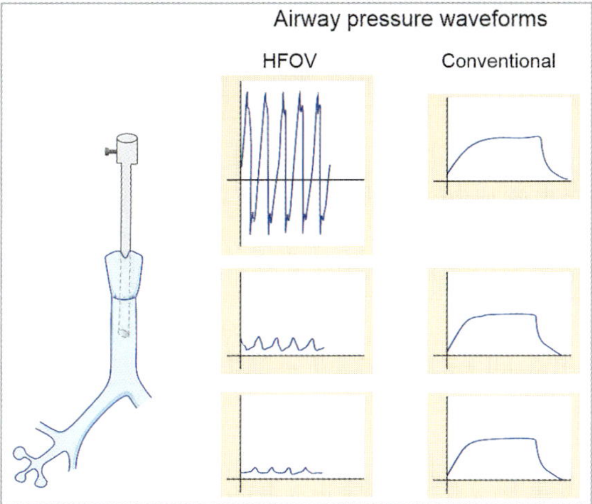

Fig. 2: Comparison of proximal airway pressure transmission to distal alveolar units in conventional mechanical ventilation (CMV) as compared to high-frequency oscillatory ventilation (HFOV).

but significantly decreases till it reaches the distal alveolar unit as shown in **Figure 2**. Additionally, the transmission or attenuation of proximal airway pressure is also not uniform across different areas of the lung and depends on their physical location in the respiratory system and the disease state. Due to the lack of transmission of uniform pressure or volume to the different segments of the lungs it becomes difficult to determine the pressure-volume curves as is the case in CMV, a crude way to assess adequate lung inflation is with the help of chest radiographs to look for lung expansion.

Ventilation

The two most important players of oxygenation are amplitude (most important) and frequency.

In CMV alveolar ventilation (CO_2 elimination) is a linear function of ventilator rate (f) and tidal volume (Vt). However, in HFOV, it is largely dependent on tidal volume (Vt) as compared to frequency (f) as given in the following formula:

$$\text{Alveolar ventilation in CMV} = f \times Vt$$
$$\text{Alveolar ventilation in HFOV} = f \times Vt^2$$

This said difference is due to the fact that during HFOV, Vt is determined by the stroke volume the ventilator applies to the system which is represented by the area under the volume-time curve as demonstrated in the **Figure 3**.

Amplitude: It is the most important parameter to control ventilation in HFV. It represents the "force" with which the piston moves and is measured in "cmH_2O". While setting the amplitude it is important to initially achieve

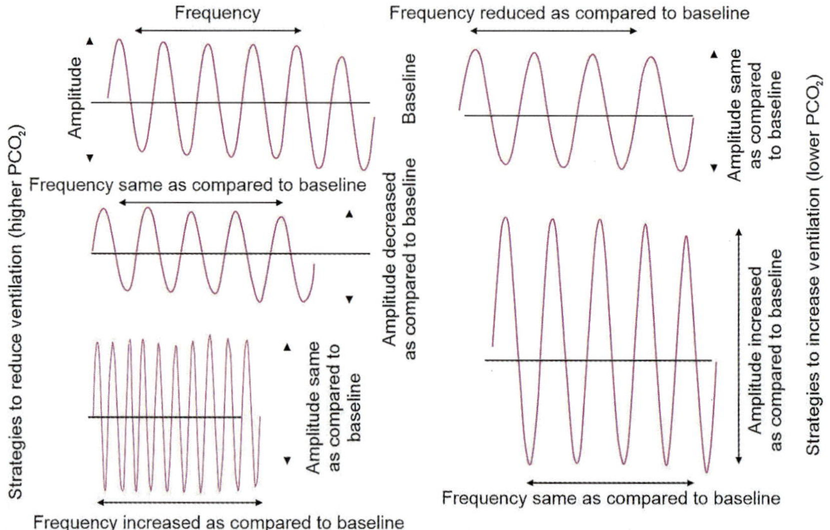

Fig. 3: Volume time curves in high-frequency ventilation (HFV) showing the effect on partial pressure of carbon dioxide (PCO_2) due to changes in the amplitude and frequency.

adequate lung recruitment by optimizing the MAP. The best way to assess adequacy of the amplitude is by visualizing the chest wiggle which should not cross the umbilicus. A rough estimate for setting the initial amplitude is twice the MAP. Any further changes in amplitude will, thereafter, depend on the extent of visualization of wiggles and partial pressure of arterial carbon dioxide ($PaCO_2$) values.

Frequency: The frequency controls the time allowed for the piston to move. The lower the frequency is set, the greater the volume displacement by piston is achieved, and hence, greater removal of CO_2 [low partial pressure of carbon dioxide (PCO_2)] and vice versa.

The most important aspect in setting the optimal frequency is the time constant (compliance X resistance). In general, patients with short time constants [e.g., respiratory distress syndrome (RDS)] can be ventilated effectively at higher frequencies than those with longer time constants [e.g., meconium aspiration syndrome (MAS) and BPD].

The control parameters of HFV, their typical range, target values, changes produced in blood gas values due to their manipulations, and side effects, are depicted in **Table 1**.

INDICATIONS OF HIGH-FREQUENCY VENTILATION

The various indications for using HFV in neonatal disease conditions are shown in **Table 2**.

TABLE 1: HFV control parameters, typical range, target values, changes in blood gas values due to their alteration, and side effects.

Control parameter	*Typical range*	*Target*	*Changes in blood gas values*	*Side effects*
Mean airway pressure (MAP)	10–25 cmH_2O	• Adequate lung recruitment as seen by the reduction in FiO_2 requirement • Adequate lung inflation on chest X-ray till 8–10 posterior ribs	• Increase: ↑PaO_2 • Decrease: ↓PaO_2	• Too high: Decreases cardiac output, barotrauma • Too low: De-recruitment
Fraction of inspired oxygen (FiO_2)	21–100%	SpO_2 between 90 and 95%	• Increase: ↑PaO_2 • Decrease: ↓PaO_2	$FiO_2 > 0.6–0.7$ increases the risk of oxytrauma
Amplitude	15–100%	$PaCO_2$ in target range of 45–55 mm Hg	• Increase: ↓$PaCO_2$ • Decrease: ↑$PaCO_2$	• High: Hypocarbia • Low: Hypercarbia
Frequency	5–15	Same as above	• Increase: ↑$PaCO_2$ • Decrease I:E: ↓$PaCO_2$	Changes have modest effect on gas exchange
Inspiratory time or I:E	1:1–1:3	Same as above	↑PaO_2	

(HFV: high-frequency ventilation; I:E: inspiratory to expiratory ratio; $PaCO_2$: partial pressure of arterial carbon dioxide; PaO_2: partial pressure of arterial oxygen; SpO_2: oxygen saturation)

TABLE 2: Indications of high-frequency ventilation in neonates.

Established	*Other*
• Air leak • Severe respiratory failure refractory to conventional ventilation [high PIP (22–24 in PT, 25–28 in term)] • Pulmonary hypoplasia • Adjunct to iNO	• Persistent pulmonary hypertension • Meconium aspiration syndrome • Congenital diaphragmatic hernia

(iNO: inhaled nitric oxide; PIP: peak inspiratory pressure)

MODES OF HIGH-FREQUENCY VENTILATION

Based on exhalation characteristics (active/passive/hybrid) and source of generation, high-frequency ventilation has been classified into three categories as shown in **Table 3**:

1. HFOV
2. High-frequency jet ventilation
3. High-frequency flow interrupter

TABLE 3: Types of high-frequency ventilation devices available and their characteristics.

Variables	*HFOV*	*HFJV*	*HFFI*
High-frequency pulses generated by	Piston or other means	Pinch valve, injector cannula	Solenoid valve
Tidal volume	< dead space	> or < dead space	> or < dead space
Frequency	5–15 Hz	5–10 Hz	8–12 Hz
Expiration	Active	Passive	Passive
I:E	1:1 or 1:2	1:4 to 1:8	1:3 to 1:6
Ability to superimpose a sigh	No (SensorMedics) Yes (Draeger)	Yes	Yes
Entrainment	None	Possible	None
Waveform	Sine	Triangular	Triangular

(HFFI: high-frequency flow interrupter; HFJV: high-frequency jet ventilation; HFOV: high-frequency oscillatory ventilation; I:E: inspiratory to expiratory ratio)

OPTIMIZING MEAN AIRWAY PRESSURE IN HIGH-FREQUENCY VENTILATION IN DIFFERENT PULMONARY CONDITIONS

Setting Mean Airway Pressure

High-volume Open Lung Strategy

This strategy is used during ventilation of lungs with low compliance (e.g., RDS and atelectatic form of MAS). This is based on the principle of open lung strategy which encompasses lung volume recruitment and avoidance of volutrauma. In this method, lung volume optimization is done by inflating the lung to near-maximum volume with stepwise increases in MAP. The lung is considered fully inflated when FiO_2 can be weaned to under 0.40 or when FiO_2 starts to increase to maintain target SpO_2. It is then deflated to the closing volume that is manifested by again an increase in FiO_2. The lung is then reinflated to a point just above closing volume as depicted in **Flowchart 1**. This technique allows ventilation to move from the inspiratory limb of the P-V curve to the expiratory limb, allowing effective ventilation and oxygenation at lower airway pressures.

Low-volume Lung Strategy

This strategy is used during ventilation of lungs with air leaks, pulmonary hypoplasia, and nonhomogenous lung disease to minimize the risk of further lung injury whereas maintaining optimum lung ventilation. In this strategy, the set MAP should be same as that on conventional ventilation. Other principle used in this strategy includes a lower frequency, permissive hypercapnia, and higher FiO_2.

Flowchart 1: Recruitment maneuver in HFV in low compliance disease states.

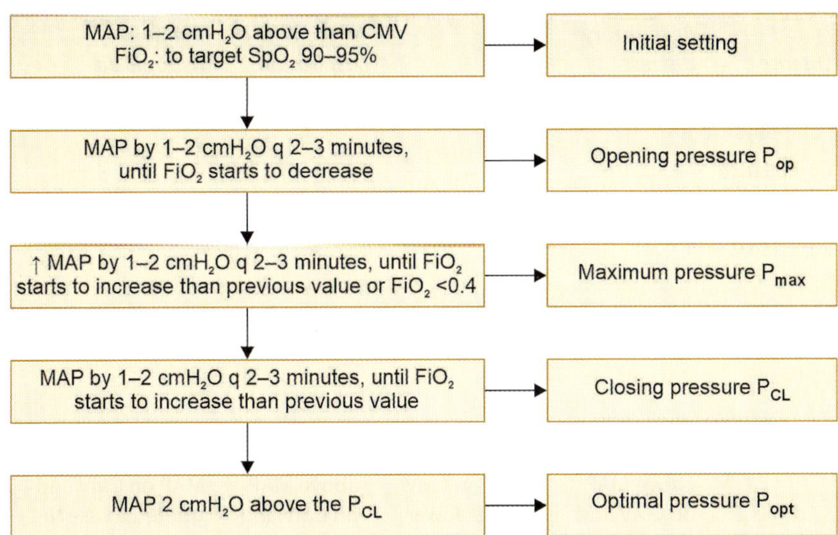

(CMV: conventional mechanical ventilation; FiO_2: fraction of inspired oxygen; HFV: high-frequency ventilation; MAP: mean airway pressure; SpO_2: oxygen saturation)
Source: De Jaegere A, van Veenendaal MB, Michiels A, van Kaam AH. Lung recruitment using oxygenation during open lung high-frequency ventilation in preterm infants. Am J Respir Crit Care Med. 2006;174(6):639-45.

DISEASE SPECIFIC VENTILATION SETTINGS

The pathophysiology, initial ventilation setting, and titration is as shown in **Table 4**.

OPTIMIZATION OF INITIAL VENTILATION SETTINGS

The target for optimal ventilation is decided based on the clinical and radiological assessment coupled with the blood gas parameters as shown in **Tables 5 and 6**.

Subsequent monitoring should be done based on clinical assessment, any change in ventilatory parameters

GUIDE FOR ADJUSTMENT OF VENTILATOR SETTINGS TARGETING BLOOD GAS PARAMETER

Adjustment of HFV settings based on blood gas values is given in **Table 6**.

SUPPORTIVE CARE

The supportive care of neonate on HFV is summarized in **Box 1**.

TABLE 4: High-frequency ventilation settings for different disease conditions.

Disease condition	*Respiratory distress syndrome*	*Air leak*	*Meconium aspiration syndrome*	*Pulmonary hypoplasia (e.g., CDH)*
Pathophysiology				
Compliance	↓	↓	↓	↓
Resistance	N/↑	N/↑	↑↑	N
Functional residual capacity	↓	N	↑	↓
Time constant	↓	N/↓	↑	↓
Initial settings and titration				
MAP	2 cmH_2O above MAP on CMV and titrated based on high volume open lung strategy	Same as that of MAP on CMV. Stay at lower MAP, accept higher FiO_2. May consider volume targeting with target tidal volume of 1.5–2 mL/kg.	2 cmH_2O above MAP on CMV and titrated based on high volume open lung strategy (atelectatic form) For hyperinflation type low volume lung strategy may be employed	2 cmH_2O above MAP on CMV and titrated to use the lowest MAP that will achieve adequate lung inflation by the appearance of the lung fields, heart size, and diaphragms, not just the rib count to avoid MAP that worsens pulmonary hypertension
FiO_2	Titrated to achieve target saturation	Titrated to achieve target saturation	Titrated to achieve target saturation	Titrated to achieve target saturation
Frequency	10–15 Hz	5–8 Hz	6–8 Hz	8–10 Hz
Amplitude	Set at twice the set MAP (or 20–25 cmH_2O). Adjust in increment of 2–5 to achieve adequate chest wall movement or "wiggle"	Set at twice the set MAP (or 20–25 cmH_2O). Adjust to achieve adequate chest wall movement or "wiggle". However, permissive hypercapnia is desired	Set at twice the set MAP (or 20–25 cmH_2O). Adjust in increment of 2–5 to achieve adequate chest wall movement or "wiggle"	Set at twice the set MAP (or 20–25 cmH_2O). Adjust to achieve adequate chest wall movement or "wiggle". However, permissive hypercapnia is desired

Contd...

Contd...

Disease condition	*Respiratory distress syndrome*	*Air leak*	*Meconium aspiration syndrome*	*Pulmonary hypoplasia (e.g., CDH)*
I:E	1:2	1:2 or 1:3	1:2	1:2
Chest X-ray	8–9 posterior rib inflation above diaphragm	6–8 posterior rib inflation above diaphragm	Atelectatic form: 8–9 posterior rib inflation above diaphragm Hyperinflation form: 6–8 posterior rib inflation above diaphragm	8–9 posterior rib inflation above diaphragm of the contralateral lung

(CDH: congenital diaphragmatic hernia; CMV: conventional mechanical ventilation; FiO_2: fraction of inspired oxygen; I:E: inspiratory to expiratory ratio; MAP: mean airway pressure)

TABLE 5: Target for initial HFV settings based on clinical assessment, radiological evaluation, and blood gas parameters.

Clinical (most important)		*Blood gas*	*Radiological*
• Baby should be breathing comfortably • Chest wall wiggle or movement should not cross the umbilicus • Absent or minimal retractions	• *Color:* Pink, capillary filling time: <3 seconds, normal blood pressure, adequate urine output • *Saturation:* 90–95%	• pH: 7.35–7.45 • PCO_2: 45–55 mm Hg • PO_2: 50–80 mm Hg • BE: ±5 • Bicarb: 20–24 mEq/L	• ET tube should be at the level of T2–T4 vertebrae • *Lung inflation:* – High volume open lung strategy: 8–9 posterior rib inflation above diaphragm – Low volume lung strategy: 6–8 posterior rib inflation above diaphragm • May require serial chest radiograph for optimization of setting

(ET: endotracheal; HFV: high-frequency ventilation; PCO_2: partial pressure of carbon dioxide)

TABLE 6: Adjustment of HFV settings based on blood gas values.

High $PaCO_2$	• Review patient and assess chest "wiggle", DCO_2, clinical events and last CXR (lung inflation) • Is the ET tube patent and correctly positioned? • Consider in-line ET suction • Consider increasing VThf • Consider adding volume target if not already in use • Reassess in 20–30 minutes with repeat blood gas and consider a repeat CXR • If not improving, despite open lung and ET tube patency, consider a change in frequency
Low $PaCO_2$	• Review patient and assess "wiggle" • Consider reducing VThf • Consider addition of volume target if not already being used • Review overall ventilation strategy and readiness for weaning based on PaO_2 and clinical status
Low PaO_2	• Increase FiO_2 • Review lung inflation and circulatory status • Consider increasing MAP by 1–2 cmH_2O • Consider a recruitment maneuver if loss of volume is likely, e.g., postsuction • Consider CXR to review lung inflation; if over expanded reducing MAP may improve PaO_2 • Consider factors associated with pulmonary hypertension as well as need for adjuncts such as surfactant and nitric oxide • Consider the possibility that the MAP is excessive, leading to impairment of pulmonary blood flow
High PaO_2	• Decrease FiO_2 till <0.4 for high volume lung strategy followed by MAP by 1–2 • For low volume lung strategy reduce MAP by 1–2 cmH_2O followed by FiO_2

(CXR: chest X-ray; DCO_2: diffusion coefficient of carbon dioxide; ET: endotracheal; HFV: high-frequency ventilation; MAP: mean airway pressure; $PaCO_2$: partial pressure of arterial carbon dioxide; PaO_2: partial pressure of arterial oxygen; VThf: high-frequency expired tidal volume)

WEANING AND EXTUBATION

Weaning can be considered once the FiO_2 is <0.4 and baby remains stable for at least 6–8 hours on same settings. Each change should be made gradual with careful attention to the clinical parameters, i.e., heart rate, SpO_2, and blood pressure (BP). Routine blood gas may be avoided but can be considered if there is clinical deterioration.

MAP: It may be weaned in steps of 1 cmH_2O every 4–6 hours decided based on SpO_2.

BOX 1: Supportive care in neonates on high-frequency ventilation (HFV).

Humidification of inspiratory gases: Warmed to 37°C and fully saturated [100% relative humidity (RH) or 44 mg/L of vapor] when they reach the airway

Endotracheal suctioning:
- Strict asepsis with stepwise protocol
- Suctioning should be done only if there are visible secretions/desaturations and/or decreased breath sounds
- Routine normal saline irrigation prior to the suctioning should not be done

Prevention of ventilator associated pneumonia:
- Elevation of head end of bed to 30°
- Strict asepsis during handling and performing procedure
- Avoid breaking into respiratory circuit
- Oral suction must follow and not precede endotracheal (ET) suction or else separate ET and oral suctioning tubing
- Sterile water in humidification systems
- Periodic drainage of condensate from breathing circuits
- The tubing should remain in dependent position as compared to the ET adapter
- Daily assessment for extubation readiness

Positioning and physiotherapy:
- Change position every 6–8 hours
- Physiotherapy has a therapeutic role in presence of chest X-ray consistent with collapse
- Should not be done in very preterm infants during the first week of life

Follow-up:
- Neuroimaging
- Retinopathy of prematurity (ROP) screening as indicated
- Hearing assessment
- Neurodevelopmental assessment

Amplitude: If volume targeting is being used, the amplitude will "autowean". However, in the absence of volume targeting amplitude may be weaned in steps of 1–2 cmH_2O every 4–6 hours guided by DCO_2.

Frequency: Kept same

Babies can be successfully weaned to conventional ventilation or extubated from HFOV.

Typical settings for extubation are:
- MAP: 9–10 cmH_2O
- FiO_2: <0.4
- Amplitude: 15–20 cmH_2O

Periextubation care:
- Feeding is stopped 3–4 hours prior to the extubation
- In babies <1.5 kg, loading dose of caffeine is used to improve the respiratory drive

Flowchart 2: Algorithm for acute deterioration of a baby on high-frequency ventilator.

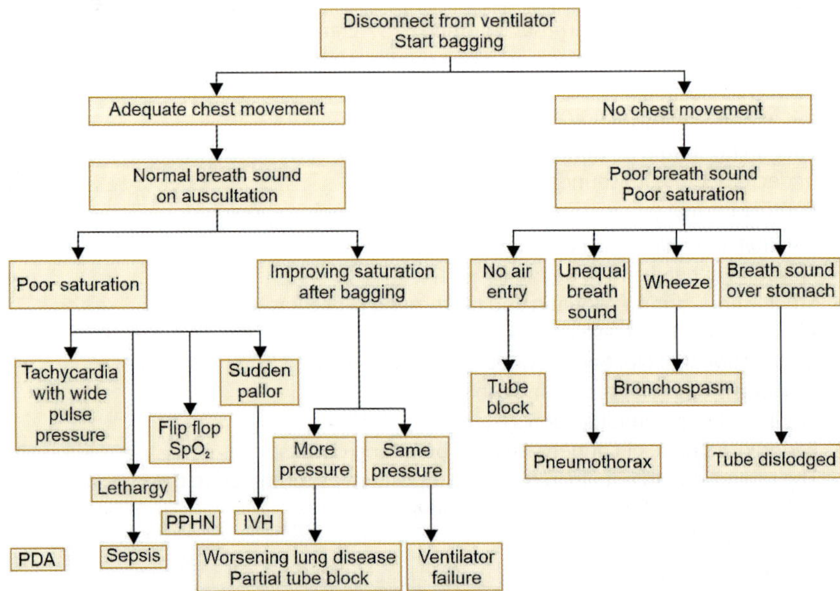

(IVH: intraventricular hemorrhage; PDA: patent ductus arteriosus; PPHN: pulmonary hypertension of the newborn; SpO_2: oxygen saturation)

Postextubation care:

- Humidification, nebulization, and frequent position change should be done.
- Meticulous monitoring for respiratory distress and vitals should be done

PRINCIPLES OF SUPPORTIVE CARE AND BEDSIDE BEST PRACTICES FOR VENTILATED BABY

Principles of supportive care are presented in **Box 1**.

ACUTE DETERIORATION OF A BABY ON VENTILATOR

Acute deterioration of a baby on high-frequency ventilator is depicted in **Flowchart 2**.

CONCLUSION

High-frequency ventilation (HFV) represents an important advancement in neonatal respiratory support, offering an effective alternative to conventional mechanical ventilation (CMV) in selected conditions. By delivering very small tidal volumes at rapid frequencies, HFV reduces ventilator-induced lung injury while maintaining optimal gas exchange. Its utility lies in the ability to independently control oxygenation through mean airway pressure (MAP) and FiO_2, and ventilation primarily through amplitude and frequency adjustments. The open lung and low-volume strategies allow tailoring of ventilation according to disease pathophysiology, thereby optimizing lung recruitment while minimizing barotrauma and volutrauma.

Clinical application of HFV is especially beneficial in severe respiratory failure, air-leak syndromes, pulmonary hypoplasia, and conditions refractory to CMV. Successful use requires meticulous attention to ventilator settings, radiographic and blood gas monitoring, and integration of supportive care measures to reduce complications. With careful weaning protocols and structured peri extubation care, HFV can facilitate better outcomes and reduce long-term morbidity such as bronchopulmonary dysplasia. Overall, HFV is a powerful modality in neonatal intensive care that, when judiciously applied, significantly enhances the safety and efficacy of respiratory management in critically ill neonates.

SUGGESTED READING

1. Ackermann BW, Klotz D, Hentschel R, Thome UH, van Kaam AH. High-frequency ventilation in preterm infants and neonates. Pediatr Res. 2023;93(7):1810-8.
2. Keszler M, Suresh GK. Goldsmith's Assisted Ventilation of the Neonate: An Evidence-based Approach to Newborn Respiratory Care, 7th edition. Philadelphia, PA: Elsevier; 2022.
3. Rajiv PK, Vidyasagar D, Satyan L. Essentials of Neonatal Ventilation, 1st edition. Gurugram, India: Elsevier; 2019.
4. Sánchez-Luna M, González-Pacheco N, Santos-González M, Tendillo-Cortijo F. High-frequency Ventilation. Clin Perinatol. 2021;48(4):855-68.

SECTION

Persistent Pulmonary Hypertension of Newborns and Inhaled Nitric Oxide Treatment

CHAPTER

Persistent Pulmonary Hypertension of Newborns and Inhaled Nitric Oxide Treatment

Kiran More

INTRODUCTION

Persistent pulmonary hypertension of the newborn (PPHN) which is also called persistent fetal circulation (PFC), occurs due to failure of the lung circulation to achieve or sustain the normal drop in pulmonary vascular resistance (PVR) at birth. Severe hypoxic respiratory failure (HRF) is the result of the pulmonary to systemic shunting of deoxygenated blood caused by this state of chronic elevated PVR. PPHN affects 0.2% of all live births and is a significant contributor to the mortality and morbidity (5–10%) in term and near-term infants.

Abnormally constricted pulmonary vasculature due to parenchymal diseases (maladaptation), hypoplastic pulmonary vasculature (under-development), or normal parenchyma with remodeled pulmonary vasculature (maldevelopment), are the most common etiopathological causes of PPHN **(Table 1)**. Abnormal ventilation perfusion mismatches can also cause pulmonary hypertension (PH) in newborns. These mismatches can be caused by excessive blood flow in certain situations, such as congenital heart defects with left-to-right shunting, or by pulmonary venous hypertension, such as congenital heart disease (CHD) with left arterial hypertension and mitral or aortic valve disease. Differentiating between these etiologies is crucial since management may change as pulmonary vasodilators are used effectively in the former conditions, however, should be avoided in the latter.

The PPHN causes pulmonary to systemic shunting, right ventricular (RV) dilatation and failure, decreased oxygenation, and increasing metabolic acidosis, all of which exacerbate PVR and feed the vicious cycle. The causes are comparable in premature infants, whose pulmonary vasculature is either maladapted, maldeveloped, or undeveloped. PH is typically caused by pulmonary vascular immaturity.

Neonatologist performed echocardiography (NPE) or bedside/point of care functional echocardiography (fECHO) is an important tool for ruling out structural heart disease, confirming the diagnosis and grading of PPHN, objective selection of specific therapies, and titrating and monitoring response to treatment strategies. Management of PPHN is challenging

TABLE 1: Etiologies of persistent pulmonary hypertension of the newborn (PPHN)/ pulmonary hypertension (PH).

A. PH with increased pulmonary vascular resistance (PVR)	
• Maladaptation of pulmonary vasculature (abnormal, "reactive" pulmonary vasoconstriction)	• Parenchymal lung diseases-meconium aspiration syndrome (MAS), respiratory distress syndrome (RDS), hypoventilation, and pneumonia • In response to certain stimuli, such as hypothermia, sepsis, stress, hypercapnia, hypoxemia, acidosis, and hyperviscosity • Exposure to maternal medications [maternal selective serotonin reuptake inhibitor (SSRI) use]
• Maldevelopment of pulmonary vasculature (remodeling of pulmonary vasculature)	• In utero closure of ductus arteriosus (e.g., maternal cyclooxygenase inhibitor use) • Pulmonary hyperperfusion in congenital heart disease with large left-to-right shunt • Infants with fetal growth restriction
• Underdevelopment of pulmonary vasculature (hypoplastic pulmonary vessels; decreased cross-sectional area)	• Congenital diaphragmatic hernia • Pulmonary hypoplasia (premature prolonged rupture of membranes, oligohydramnios, etc.)
B. PH with ventilation perfusion mismatch	
1. Excessive blood flow	• Congenital heart defects with left-to-right shunting, e.g., ventricular septal defect (VSD), atrial septal defect (ASD), patent ductus arteriosus (PDA) etc.
2. Pulmonary venous hypertension	• Congenital heart disease (CHD) with left arterial hypertension, mitral or aortic valve disease

as it is a complex interplay of optimum ventilation strategies, appropriate choice and usage of inotropes, and pulmonary vasodilators based on the phenotypes of presentation. In this chapter, we shall try to address concepts of pathophysiology and management principles of PPHN.

DIAGNOSIS OF PERSISTENT PULMONARY HYPERTENSION OF THE NEWBORN

Suspicion and clinical diagnosis of PPHN can be made based on differential saturation of >5–10% between preductal and postductal values and the presence of clinical lability with desaturation events **(Fig. 1)**. Arterial blood analysis confirms severe hypoxemia by calculating oxygen index (OI) which can classify PPHN into mild (OI < 15), moderate (OI 15–25), and severe (OI 25–40); however, confirmation of diagnosis can be made only on bedside echocardiography.

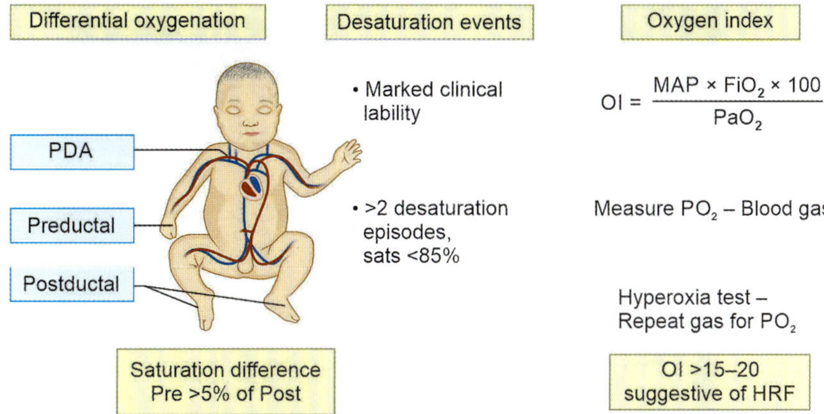

Fig. 1: Clinical diagnosis of PPHN. (FiO_2: fraction of inspired oxygen; HRF: hypoxic respiratory failure; MAP: mean airway pressure; OI: oxygen index; PaO_2: partial pressure of arterial oxygen; PDA: patent ductus arteriosus; PO_2: partial pressure of oxygen; PPHN: persistent pulmonary hypertension of the newborn)
Source: Clark Rh et al. N Engl L Med. 2000.

Table 2 gives a summary of echocardiographic parameters used for the assessment of PH systematically.

MANAGEMENT OF PERSISTENT PULMONARY HYPERTENSION OF THE NEWBORN

Presentation and ventilation strategies for PPHN based on various phenotypes **(Table 1; Figure 2)**:

- *Maladaptation of pulmonary vasculature:* Characterized by an otherwise structurally normal vasculature but marked by exaggerated vasoreactivity often due to asphyxia or sepsis, or associated with parenchymal lung diseases like meconium aspiration syndrome (MAS) or pneumonia. In conditions with normal lung compliance, lung protective strategies to avoid volutrauma will work so less invasive ventilation strategies combined with inhaled nitric oxide (iNO) or gentle cytomegalovirus (CMV) with low to moderate positive end-expiratory pressure (PEEP) helps maintain alveolar recruitment without causing overdistension. This strategy, alongside iNO, can effectively reduce pulmonary arterial pressure by reversing transient pulmonary vasospasm Studies show that achieving optimal oxygenation saturation (SpO_2) targets of 91–95% minimizes oxidative stress without compromising pulmonary circulation.

Conditions with poor lung compliance such as respiratory distress syndrome, MAS, or pneumonia have poor lung compliance so ventilation should aim at adequate lung recruitment. Open lung ventilation strategies with higher PEEPs, higher tidal volumes, or the use of high-frequency

TABLE 2: Echocardiographic assessment of pulmonary hypertension.

No	*ECHO parameter*	*View*	*Image acquisition*	*Comment*	*ECHO image*
Step 1: Rule out congenital heart disease and other potential associated conditions					
1	Situs view	Subcostal	Situs view	Confirmation of situs solitus	
	Great arteries arising from ventricles	• Subcostal • Parasternal short axis (PSAX) view	Visualize great vessels arising from both ventricles and crossing each other	Rule out transposition of great vessels	
	Venous return	Suprasternal/ crab view	Visualize all four veins draining into left atrium	Rule out total anomalous pulmonary venous connection (TAPVC)	
Step 2: Is there persistent pulmonary hypertension of the newborn (PPHN) and how severe it is?					
2	*2.1 Estimation of pulmonary artery pressures*				
	• 2.1.1 Peak TR velocity (TRV) • Pulmonary arterial systolic pressure (PASP)~right ventricular systolic pressure (RVSP)	• Apical four chamber (A4C) • Parasternal long axis (PLAX) (inflow) • PSAX • Subcostal • Modified PSAX and A4C	• Peak TRV measured by CW Doppler across the tricuspid valve • Ensure the CW Doppler to flow angle is correctly aligned	• The angle of insonation should be <20° to achieve a reliable measurement • Even small errors in the absolute measurement of TRV can result in significant changes to the estimate of RVSP	

Contd…

Contd…

No	ECHO parameter	View	Image acquisition	Comment	ECHO image
	RVSP = 4 × (Vmax TR)^2 + RAP (RAP = 3–5 mm Hg)		• Measure from a complete TR envelope. Choose the highest velocity • Eccentric jets can lead to incomplete Doppler envelopes and underestimation of TR velocity • Velocity can be under estimated in severe/free TR and should be stated in the report • A TRV <2.5 m/s is considered normal	Limitation: • Not reliable in presence of right ventricular failure or right ventricular outflow tract obstruction or presence of valvular incompetence • TR cannot always be observed and maybe absent in 15–40% of patients with PPHN	
	2.1.2 Peak pulmonary regurgitation (PR) velocity Mean pulmonary arterial pressure (MPAP) = 4 × (Vmax PR)^2 + RVdP (RVdP; right ventricular diastolic pressure RVdP = 2–5 mm Hg)	• PLAX (outflow) • PSAX • Subcostal	• A CW Doppler measurement through the pulmonary valve in line with the PR jet • The peak (early/beginning of diastole) PR velocity (PRVBD) value is measured • An early PR velocity >2.2 m/s is considered a marker of raised MPAP	• PR cannot always be observed in patients with PPHN • This may have additional value when TRV cannot be used or relied upon • *Limitation:* Not reliable in presence of valvular incompetence	

Contd…

Contd…

No	*ECHO parameter*	*View*	*Image acquisition*	*Comment*	*ECHO image*
	2.1.3 IVS configuration/LV eccentricity index. (LVsEI)	• PSAX • PSAX	• Measure from PSAX view at mid LV level between papillary muscle and tips of mitral valve leaflets. End systole is taken as the frame with the smallest LV cavity; end diastole is measured on the peak of the R-wave • Interpretation based on shape: – O shaped is <50% of LVP – D shaped is 50–100% – Crescent shaped is >100% • *LVsEI:* The ratio of the minor axis dimensions as shown in the image (D2/D1) measured at end systole and end diastole • D1 = left ventricular diameter perpendicular to the septum • D2 = left ventricular diameter parallel to the septum	• LV diastolic EI is more a marker of volume overloaded right ventricle; for clinical conditions such as PPHN, pressure overload predominates, and hence the usefulness of the systolic eccentricity index (EI) • Left ventricular EI >1.1 is considered abnormal. *Limitations:* • Off-axis PSAX images may cause artefactual eccentricity • RV pressure and volume overload can lead to an abnormal shape and function of the interventricular septum, resulting in flattening	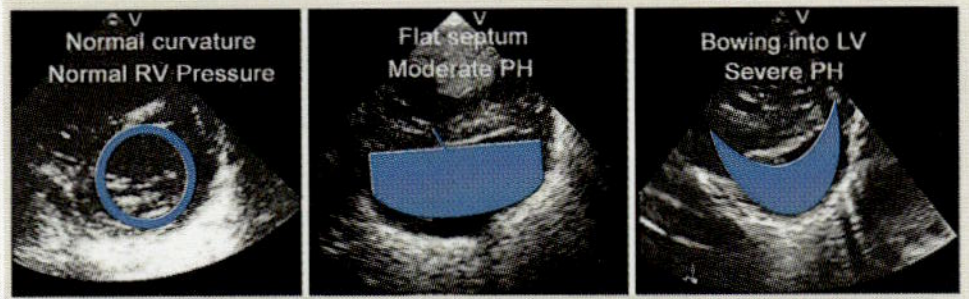 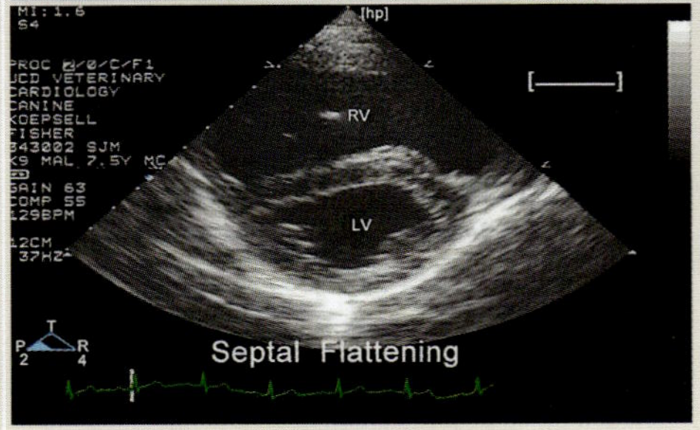 Septal Flattening 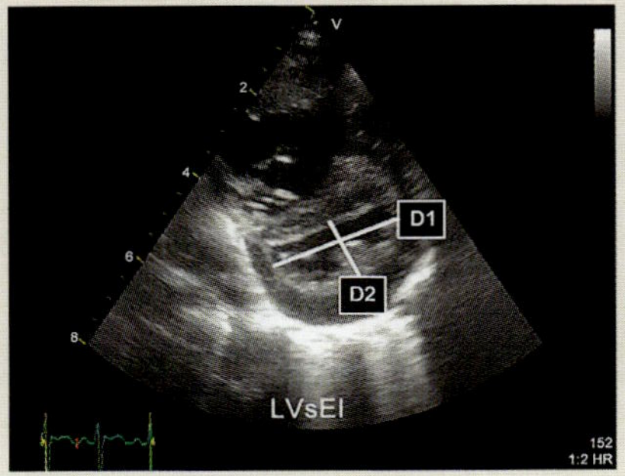

Contd…

Contd...

No	*ECHO parameter*	*View*	*Image acquisition*	*Comment*	*ECHO image*
	Peak transductal right-to-left velocity SPAP = 4 × $(VmaxDA)^2$ + SSAP	• Ductal view • Subcostal • PSAX	PW or CW Doppler of transductal right-to-left blood flow can be used to estimate SPAP, when it lasts ≥30% of the heart cycle, by measuring its peak velocity	• A ductal right-to-left or bidirectional shunt is observed in 73–91% of the patients with PPHN • Measurement of PAP via ductal flow is often not reliable. Assessment of the direction of transductal blood flow is more useful and will indicate the relation between pulmonary and systemic pressures	
	2.2 Pulmonary vascular resistance:				
	PVR = PAAT/RVET ratio	• PLAX (outflow) • PSAX • Subcostal	PAAT is validated as a feasible and reproducible, noninvasive echocardiographic imaging marker, for detection of pulmonary vascular disease and PH in neonates and children	It is only a surrogate marker and does not give estimation of PAH	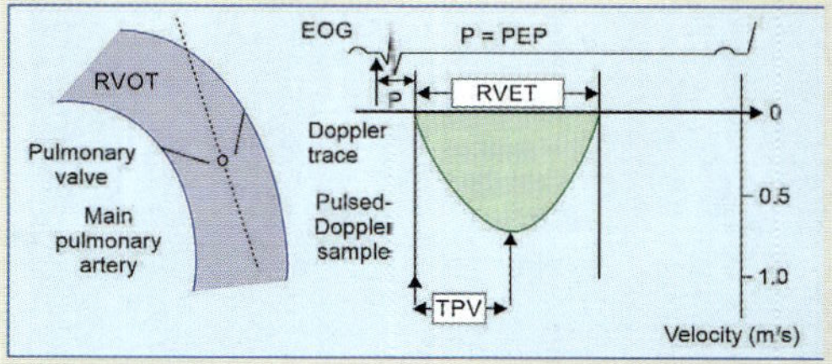

Contd...

Contd…

No	*ECHO parameter*	*View*	*Image acquisition*	*Comment*	*ECHO image*
			• PAAT cutoff value of <90 ms reliably detects pulmonary vascular disease, <40 ms detects pulmonary vascular disease in its most severe form of PH • The normal PAAT:RVET ratio is ~0.31 or greater. PAAT: RVET <0.23 is indicative of increased PAP		
	TRV/VTI (RVOT)	• PLAX (outflow) • PSAX	• PVR can be estimated by calculating the TRV: VTI ratio, which is the ratio between TRV and the VTI of blood flow through the RVOT using pulsed-wave Doppler • TRV:VTI ratio have been shown to correlate well with PVR in children and a cut off value of 0.14 provided high predictive values	Paucity of data in neonates	
	Pulmonary artery compliance CdynPA = [(Ds-Dd)/(Dd × SPAP)] × 10^4	• PLAX (outflow) • PSAX	• Dynamic pulmonary artery compliance (CdynPA) can be calculated by measuring pulmonary diameter in systole (Ds) and diastole (Dd) and analyzing the TR jet to calculate SPAP • Lower CdynPA is found in children with PH	Paucity of data in neonates	

Contd…

Contd…

No	ECHO parameter	View	Image acquisition	Comment	ECHO image
	2.3 Assessing direction of Shunts-PDA, PFO				
	Transductal shunt—PDA	• Ductal view • Subcostal • PSAX	• In 73–91% of patients with PPHN, a transductal right-to-left or bidirectional shunt can be observed. A bidirectional shunt with a systolic right-to-left duration ≥30% of the total heart cycle is considered non-physiologic and likely to represent PPHN • An exclusive right-to-left transductal shunt in patients with PPHN is associated with an increased risk of mortality	Measurement of pulmonary artery pressure via ductal flow is often not reliable	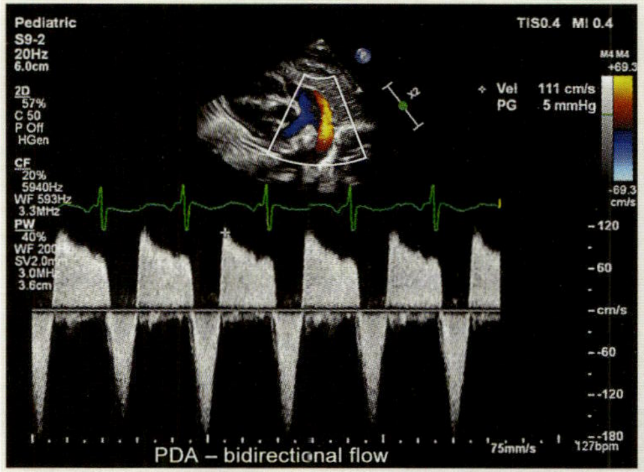 PDA – bidirectional flow
	Interatrial—PFO	Subcostal	An atrial bidirectional or right-to-left shunt is detected in 73–100% of PPHN patients. Also, left-to-right shunting over the interatrial septum is possible, since in PPHN diastolic pulmonary artery pressure is generally sub-systemic with suprasystemic SPAP		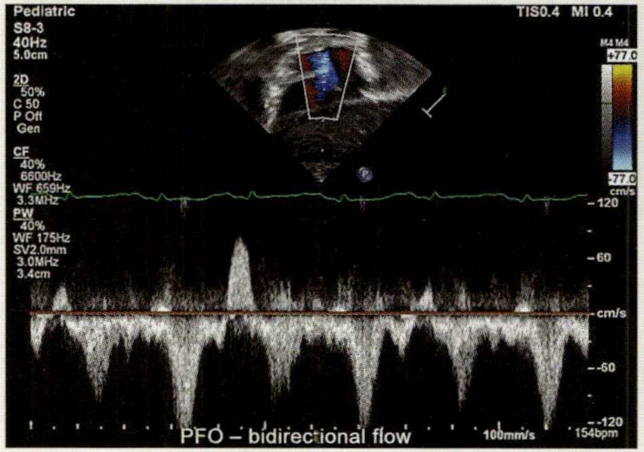 PFO – bidirectional flow

Contd…

Contd…

No	*ECHO parameter*	*View*	*Image acquisition*	*Comment*	*ECHO image*
3.	*Step 3: Is there associated right or left or bi- ventricular dysfunction?*				
	3.1 Objective assessment of RV function:				
	3.1.1 Fractional area change (FAC)	• A4C • 2-D	• RV dimensions measured in 2-D by manual tracing of the endocardial border of the right ventricle • Trabeculations should be included within the cavity while tracing the area • RV-FAC = Area at the end of diastole (cm^2) – area at the end of systole (cm^2)/area at the end of diastole (cm^2)	• Normal values range from 25 to 45% • Median RV-FAC value of 19% is considered abnormal and associated with need for extracorporeal membrane oxygenation (ECMO) or death; • RV-FAC ≤33% is a major criterion in cardiomyopathy/ dysplasia/akinesia or dyskinesia and • RV-FAC >33% and <40% is a minor criterion cardiomyopathy/ dysplasia/akinesia or dyskinesia	RVA_D = 25 cm^2 RVA_s = 10 cm^2 ((25 cm^2 – 10 cm^2) /25 cm^2 × 100) = 60% RVFAC

Contd…

Contd...

No	*ECHO parameter*	*View*	*Image acquisition*	*Comment*	*ECHO image*
	Tricuspid annular plane systolic excursion (TAPSE)	A4C	• To assess RV longitudinal function and obtained from the 4-chamber view using the M-Mode with the cursor aligned along the direction of the lateral annulus • TAPSE is both angle and load dependent	• Normal value in babies 1,500–2,500 g is 0.45 ± 0.03 cm • In babies 2,500–3,600 g is 0.8 ± 0.16 cm. • Diminished values below 4 millimeters are predictive of the need for ECMO and death in infants with PPHN	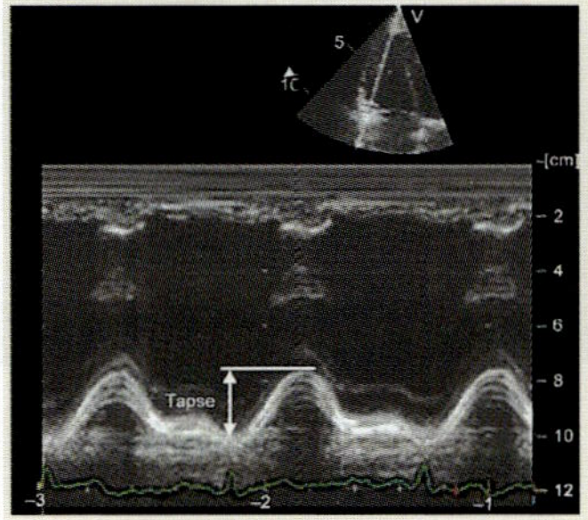
	MPI via TDI	• A4C • Tissue Doppler or pulsed wave Doppler	• MPI is an index of global RV performance. • The isovolumic contraction time (IVCT), isovolumic relaxation time (IVRT) and ejection time intervals can be measured using • MPI = (IVET + IVRT)/RVET • *IVET; isovolumic ejection time; IVRT; isovolumic relaxation time; RVET; right ventricular ejection time* • Tissue Doppler is preferred as it is derived from a single sample	• Normal MPI in term infants is 0.42 (0.15). • RV MPI in term infants decreases from 0.42 (0.14) on day 1 of life to 0.29 (0.09) after PDA closure and 0.22 (0.09) on 28th day of life • MPI >0.43 by pulsed wave Doppler or >0.54 by tissue Doppler indicates RV dysfunction • Tissue Doppler values >0.64 are associated with worse prognosis	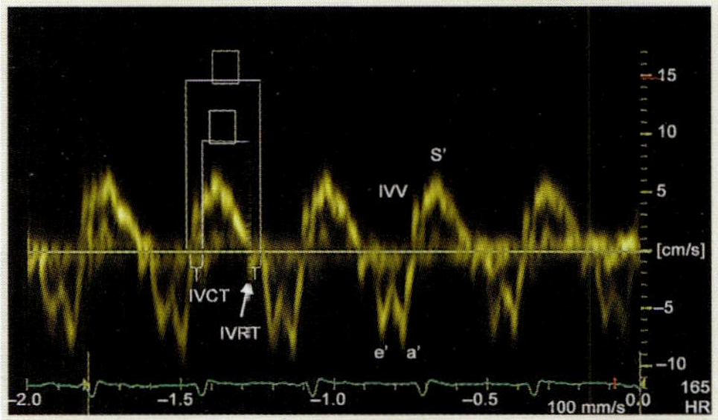

Contd...

Contd…

No	*ECHO parameter*	*View*	*Image acquisition*	*Comment*	*ECHO image*
	Objective assessment of LV function:				
	LV dimensions	PLAX or PSAX	• LV dimension measured by 2-dimensional M-mode echocardiography at the level of the papillary muscles in PLAX or PSAX • Following measurements are taken: – Left-ventricular end-diastolic dimension (LVEDD), – Left-ventricular end-systolic dimension (LVESD), – Interventricular septal thickness at end diastole (IVSd) and end systole (IVSs) – Left ventricular posterior wall thickness at end diastole (LVPWd) and end systole (LVPWs)		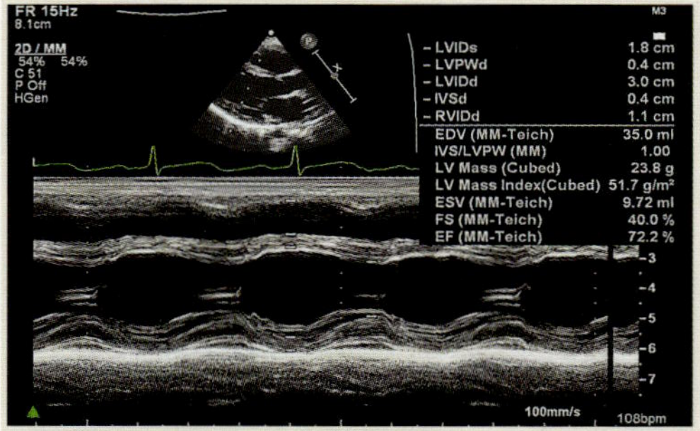
	Shortening fraction (FS%)		Measured by 2D or M-mode: Shortening fraction (FS%) is a measure of global LV systolic function $FS\% = \frac{(LVEDD - LVESD)}{LVEDD} \times 100$		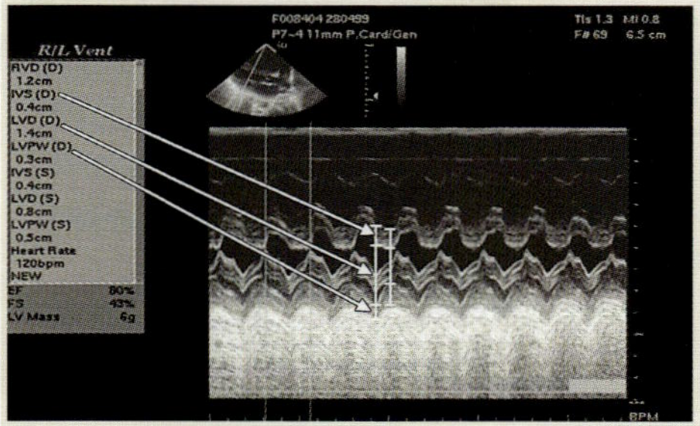

Contd…

Contd…

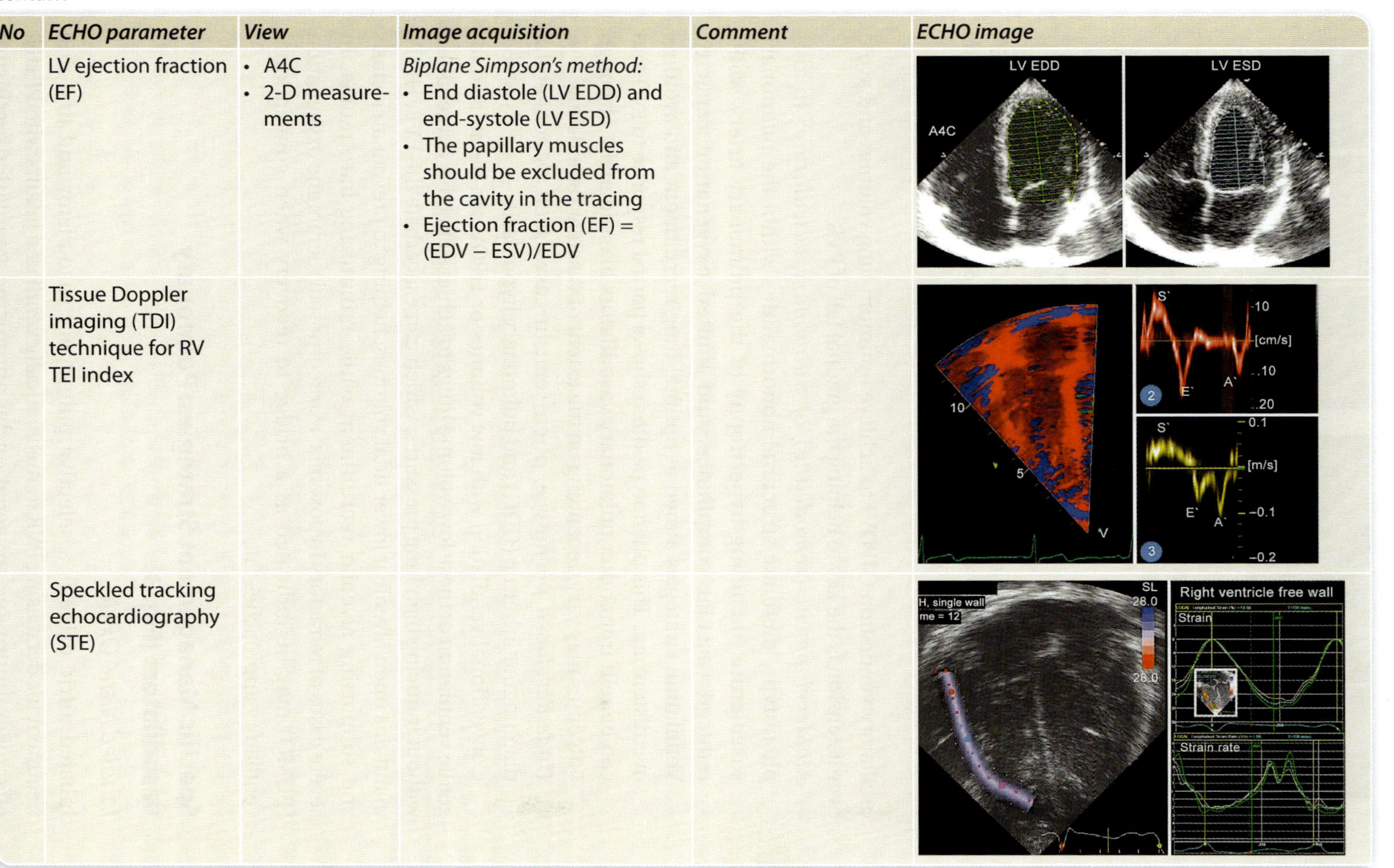

No	ECHO parameter	View	Image acquisition	Comment	ECHO image
	LV ejection fraction (EF)	• A4C • 2-D measurements	*Biplane Simpson's method:* • End diastole (LV EDD) and end-systole (LV ESD) • The papillary muscles should be excluded from the cavity in the tracing • Ejection fraction (EF) = (EDV – ESV)/EDV		
	Tissue Doppler imaging (TDI) technique for RV TEI index				
	Speckled tracking echocardiography (STE)				

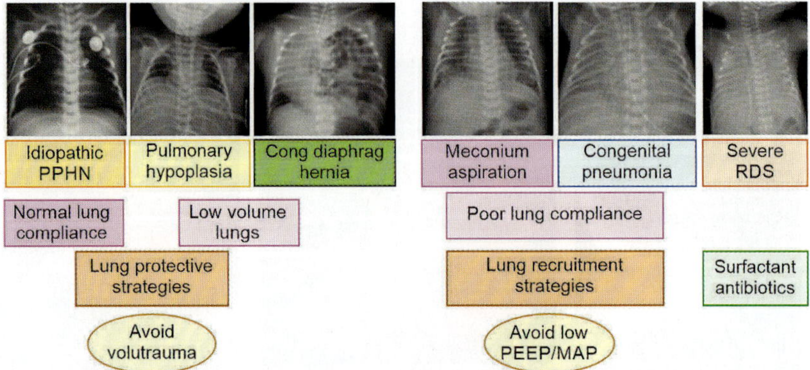

Fig. 2: Ventilation strategies based on etiology. (MAP: mean airway pressure; PEEP: positive end-expiratory pressure; PPHN: persistent pulmonary hypertension of the newborn; RDS: respiratory distress syndrome)

oscillatory ventilation (HFOV) to achieve optimum lung volumes and avoid overdistension is the key to helping the gradual fall of PVR.

- *Maldevelopment (remodeling) of pulmonary vasculature*: In this phenotype, there are structural abnormalities within the pulmonary vasculature, including hypertrophy of the pulmonary artery walls, reduced vascular compliance, and limited oxygenation capacity. Ventilation strategies aimed at optimal lung recruitment and avoiding overdistension. This phenotype often shows partial response to iNO and can benefit from other pulmonary vasodilators like sildenafil, although outcomes may vary depending on the extent of vascular remodeling.
- *Underdeveloped phenotype*, often seen in cases such as congenital diaphragmatic hernia (CDH) and pulmonary hypoplasia.

Conventional ventilation with low volumes or HFOV can be utilized for gentle ventilation of these low-volume lungs to achieve effective oxygenation without inducing high lung pressures, which can exacerbate the PVR. HFOV maintains open alveoli at lower tidal volumes, helping to prevent atelectasis and supporting alveolar recruitment while minimizing barotrauma. In severe cases of refractory hypoxemia, extracorporeal membrane oxygenation (ECMO) may be indicated as a bridge to recovery when conventional ventilatory approaches fail.

Specific Management Strategies: Pulmonary Vasodilators (Fig. 3)

Inhaled Nitric Oxide

Inhaled nitric oxide is a selective pulmonary vasodilator and first-line treatment for decreasing PVR in mechanically ventilated infants with PPHN, effectively improving oxygenation by optimizing ventilation-perfusion

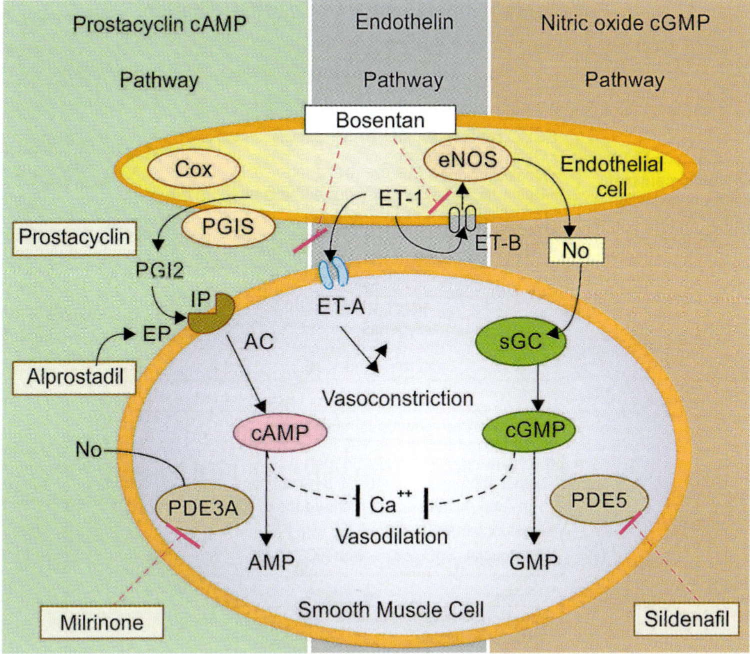

Fig. 3: Mechanisms of actions of various pulmonary vasodilators.

matching. Clinical trials have shown that iNO reduces the need for ECMO in term neonates, and it is the only Food and Drug Administration (FDA)-approved therapy for hypoxemic respiratory failure in infants over 34 weeks gestation. A starting dose of 20 ppm is recommended to maximize oxygenation while minimizing adverse effects like increased nitrogen dioxide and methemoglobin levels.

Inhaled nitric oxide should be started early, with methemoglobin levels monitored at 2 hours, 8 hours, and daily thereafter. For weaning from iNO, we are sharing an evidence-based protocol that will help in using iNO effectively. Unresponsiveness or failed weaning risks dependence. Echocardiography is essential early on, especially for nonresponders or those worsening after iNO initiation **(Flowchart 1)**.

Sildenafil

It is a phosphodiesterase 5 (*PDE5)* inhibitor that increases cGMP levels to cause pulmonary vasodilation and is recommended for infants who either do not respond to iNO or when iNO is unavailable. It is preferably given intravenously in critically ill neonates but requires close blood pressure (BP) monitoring due to the risk of systemic hypotension. Echocardiography is advised before starting sildenafil, especially to assess right-to-left shunts across the patent foramen ovale (PFO) or patent ductus arteriosus (PDA).

Flowchart 1: Inhaled nitric oxide (iNO) initiation.

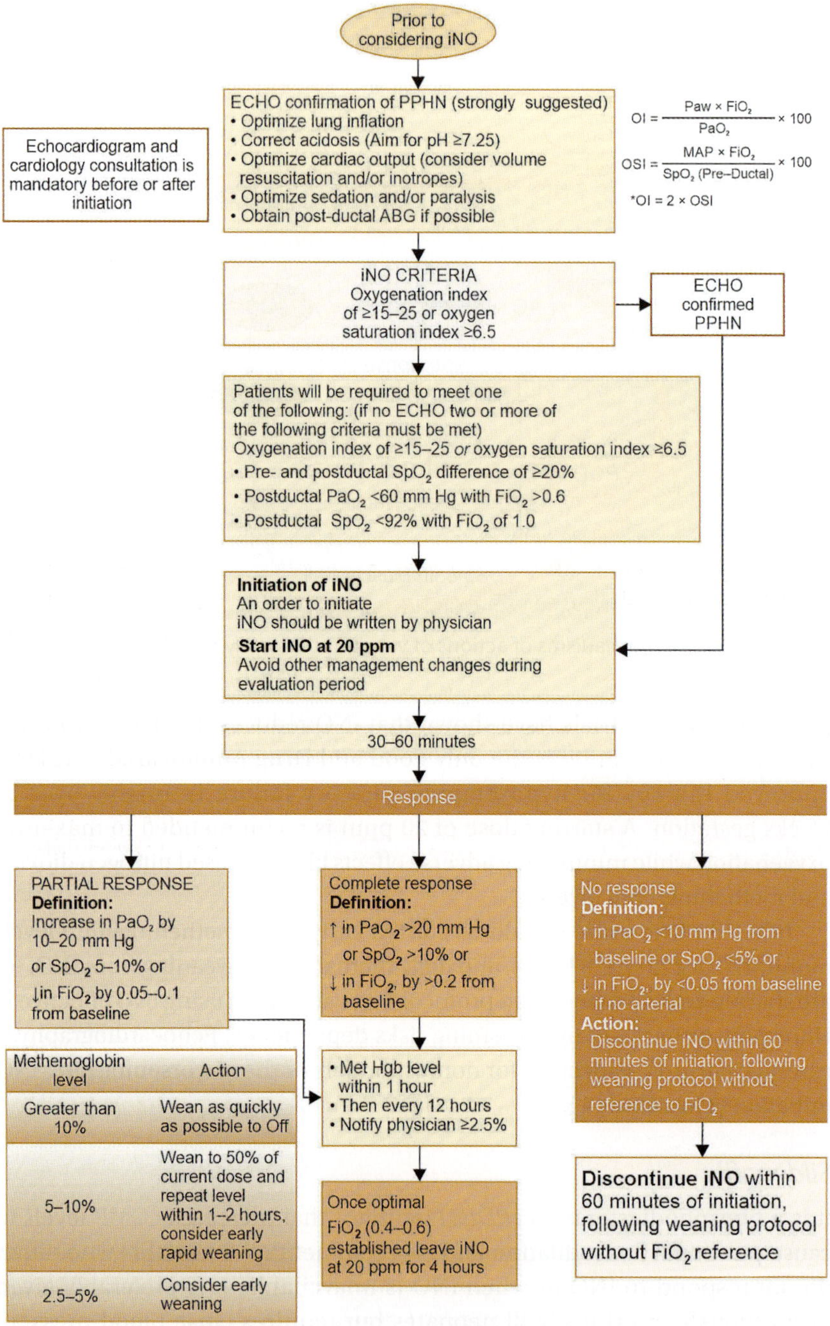

Prior to considering iNO

ECHO confirmation of PPHN (strongly suggested)
- Optimize lung inflation
- Correct acidosis (Aim for pH ≥7.25)
- Optimize cardiac output (consider volume resuscitation and/or inotropes)
- Optimize sedation and/or paralysis
- Obtain post-ductal ABG if possible

Echocardiogram and cardiology consultation is mandatory before or after initiation

$$OI = \frac{Paw \times FiO_2}{PaO_2} \times 100$$

$$OSI = \frac{MAP \times FiO_2}{SpO_2 \text{ (Pre–Ductal)}} \times 100$$

*OI = 2 × OSI

iNO CRITERIA
Oxygenation index of ≥15–25 or oxygen saturation index ≥6.5

ECHO confirmed PPHN

Patients will be required to meet one of the following: (if no ECHO two or more of the following criteria must be met)
Oxygenation index of ≥15–25 *or* oxygen saturation index ≥6.5
- Pre- and postductal SpO_2 difference of ≥20%
- Postductal PaO_2 <60 mm Hg with FiO_2 >0.6
- Postductal SpO_2 <92% with FiO_2 of 1.0

Initiation of iNO
An order to initiate iNO should be written by physician
Start iNO at 20 ppm
Avoid other management changes during evaluation period

30–60 minutes

Response

PARTIAL RESPONSE
Definition:
Increase in PaO_2 by 10–20 mm Hg or SpO_2 5–10% or ↓in FiO_2 by 0.05–0.1 from baseline

Methemoglobin level	Action
Greater than 10%	Wean as quickly as possible to Off
5–10%	Wean to 50% of current dose and repeat level within 1–2 hours, consider early rapid weaning
2.5–5%	Consider early weaning

Complete response
Definition:
↑ in PaO_2 >20 mm Hg or SpO_2 >10% or ↓ in FiO_2, by >0.2 from baseline

- Met Hgb level within 1 hour
- Then every 12 hours
- Notify physician ≥2.5%

Once optimal FiO_2 (0.4–0.6) established leave iNO at 20 ppm for 4 hours

No response
Definition:
↑ in PaO_2 <10 mm Hg from baseline or SpO_2 <5% or ↓ in FiO_2, by <0.05 from baseline if no arterial
Action:
Discontinue iNO within 60 minutes of initiation, following weaning protocol without reference to FiO_2

Discontinue iNO within 60 minutes of initiation, following weaning protocol without FiO_2 reference

(ABG: arterial blood gas; ECHO: echocardiography; FiO_2: fraction of inspired oxygen; OI: oxygen index; PaO_2: partial pressure of arterial oxygen; PPHN: persistent pulmonary hypertension of the newborn; SpO_2: oxygen saturation)

Although, oral sildenafil has been shown to improve oxygenation and reduce mortality in settings where iNO is unavailable, caution is advised due to the FDA safety warnings based on trials indicating higher risk of mortality especially, while using higher doses.

Milrinone

It is a phosphodiesterase 3 (PDE3A) inhibitor that increases cAMP levels, providing both pulmonary vasodilation and inotropic support, making it suitable for infants with normal BP but ventricular dysfunction or in cases where iNO is contraindicated, such as with left ventricular (LV) dysfunction and pulmonary venous hypertension. It should be infused intravenously without a loading dose to minimize systemic hypotension, and precautions like optimal cardiac filling or low-dose epinephrine may be necessary before administration.

Prostacyclin Agents

Inhaled *PGI2 (iloprost)* can be used for iNO-resistant PPHN, although intravenous (IV) formulations like epoprostenol are generally avoided due to the risk of hypotension in neonates. Prostaglandin E1 can be used to maintain ductus arteriosus patency, reducing RV afterload and aiding in right-to-left shunting for infants with persistent PH and failing RV, with echocardiography guiding its use.

Endothelin-1 Receptor Antagonist

Vasoconstriction is facilitated by endothelin-1 (ET-1) signaling via ET-A receptors. Although its effectiveness in neonates varies, but limited evidence of using bosentan in resistant PPHN indicates promise and can be considered, especially in resource poor settings.

Utility of NPE in the Management of PPHN (Figs. 4A and B)

Decision-making Based on Blood Pressure and Cardiac dysfunction

- *Normal BP and good cardiac function*: iNO, if available, otherwise IV or oral sildenafil can be used. If BP starts dropping, consider fluid boluses and low dose epinephrine or norepinephrine, and the use of vasopressin is also on the rise. Hydrocortisone can often be started early as it takes some time to act.
- *Normal BP but cardiac dysfunction on echo*: Consider low-dose epinephrine or dobutamine to optimize cardiac function and use iNO once cardiac function is stable. However, if the BP drops then one should avoid IV sildenafil as it may worsen hypotension. Cardiac dysfunction requires optimization with epinephrine along with Milrinone, provided BP improves. In severe cases, early consideration of ECMO should be undertaken.

BP and Echo

	BP normal	BP low
Cardiac dysfunction	**Treatment:** Standard management plus iNO if available/Sildenafil (IV) If no INO • Milrinone +/- low dose Adenaline • Dobutamine-HIE	**Treatment:** Standard management iNO if available/(Sildenafil-caution) • Adrenaline + Milrinone • Milrinone + Vasopressin • Hydrocortisone • **Explore ECMO options**
Cardiac function normal	**Treatment:** Standard management plus • iNO if available • If no iNO • Sidenafil – IV or oral • Inhaled PG12	**Treatment:** Standard management INO if available If no iNO • A Fluid bolus • Dopamine up to 10 mic (Risk ↑PVR) • Adrenaline up to 0.05 to 0.2 mic/k/min • Nor-adrenaline • Vasopressin very low dose • Hydrocortisone

A

Echo shunts

	R-L shunt PDA level	Shunt R-L shunt
R-L shunt Atrial level shunt	Duct dependent pulmonary circulation *Treatment:* Prostaglandin E1 infusion	**PPHN** *Treatment:* • Ventilation and Oxygen • iNO • Sildenafil IV/PO • Milrinone + Adrenaline
L-R shunt	• Normal • Lung dz and no PPHN *Treatment:* • Ventilation • Surfactant	• LV dysfunction and PV HTN • RV dependent systemic circulation *Treatment:* • Milrinone +/- Inotrope • Prostaglandin E1 infusion • Nitric contraindicated

B

Figs. 4A and B: ECHO-based management approach. (BP: blood pressure; ECHO: echocardiography; ECMO: extracorporeal membrane oxygenation; iNO: inhaled nitric oxide; IV: intravenous; LV: left ventricular; PDA: patent ductus arteriosus; PPHN: persistent pulmonary hypertension of the newborn; PV HTN: pulmonary vein hypertension; PVR: pulmonary vascular resistance)

Decision-making Based on Shunting at the Level of PDA and Interatrial Septum (PFO)

- *Left to right shunting across PDA and PFO*: Conservative and supportive management as no or minimal PPHN.
- *Right to left shunting at PFO and left to right across PDA:* It is always abnormal, and it might suggest duct-dependent pulmonary circulation or suprasystemic pulmonary pressures, so one can safely start prostaglandins pending confirmation from the cardiologist about structural abnormality.
- *Right to left shunting at the PDA but left to right at PFO:* This could suggest a different physiology of LV dysfunction along with PH. Here one needs to support the heart with milrinone and or epinephrine and might consider prostaglandins. In this situation, iNO is relatively contraindicated as it might make things worse by worsening pulmonary venous hypertension.
- *Right to left shunting at the PDA and PFO*: This means suprasystemic PH, hence iNO, sildenafil, and other pulmonary vasodilators with inotropes (if cardiac dysfunction) should be used to optimize pulmonary and systemic hemodynamics.

Algorithm-based Management of PPHN in Centers with or without Availability of Inhaled Nitric Oxide (Flowcharts 2 and 3)

Centers where iNO is available: Initiating iNO early to reduce PVR helps, with echocardiography guiding further interventions. If oxygenation improves, iNO is gradually weaned. In nonresponders or those with LV dysfunction, adjunctive therapies like milrinone or sildenafil are considered, and ECMO is considered for refractory cases.

Centers where iNO is unavailable: Initial management should focus on optimizing ventilation and systemic BP. Sildenafil is employed as the primary pulmonary vasodilator. Supportive care, including fluid management and inotropes, is tailored to cardiac function, with ECMO as a last resort for severe hypoxemia.

INHALED NITRIC OXIDE GUIDELINES

Inhaled nitric oxide should be started early, with regular monitoring of methemoglobin levels, and carefully weaned using a gradual approach protocol to prevent rebound PH, by following the weaning protocol as described in **Flowchart 4**. Echocardiographic assessment is essential, especially for iNO nonresponders or those who worsen, to identify any underlying cardiac conditions.

Flowchart 2: Management of PPHN in centers with availability of inhaled nitric oxide (iNO).

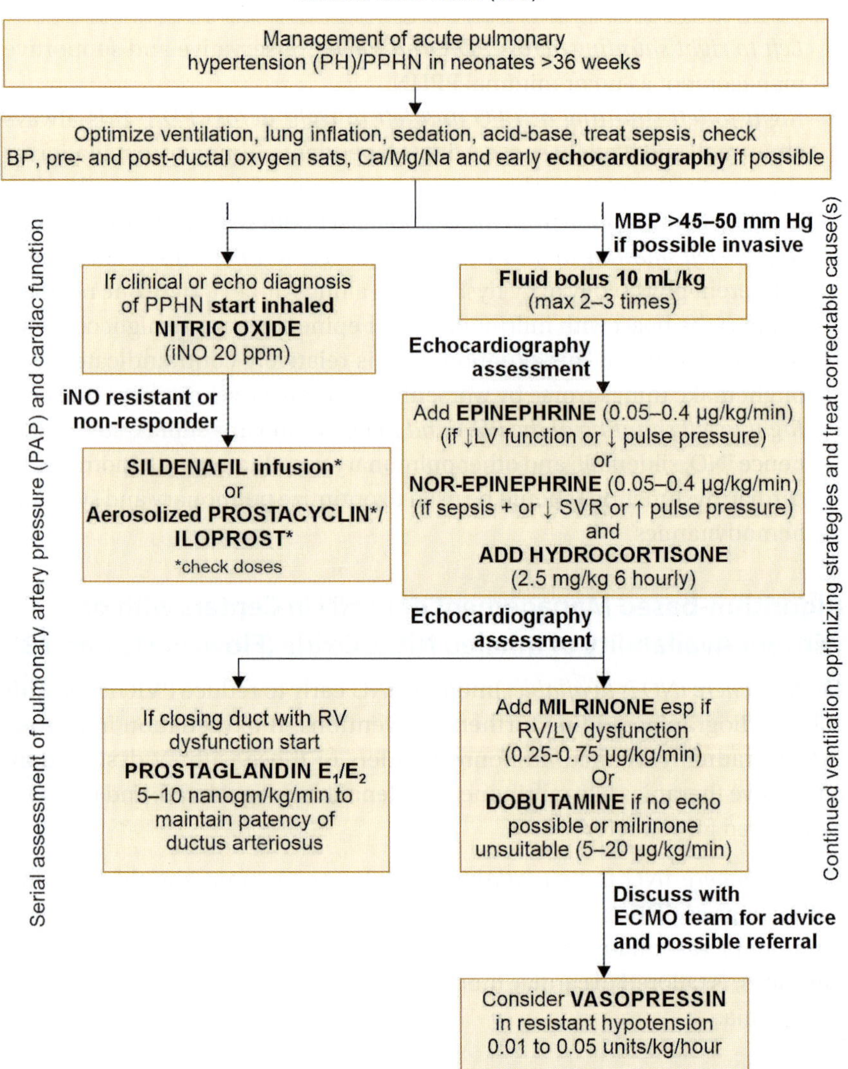

(BP: blood pressure; ECMO: extracorporeal membrane oxygenation; LV: left ventricular; MBP: mean blood pressure; PPHN: persistent pulmonary hypertension of the newborn; RV: right ventricular)

Flowchart 3: Management of PPHN in centers without availability of inhaled nitric oxide (iNO).

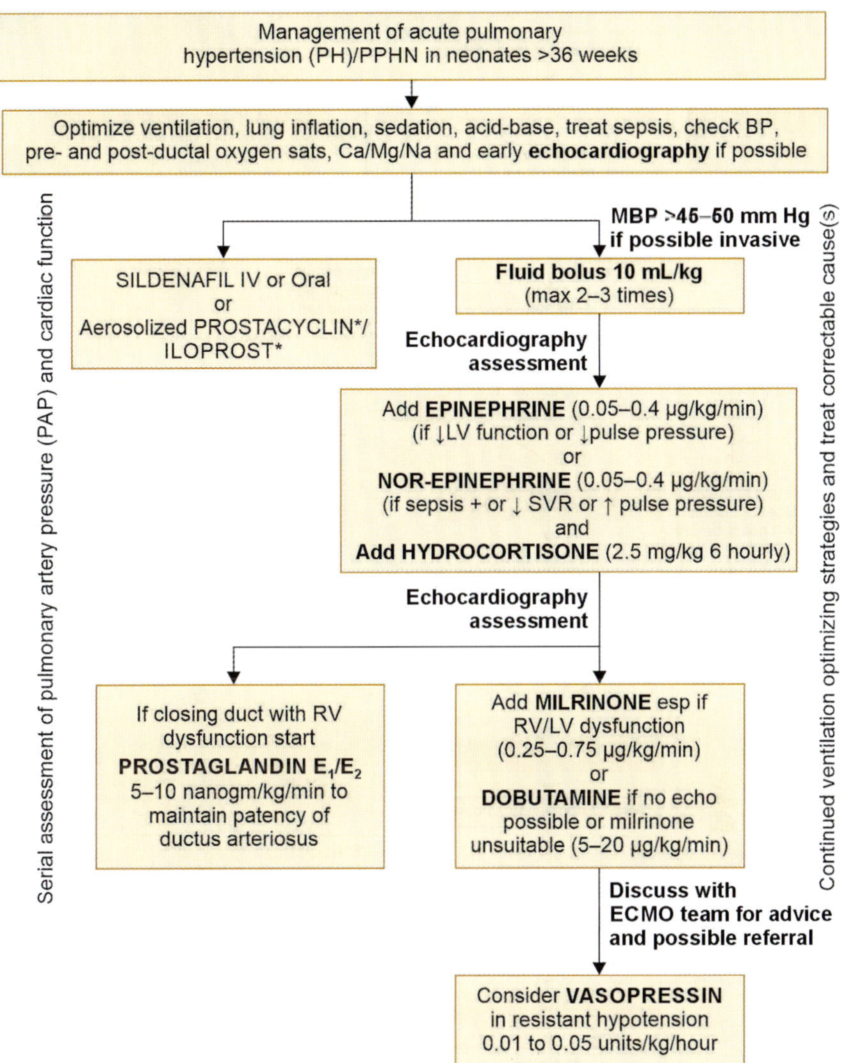

(BP: blood pressure; ECMO: extracorporeal membrane oxygenation; LV: left ventricular; MBP: mean blood pressure; PPHN: persistent pulmonary hypertension of the newborn; RV: right ventricular)

Flowchart 4: Inhaled nitric oxide (iNO) weaning protocol.

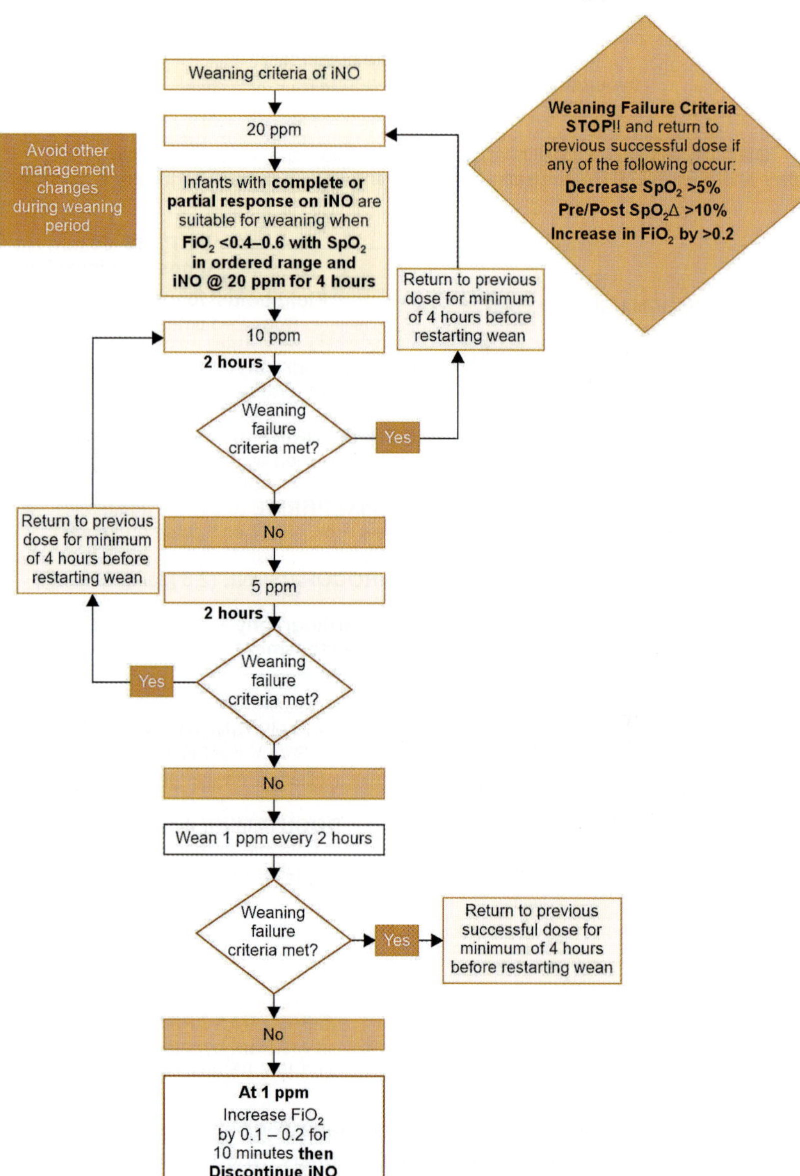

(FiO_2: fraction of inspired oxygen; SpO_2: oxygen saturation)

CONCLUSION

Effective management of PPHN requires timely intervention with specific therapies such as iNO and adjunctive pulmonary vasodilators, guided by echocardiography. Despite advancements, challenges persist in reducing mortality and long-term morbidity in such cases, necessitating ongoing research into novel treatment strategies and optimization of existing therapies, including comprehensive ventilatory support and pharmacological interventions.

SUGGESTED READING

1. Dakshinamurti S. Pathophysiologic mechanisms of persistent pulmonary hypertension of the newborn. Pediatr Pulmonol. 2005;39(6):492-503.
2. de Boode WP, Singh Y, Molnar Z, Schubert U, Savoia M, Sehgal A, et al. Application of Neonatologist Performed Echocardiography in the assessment and management of persistent pulmonary hypertension of the newborn. Pediatr Res. 2018;84:68-77.
3. Elmekkawi A, More K, Shea J, Sperling C, Da Silva Z, Finelli M, et al. Impact of Stewardship on Inhaled Nitric Oxide Utilization in a Neonatal ICU. Hosp Pediatr. 2016;6(10):607-15.
4. Mathew B, Lakshminrusimha S. Review persistent pulmonary hypertension in the newborn. Children (Basel). 2017;4(8):63.
5. More K, Athalye-Jape G, Rao SC, Patole SK. Endothelin receptor antagonists for persistent pulmonary hypertension in term and late preterm infants. Cochrane Database Syst Rev. 2016;2016(8):CD010531.
6. More K, Soni R, Gupta S. The role of bedside functional echocardiography in the assessment and management of pulmonary hypertension. Semin Fetal Neonatal Med. 2022;27(4):101366.
7. Puthiyachirakkal M, Mhanna MJ. Pathophysiology, management, and outcome of persistent pulmonary hypertension of the newborn: A clinical review. Front Pediatr. 2013;1:23.
8. Singh Y, Lakshminrusimha S. Pathophysiology and Management of Persistent Pulmonary Hypertension of the Newborn. Clin Perinatol. 2021;48(3):595-618.

SECTION 9

Extracorporeal Membrane Oxygenation

CHAPTER 9

Extracorporeal Membrane Oxygenation

Rohit Anand

INTRODUCTION

Extracorporeal membrane oxygenation (ECMO) is considered the standard of care for neonates with respiratory and cardiac failure refractory to conventional treatment. Neonates with respiratory failure have the highest survival across all patient with indications of ECMO.

INDICATIONS

The main criterion is that the disease must be reversible, usually within 2–4 weeks. Respiratory failure remains the number one indication for neonatal ECMO (77%), and the use of ECMO for cardiac indications is growing. Any neonate with respiratory failure with oxygenation index (OI) >25 should be cared for in an ECMO center. The indications and contraindications of neonatal ECMO is as shown in **Flowchart 1**.

Flowchart 1: Indications and contraindications of neonatal extracorporeal membrane oxygenation (ECMO).

Indication

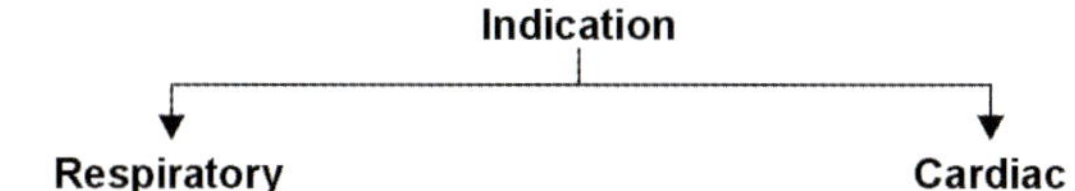

Respiratory	**Cardiac**
Severe hypoxemic respiratory failure: • Oxygenation index >40 • Lack of response to mechanical ventilation and other forms of rescue therapy • Elevated ventilator pressures and/or signs of barotrauma	*For cardiac ECMO:* Neonates having poor oxygen delivery and organ perfusion despite the use of two medications and low cardiac output, oxygen saturations <50%, or persistent lactate >4.0

Contraindications

• Weight <2 kg • Lack of consent • Gestational age <35 weeks • Intracranial hemorrhage grade III or IV • Contraindications to anticoagulation	• Lethal genetic conditions • History of severe asphyxia or severe global cerebral ischemia • Prolonged mechanical ventilation longer than 7–14 days • Untreatable congenital cardiac malformation or diseases

Flowchart 2: Comparison of venovenous (VV) and venoarterial (VA) extracorporeal membrane oxygenation (ECMO) in neonates.

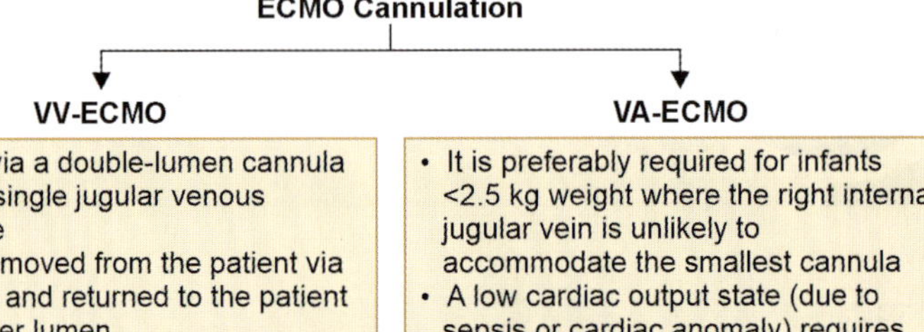

EXTRACORPOREAL MEMBRANE OXYGENATION CANNULATION

There are two approaches: Venovenous (VV) or venoarterial (VA) as shown in **Flowchart 2**. Many centers prefer the VV-ECMO approach nowadays.

In babies with congenital diaphragmatic hernia conventionally VA-ECMO support is used as they are often unstable at the time of cannulation as well as due to other anatomical reasons.

EXTRACORPOREAL MEMBRANE OXYGENATION CIRCUIT AND COMPONENTS

An ECMO circuit consists of a mechanical blood pump, a gas exchange device (membrane oxygenator), and a heat exchanger, all connected to the circuit tubing between the venous access cannula and the venous (VV) or arterial (VA) infusion cannula. The pump is an important component, and novel centrifugal pumps are used nowadays. The membrane oxygenator adds oxygen and removes carbon dioxide from the blood. The ECMO circuit is primed with packed red blood cells (PRBCs) and fresh frozen plasma (FFP) to a hematocrit of 35–45%. The blood prime is heparinized; due to citrate anticoagulation, calcium is also added to correct hypocalcemia and acidosis is corrected by adding sodium bicarbonate as a buffer.

The blood prime should be warmed to 37°C, while in babies undergoing hypothermia, it should be warmed up to 34°C. Once ECMO is initiated, pump flow should be increased over time to determine the maximal flow that can be achieved. The pump flow can range from 80 to 150 mL/kg/min. The medical gas flow is initiated in a 1:1 blood flow ratio to gas flow. If the pump flow is 100 mL/kg/min then sweep flow is 0.1 L/min. Sweep flow is adjusted to target an arterial PCO_2 of 40–50 mm Hg as hypocapnia is associated with cerebral vasoconstriction and periventricular leukomalacia.

MONITORING OF ANTICOAGULATION IN NEONATAL EXTRACORPOREAL MEMBRANE OXYGENATION

The immaturity of the anticoagulation system and the risk of intracranial hemorrhage (ICH) make using anticoagulation challenging in neonates. Unfractionated heparin (UNFH) has been the anticoagulation of choice for ECMO. Some of the ECMO centers have their protocols regarding the UNFH rate. The activated clotting time (ACT) is an available rapid bedside test to measure the anticoagulant activity of UNFH for ECMO. The anti-factor Xa assay is another important and specific tool for titrating UNFH for ECMO. The ACT is influenced by coagulopathy, thrombocytopenia, and dilution while the anti-factor Xa assay is specific to the anticoagulation effect and not influenced by such factors.

HEMATOLOGICAL MONITORING

For the patients on ECMO, the platelets counts should be maintained above 80,000, hematocrit >35–40%, fibrinogen >150 mg/dL, and normal prothrombin time-international normalized ratio (PT-INR). The platelet count, hematocrit, and coagulation factors should be monitored and deficiencies should be corrected.

RESPIRATORY SUPPORT AND MONITORING

On ECMO, the lungs are allowed to rest and recover from the underlying lung disease. The ventilation settings on VV-ECMO are higher than on VA-ECMO. The patient's arterial blood gases, along with pre- and postoxygenator blood gases, are obtained every 6–12 hours. Daily chest radiographs are obtained to confirm ECMO catheter and tube positions, to assess lung volume changes, and to diagnose air leak syndromes. Endotracheal suctioning is recommended every 4–6 hours, and there should be a watch for blood-tinged secretions to monitor for pulmonary hemorrhage.

CARDIOVASCULAR SUPPORT AND MONITORING

The neonates on ECMO often require inotropic or vasopressor support. Studies have shown that the patients with decreased cardiac function may still be considered for VV-ECMO. Hypertension is one of the common complications as per available datasets. Echocardiography may be a useful tool to detect underlying cardiac pathology before cannulation and thereafter to assess and monitor cannula position.

NEUROLOGIC SYSTEM AND NEUROMONITORING

Neonatal ECMO patients are at high risk of brain injury, and regular assessment of the neurological system should be done via neurological examination, daily cranial ultrasound (CUS), and other diagnostic modalities such as amplitude-integrated electroencephalogram (aEEG) and near-infrared spectroscopy (NIRS). ICH is the most significant complication in neonates on ECMO, and as per the available dataset, gestational age is the strongest predictor of ICH in neonates on ECMO.

Timing of Cranial Ultrasound

The CUS should be done before the initiation of ECMO, and then daily after 12–24 hours after cannulation. Evidence suggests that 90% of the ICH occurs in the first 5 days of ECMO therapy and thereafter chances are less. Early detection of neurological injury is important for early therapeutic intervention to improve outcomes.

Role of Amplitude-integrated Electroencephalogram and Near-infrared Spectroscopy

The use of aEEG can predict death or moderate to severe intracranial injury. NIRS monitoring helps to identify poor cerebral oxygen delivery and infants with a high risk of adverse developmental outcomes.

FLUID, ELECTROLYTES, AND NUTRITION

The usual neonatal ECMO patients are edematous due to fluid overload before cannulation, and the initial fluid intake on ECMO is limited to 60–100 mL/kg/day. The ECMO patients achieve natural diuresis once the cardiac output improves and the capillary leak resolves. As per the literature, VV-ECMO is associated with positive fluid balance and lower urine output in the first 96 hours of bypass. Diuretics are used following ECMO initiation and sometimes continuous renal replacement therapy (CRRT) is used if urine output does not improve.

Neonates on ECMO are not fed enterally due to concerns of intestinal ischemia and the risk of necrotizing enterocolitis (NEC). There is emerging evidence of enteral feeding in neonates on ECMO.

INFECTION

Infections are common during ECMO, which can lead to a negative impact on survival as well as significantly increases the duration of ECMO. It is mandatory to practice the strategies to prevent catheter-related infections and ventilator-associated infections in these neonates.

WEANING EXTRACORPOREAL MEMBRANE OXYGENATION

Weaning of ECMO is indicated with the improvement of the patient's condition.

- The pump flow is decreased by 5–10 mL/kg/h every 2–4 hours maintaining the arterial saturation >90% until 50 mL/kg/min flow is reached. On VV-ECMO, the pump flow is weaned to a minimum of approximately 30 mL/kg/min while on VA-ECMO it can be weaned to 20 mL/kg/min.
- The sweep flow can be weaned until off, ventilator rate and fraction of inspired oxygen (FiO_2) may be increased.

For patients who require ECMO for a long duration, it may be necessary to use high-frequency ventilation, surfactant, inotropes, and inhaled nitric oxide (iNO) to wean off.

LONG-TERM MORBIDITIES AND FOLLOW-UP

The ECMO-survived neonates are at high risk for long-term outcomes, which ultimately depend upon the primary underlying condition and adverse events arising during the ECMO course. Morbidities such as bilateral sensorineural hearing loss, motor problems, learning difficulties, behavior disorders, and cognitive and neuropsychological impairments require specific assessment and a multidisciplinary approach to management.

FUTURE DIRECTIONS

Over a while, the use of ECMO has improved and the now ECMO use may be extended to more premature infants in the next few years. There is a new development related to experimental models of artificial placenta. An ideal artificial placenta provides ECMO through the umbilical vessels, thus preserving major fetal blood vessels from cannulation. A trial using an artificial placenta in preterm lambs showed increased survival compared to mechanical-ventilated lambs. Advances in technology would help to reduce ECMO-related complications.

CONCLUSION

Extracorporeal membrane oxygenation (ECMO) has emerged as a vital rescue therapy for neonates with severe respiratory and cardiac failure unresponsive to conventional management. Advances in circuit design, anticoagulation monitoring, and neuroprotection strategies have significantly improved survival, though risks such as intracranial hemorrhage, infection, and long-term neurodevelopmental morbidity remain substantial. Careful patient selection, vigilant monitoring, and structured follow-up are essential to optimize outcomes. With ongoing innovations—including the concept of artificial placenta—ECMO is poised to expand its role in neonatal care, offering new hope for critically ill infants.

SUGGESTED READING

1. Amodeo I, Di Nardo M, Raffaeli G, Kamel S, Macchini F, Amodeo A, et al. Neonatal respiratory and cardiac ECMO in Europe. Eur J Pediatr. 2021;180(6):1675-92.
2. Arensman RM, Short BL, Koo N, Mudreac A. Extracorporeal membrane oxygenation. In: Keszler M, Gautham KS (Eds). Goldsmith's Assisted Ventilation of the Neonate, 7th edition. Philadelphia: Elsevier; 2022.
3. Rajiv PK, Lakshminrusimha S, Vidyasagar D (Eds). Essentials of Neonatal Ventilation, 1st edition. Elsevier Health; 2018.
4. Van Ommen CH, Neunert CE, Chitlur MB. Neonatal ECMO. Front Med. 2018;5:289.

SECTION

Nursing Care in Babies on Noninvasive and Invasive Ventilation, Transportation of Neonate on Assisted Ventilation

CHAPTER

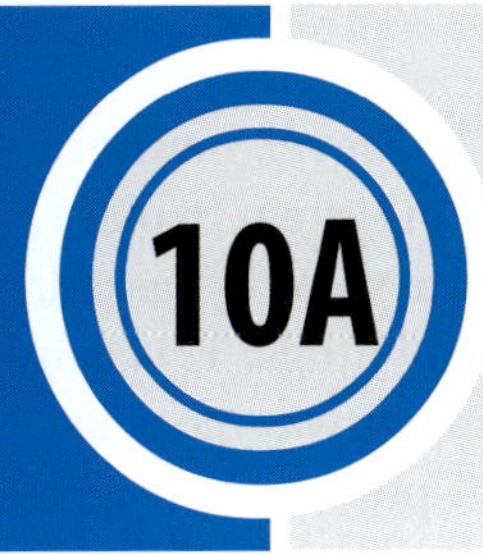

Respiratory Gas Conditioning in Neonatal Ventilation

Anish Pillai

INTRODUCTION

Humidification of ventilatory gas is an important component in the respiratory care of newborn babies requiring any form of respiratory support. Newborn babies, especially those born premature, have immature lungs and fragile airway mucosa, which makes them prone to respiratory complications. Providing warm and humidified gas to the lungs by optimizing the heating and humidification of ventilatory gas reduces the chances of airway epithelial injury and improves overall outcomes.

HUMIDIFICATION AND NEONATAL RESPIRATORY SYSTEM

The nasal cavity, pharynx, and trachea in a healthy adult are capable of warming, filtering, and humidifying inspired air. The inspired air is naturally heated and humidified gradually along the respiratory tract to a temperature of 37°C and relative humidity of 100% **(Fig. 1)**.

Around one-fourth of this heat and moisture is also recovered during expiration by the nasopharynx. This natural gas conditioning helps in

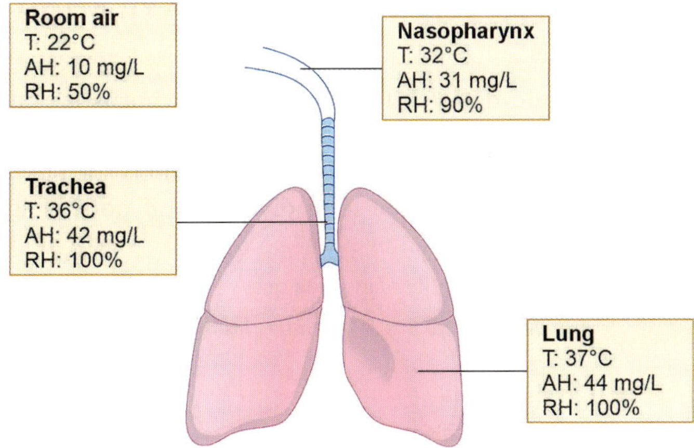

Fig. 1: Respiratory gas conditioning.

maintaining epithelial integrity and promotes healing. However, newborn infants do not have an efficient heating and humidification system in place. Also, for babies on respiratory support, the upper airways are bypassed, causing cold medical gases to be delivered directly to the lungs. This can cause issues such as airway dryness, thickened mucus, and airway blockage. This could hinder ventilation and gas exchange and predispose the baby to a prolonged need for respiratory support. Airway inflammation and epithelial injury increase the risk of respiratory infections. Cold, nonhumidified gases can cause temperature instability and hypothermia in preterm babies.

PHYSICS OF HUMIDIFICATION

Water exists in three states: Solid, liquid, and gas. The solid state of water is ice. On addition of heat or energy, ice is converted to liquid water. When further heat or energy is added, water is converted to its gaseous form, which is water vapor or steam. The amount of water vapor in the air is called humidity, which can be expressed as absolute or relative humidity. Absolute humidity is the actual amount of water vapor present in a liter of gas, expressed as mg/L. The relative humidity is the ratio of the actual amount of water vapor in a gas, compared to the maximum amount of water vapor the gas can hold at a particular temperature; expressed as a percentage. Warmer gases have a higher capacity to hold water vapor compared to cold gases. Once the gas reaches 100% relative humidity (at a particular temperature), condensation of water vapor occurs. The temperature at which the gas is at 100% relative humidity (completely saturated) is called dew point. Once the gas temperature cools below its dew point, condensation of water vapor to water will occur. The temperature and humidity values of medical gas are described in **Table 1**.

CLINICAL BENEFITS OF HUMIDIFIED VENTILATION FOR NEWBORNS

The benefits of humidified ventilatory gas for newborns are numerous and indispensable for supporting the recovery of tiny babies. Prolonged ventilation in neonates can lead to various complications such as infection, endotracheal tube block, chronic lung disease, and poor weight gain.

TABLE 1: temperature and humidity of inspired gas.

	Temperature	*Relative humidity*	*Absolute humidity*
Medical air	12–15°C	2%	0.3 mg/L
Room air	25°C	50%	9 mg/L
Lungs	37°C	100%	44 mg/L

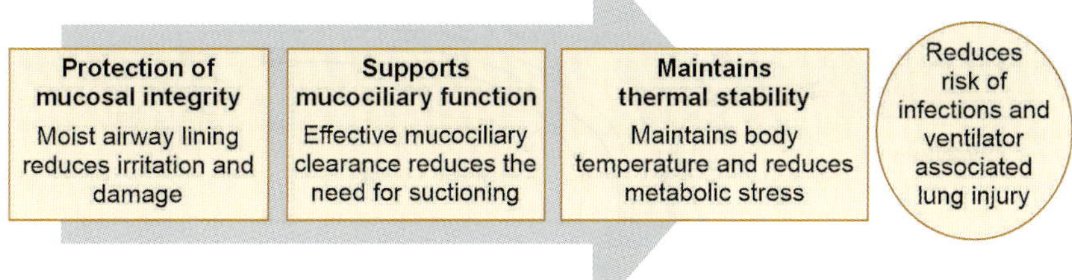

Fig. 2: Mechanisms by which humidification can improve outcomes.

The mechanisms by which heating and humidification of respiratory gases improve clinical outcomes are described in **Figure 2**.

TYPES OF HUMIDIFICATION SYSTEMS

There are two primary methods of humidification systems for patients on respiratory support: *Passive humidification* and *active humidification.*

1. *Passive humidification:* Passive humidification systems, such as heat and moisture exchangers (HMEs), capture heat and moisture from the patient's exhaled air and return it to the inspired air. However, the amount of heat and moisture trapped by these HMEs is variable and unmeasured. Neonates require higher humidity levels, as their intrinsic mucociliary mechanisms for heating and humidification are underdeveloped. Thus, HMEs are not regularly used in neonatal respiratory circuits, as they do not provide the consistent humidification needed to protect these delicate lungs.
2. *Active humidification:* Active humidification systems are the preferred option for neonates on any respiratory support. These systems use a heated water chamber to warm and humidify the inspiratory gases delivered to the baby. The humidifier is connected to the inspiratory circuit of the ventilator or noninvasive device. The humidifier maintains a specific temperature (typically around 37°C) and ensures the air is nearly fully saturated (>95% relative humidity) with water vapor at that temperature. The humidifier chamber is filled with distilled water, which is heated to 37°C and the humidity is at 44 mg/L. The inspiratory circuit extending from the humidifier to the patient has a heated wire that prevents the loss of heat as the gas travels to the patient. The heated-wire enabled circuit also additionally heats the inspired gas up to 39–40°C up to a distal point in the circuit. The inspiratory gas has to then travel a short distance in the inspiratory limb (beyond the heated-wire circuit), and then across the

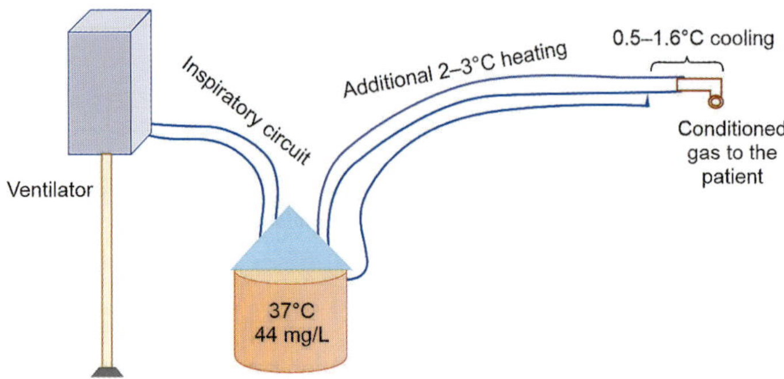

Fig. 3: Active humidification process.

endotracheal tube where it loses around 2-3°C temperature. The final assumed temperature at the level of the lung is 37°C, with close to 100% relative humidity **(Fig. 3)**.

Active humidifiers have a visible continuous temperature display ensuring stable, consistent humidification over prolonged periods of respiratory support. This makes them suitable for neonates with underdeveloped airways and lung tissue.

Further, it is also important to note that the proximal sensor of the temperature probe (patient end) should be placed outside of the heating field with an extension adapter (not having heated wire) placed inside the heated field of the radiant warmer or incubator to avoid condensation in the inspiratory limb of the respiratory circuit as shown in **Figures 4A and B**.

HUMIDIFICATION CHALLENGES AND TROUBLESHOOTING

Maintaining proper humidification in neonatal ventilation is challenging as they often require prolonged respiratory support and are prone to ventilator-associated complications. Overhumidification can lead to water droplets in the respiratory tubing, which can be a source of infection if the water enters the infant's lungs. On the other hand, underhumidification can cause dryness and mucosal erosion of the airways. Reasons for excessive water condensation include long inspiratory tubing, very cold ambient temperature, and loose or incorrectly fitting temperature sensors. High air temperature due to empty water in the humidifier chamber is also a common reason for alarm. The neonatal intensive care unit (NICU) nurses and medical team must continuously monitor the tubing, chamber, and the humidification level in the circuits, ensuring that condensation does not build up and that the air reaching the infant remains at optimal conditions. Regular checks and maintenance of the humidification equipment are essential to prevent malfunctions and maintain a sterile and effective humidification system.

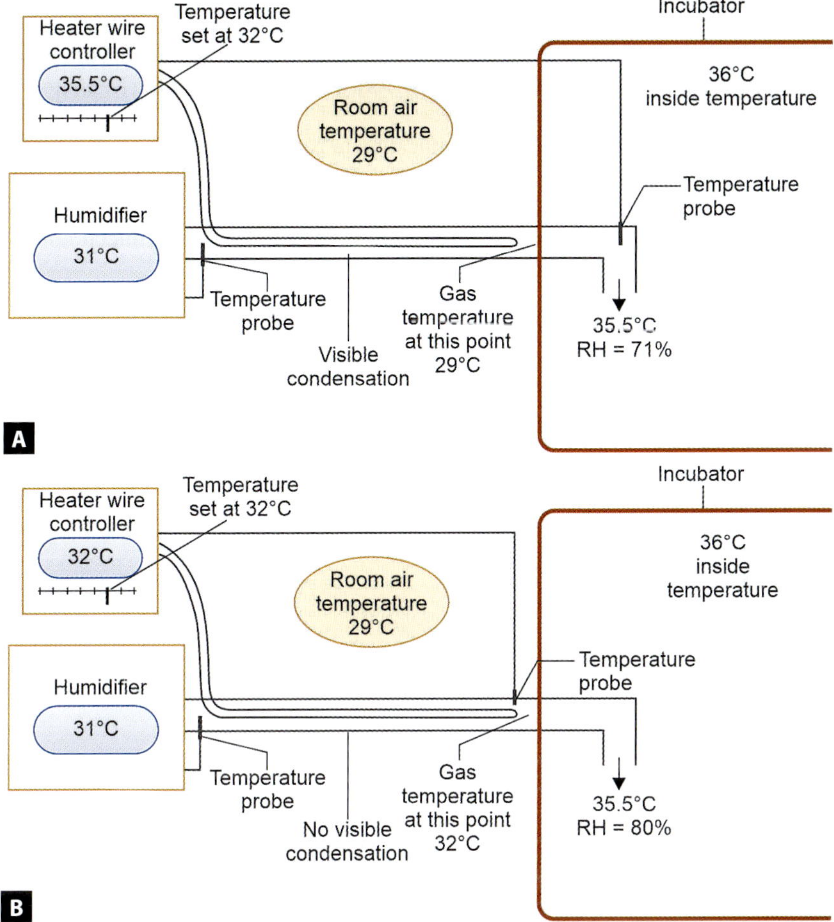

Figs. 4A and B: (A) Proximal end of the temperature probe located inside a heated field tends to indicate a heat representative of the heated field rather than of the inspiratory gas. The humidifier does not provide the heat that is being detected by the temperature probe resulting in condensation in the inspiratory limb of the circuit; (B) Proper placement of the probe. (RH: relative humidity)

Source: Chatburn RL. Principles and practice of neonatal and pediatric mechanical ventilation. Respir Care. 1991;36:560.

CONCLUSION

Humidification of ventilatory gases for newborn babies is the standard of care and essential for airway protection and physiological stability. Providing moist, warm air at the optimal temperature to the baby can enhance patient comfort and improve outcomes for these fragile babies. By conducting regular staff training, careful bedside monitoring, and the use of advanced humidification systems, the outcomes of infants dependent on respiratory support can be improved.

SUGGESTED READING

1. MacKendrick W, Slotarski K, Casserly GBS, Hawkins HS, Hageman JR. Pulmonary Care. In: Keszler M, Gautham KS (Eds). Assisted Ventilation of the Neonate, 7th edition. Amsterdam: Elsevier; 2021.
2. O'Reilly M, Schmölzer GM. Humidification in Neonatal-Pediatric Critical Care: Invasive Ventilation. In: Esquinas AM (Ed). Humidification in the Intensive Care Unit. Springer, Cham; 2023.
3. Schulze A. Respiratory gas conditioning in infants with an artificial airway. Semin Neonatol. 2002;7(5):369-77.

CHAPTER

General Care of Neonates on Assisted Ventilation

Debashish Nanda

INTRODUCTION

Nutritional management remains a crucial aspect for sick neonates. The goal of nutrition management in neonates, especially preterm infants, is achieving postnatal growth at a rate that approximates the intrauterine growth of a fetus and ensuring optimal long-term neurodevelopment. This is best achieved by the provision of enteral nutrition. However, parenteral nutrition (PN) is required when enteral nutrition is inadequate or contraindicated. Achieving adequate nutrition goals still remains challenging in neonates who are on respiratory support. In addition to respiratory care and other supportive measures, optimum nutrition would be important to facilitate recover.

PARENTERAL NUTRITION

Parenteral nutrition (PN) has to be started whenever enteral feeds are not possible. PN may be considered in premature neonates <28 weeks and/or birth weight <1,000 g or in cases where enteral feeding is expected to be delayed for >3 days.

- Begin with an initial total energy intake of around 40–60 kcal/kg/day on day 1 and gradually increase and reach up to 110–120 kcal/kg/day by day 4 or beyond in preterm neonates, and 90–100 kcal/kg/day for term neonates. Start with an amino acid intake of 1–1.5 g/kg/day and lipid (20% intralipid) of 1.5 g/kg/day and gradually increase up to 3.5 g/kg/day of both amino acid and lipid. Glucose infusion has to be adjusted between 6 and 13 mg/kg/min. Electrolytes, calcium, phosphorus, and multivitamins have to be given as per standard recommendations.
- Considering a higher incidence of gram-negative sepsis and sepsis-related mortality in developing countries, the practice of total parenteral nutrition (TPN) should be individualized in units depending on resources.

ENTERAL NUTRITION

Type of Milk

- Mother's own milk (MOM) remains the first choice. Since the baby is separated from the mother, she has to be encouraged to start early and frequent expression of milk to maintain milk supply.
- Second choice is donor human milk (DHM) if available. This is possible in the units that have a facility for a lactation management unit (LMU) or have access to comprehensive lactation management center (CLMC).

  Donor human milk may be used if MOM is not available or to supplement MOM for premature neonates <1,500 g or <32 weeks of gestation. It may be continued till the neonate reaches 34 weeks postmenstrual age (PMA) or postnatal weight of 1,800 g.
- The last choice would be formula (term/preterm).

Human Milk Fortification

For neonates with gestational age (GA) of <34 weeks or <1,800 birth weight:

- Fortification should start once the baby reaches a feed volume of 80–100 mL/kg/day.
- The standard bovine-based HMF should be added to either MOM or DHM. One gram of HMF should be mixed with 25 mL of MoM or DHM.

Assessment of Feeding

- *Emesis:*
  - If the neonate has any blood-tinged emesis or has frank bilious emesis, feeds should be stopped and the baby has to be evaluated.
  - If the neonate has emesis that looks like digested milk, continue to advance feedings per the protocol and follow clinically.
- *Gastric residuals:* Do not routinely check for gastric residuals to decide on enteral feeding.

Abdominal Examination

Abdominal girth has to be measured in neonates prior to feeds. Some neonates may develop abdominal distension while on noninvasive respiratory support. It would be a good practice to open the end of the feeding tube after 30 minutes of a feeding session to allow abdominal decompression. If abdominal girth increases by >2 cm from baseline in the presence of any of the additional clinical signs: firmness, tenderness, color change, increased aspirates, altered aspirates further feeds should be stopped and the patient has to be evaluated.

Stool Pattern

If there is blood in the stool, stop any further feeding.

Feeding Babies on Noninvasive Ventilation, Continuous Positive Airway Pressure (CPAP) [Including Humidified High Flow Nasal Cannula (HHFNC) ≥2 LPM]

- Start feedings based on birth weight if there are no contraindications [shock, surgical abdomen, moderate to severe perinatal asphyxia, seizures, and septic ileus/necrotizing enterocolitis (NEC)].
- Open orogastric (OG) tube after 30 minutes of feeding.
- Increase feeds as per usual recommendations.
- Do not rely solely on abdominal distension as a sign of feeding intolerance.

Feeding Babies with Hypotension

Based on the available evidence at this time, it is reasonable to initiate trophic feeds while the baby is stable on a single inotrope (dopamine/dobutamine ≤10 μg/kg/min).

Feeding Babies Receiving a Blood Transfusion

At this time, there is no strong evidence that withholding feeding during the transfusion of blood products is associated with a reduced incidence of transfusion-related gut injury. The National Neonatology Forum Clinical Practice Guidelines (NNF CPG, use of blood components in newborn guidelines) suggests that the enteral feeds should be withheld in preterm neonates during packed red blood cell transfusion. The feed should be withheld 3 hours prior to the end of the transfusion (weak recommendation).

SKIN CARE

Skin functions as a barrier, helps in thermoregulation, and is also important for infection prevention. Sick neonates admitted to the neonatal intensive care unit (NICU) often require multiple sampling, fixation of multiple devices (nasal interfaces, pulse oximeter probe, etc.), and receive vasoactive drugs (dopamine and adrenaline) which increases the chances of skin breakdown. Skin breakdown increases the possibility of microbial invasion. Hence, skin care is an important component of the care of sick neonates. Preterm neonatal skin possesses certain structural and functional limitations, which increases the chances of skin breakdown and also signifies the importance of skin care in this vulnerable population.

Risk Factors for Skin Injury

- Prematurity
- Using various equipment for monitoring
- Use of adhesives to secure lines, tubes, and other monitoring devices
- Increased chances of edema

- Use of sedation (during ventilation, high-frequency oscillation, etc.) which can cause pressure necrosis
- Certain medications such as vasopressors, calcium, and sodium bicarbonate increase the chances of skin breakdown
- Interfaces used during noninvasive ventilation (use of nasal prongs or masks)
- Risk of thermal injury while on radiant warmer (accidental displacement of probe), temperature of any product in contact with the skin should not be >41°C.

Assessment of Skin Injury

Skin injury and pressure ulcers are serious, yet preventable complications in premature neonates managed in the NICU. Preventing pressure ulcers is an important aspect of care in preterm infants.

The Neonatal Skin Condition Score (NSCS) is a simplified score to assess skin breakdown and can be utilized by caregivers. It was developed in 2007 for use in newborns from birth to 28 days of age as shown in **Table 1**. The scale evaluates overall skin condition and can help in deciding appropriate actions such as using emollients, oil, skin barriers, consultation with the skin team, etc.

Pressure injuries, particularly the nasal injuries observed in neonates while receiving nasal CPAP, are a common cause of skin breakdown observed in NICU. There is currently no recognized classification available to describe the severity of nasal trauma secondary to nasal CPAP in neonates.

National Pressure Ulcer Advisory Panel (NPUAP) is used for staging the severity of these injuries as shown in **Figure 1**.

- *Stage I:* Erythema not blanching, on an otherwise intact skin
- *Stage II:* Superficial ulcer or erosion, with partial thickness skin loss
- *Stage III:* Necrosis, with full-thickness skin loss.

Clinicians and nurses caring for babies who are on noninvasive respiratory support have to implement additional care to avoid pressure injuries particularly the nasal injuries in these neonates.

TABLE 1: Neonatal skin condition score (NSCS).

Score	*Dryness*	*Erythema*	*Breakdown*
1	Normal, no sign of dry skin	No evidence of erythema	None evident
2	Dry skin and visible scaling	Visible erythema, <50% body surface	Small, localized areas
3	Very dry skin and cracking/ fissures	Visible erythema, ≥50% body surface	extensive

Score 1–3 for each category: Perfect score = 3, worst score = 9.

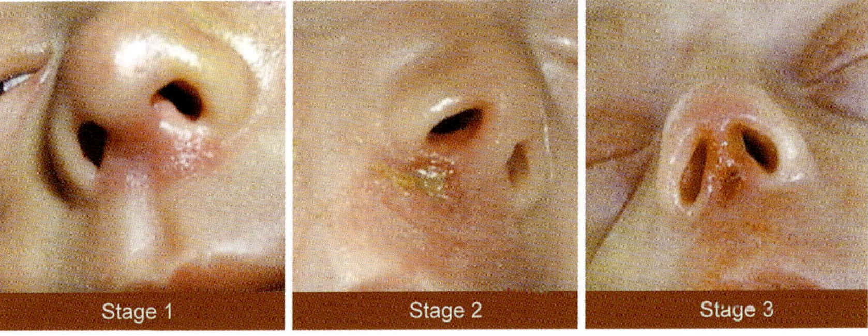

Fig 1: Severity of nasal injury in neonates on noninvasive ventilation (NIV).

- Prongs should be of appropriate size to make an effective seal but should not put additional pressure on alae nasi (there should not be any blanching of alae nasi).
- Pressure over the nares and the bridge of the nose has to be avoided.
- Intermittent inspection and suction of nostril every 4 hours.
- Normal saline is to be instilled in the nostril every 4 hours to minimize crusting.
- Properly secure the interface and use appropriate humidification.
- Barrier devices (Cannulaids) may be considered.

Use of Adhesives

Adhesives and tapes are frequently used in the NICU for securing various devices and monitoring equipment. It increases the chances of skin injury while removing. Every effort to be taken to minimize the use of adhesives and tapes. Transepidermal water loss can increase significantly upon removal of adhesives. Using nonadhesive products in conjunction with transparent dressing and double-backed tape may be encouraged. Saline wipes or moistened gauze may be used for gentle removal of tapes and adhesives. Skin injury may further be reduced by pulling the adhesive parallel to the skin surface while removing and folding the adhesive onto itself. Hydrogel- and silicone-based adhesive products have been shown to reduce skin trauma, with hydrogel having some analgesic effect on wounds. Sometimes delaying tape removal may be helpful because many adhesives attach less well to the skin when in place for over 24 hours.

Use of Emollients

Premature neonates have a compromised epidermal barrier, which increases the susceptibility to infection and hence morbidity and mortality. Oil massage that has been a traditional practice in low- and middle-income countries (LMICs), augments the mechanical barrier. In addition, it also acts as a source of essential fatty acids such as linoleic acid. Topical vegetable oils such as coconut oil, soybean oil, sunflower, sesame, and olive oil can be used as emollients. Few studies from LMICs suggest additional beneficial effects of topical emollients in reducing mortality and hospital-acquired infections significantly and a better weight gain in preterm infants.

Use of Disinfectants

Povidone iodine, isopropyl alcohol, or other alcohol-based disinfectant can cause significant tissue damage in very-low-birth-weight (VLBW) infants. Use of these products may be discouraged in VLBW infants till the stratum corneum matures. Prolonged or repeated use of iodine-containing disinfectants may affect thyroid function in premature infants. It can also cause skin irritation and tissue damage. Chlorhexidine-based preparations are recommended for use, but the solution should be completely removed after the procedure with saline to avoid systemic absorption.

Humidity

Humidified incubators may be considered for nursing premature neonates <32 weeks of gestation and/or <1,200 g. The use of an incubator in these infants is associated with a reduction in insensible water loss and fluid requirements improves skin integrity and sodium homeostasis.

Use of Transparent Plastic Covering

The use of a thin plastic transparent covering may be effective in reducing evaporative water in premature infants. It would diminish an infant's exposure to convective air currents while being nursed on an open radiant warmer bed. The occlusive wrap must be made of polyethylene rather than polyurethane because only polyethylene transmits the long wavelength energy of radiant heat.

DEVELOPMENTALLY SUPPORTIVE CARE

Developmentally supportive care (DSC) measures need to be integrated into routine clinical practice. It would reduce stress, promote growth, and provide much stimulation to the developing brain.

A sick neonate on respiratory support in the neonatal unit is often exposed to various painful and stressful events. Many times, sick neonates need frequent blood sampling and clinical assessments, which reduces the duration of sleep and induces pain and stress. A careful and individualized approach to promote sleep and evaluate and manage pain and stress in sick neonates would reduce overall exposure to pain/stress and promote a better long-term development.

Promoting Sleep

- Promote sleep by providing appropriate nesting, swaddling.
- Skin-to-skin contact needs to be promoted in hemodynamically stable neonates. Neonates on noninvasive respiratory support can be provided by Kangaroo Mother Care (KMC). If adequate supervision is ensured, KMC can be provided to hemodynamically stable neonates on invasive ventilation.
- Day-night pattern may be simulated by reducing lights at night to facilitate nocturnal sleep. All staff members including family members should be provided education on caregiving activities that promote safe sleep.
- Focused light should be used while performing various procedures.
- Ambient noise level should be minimized by:
  - Creating awareness among healthcare workers.
  - Setting proper alarm limits in monitors and promptly responding to various alarms.
  - Avoiding cross-talks during clinical work.

Managing Pain and Stress

- Caregiving activities should be adapted to minimize pain and stress. The use of adhesives should be minimized and should be removed only when it has loosened from the skin surface. Use normal saline to wet adhesive tapes prior to removal.
- A unit protocol to document and manage pain and stress should be in place. Every painful procedure should have documentation of the score before, during, and following the intervention till the return of the infant's pain scores to the preprocedural level.
- There should be use of both nonpharmacologic and/or pharmacologic measures prior to painful or stressful procedures. PIPP (Premature Infant Pain Profile) and N-PASS (Neonatal Pain Agitation and Sedation Scale) scales are useful for assessing acute pain and prolonged pain, respectively.
- Comfort measures such as skin-to-skin contact, facilitated tucking, swaddling, containment, and a quiet environment are effective strategies for pain management.
- Among the pharmacological measures, sucrose, dextrose, and paracetamol are effective for minor procedures.
- Opioids should not be used routinely in babies who are on invasive ventilation. Rather, opioids should be used selectively, when indicated by clinical judgment and evaluation of pain indicators.

Table 2 shows a suggested plan for the management of pain in neonates.

TABLE 2: Suggested approach for pain management.

Type of pain	Useful agent
Mild pain	Oral sucrose, breastmilk
Moderate pain	Oral/rectal/IV paracetamol
Severe pain	Opioids such as morphine/fentanyl
Local pain relief	Local infiltration of lignocaine/topical analgesic cream

CONCLUSION

The care of neonates on assisted ventilation extends well beyond respiratory management and requires an integrated, multidisciplinary approach. Optimal nutrition—preferably with mother's own milk and timely fortification—supports growth and neurodevelopment, while parenteral nutrition is essential when enteral feeding is not feasible. Vigilant attention to skin care, including prevention of device-related injuries and judicious use of adhesives and emollients, is vital in reducing complications and infection risk. Developmentally supportive care strategies such as promoting sleep, minimizing noise and light, practicing Kangaroo Mother Care, and effective pain and stress management significantly enhance long-term outcomes. By combining meticulous clinical monitoring with family-centered, individualized care, clinicians can improve both survival and quality of life for critically ill neonates on respiratory support.

SUGGESTED READING

1. American Association for Respiratory Care. AARC Clinical Practice Guidelines. Endotracheal suctioning of mechanically ventilated patients with artificial airways. Respir Care. 2010;55:758-64.
2. Cleminson J, McGuire W. Topical emollient for preventing infection in preterm infants. Cochrane Database Syst Rev. 2016;2016(1):CD001150.
3. DiBlasi R. Respiratory care of the newborn. In: Keszler M, Gautham KS (Eds). Goldsmith's Assisted Ventilation of the Neonate, 7th edition. Elsevier; 2022. pp. 363-83.e5.
4. Fischer C, Bertelle V, Hohlfeld J, Forcada-Guex M, Stadelmann-Diaw C, Tolsa JF. Nasal trauma due to continuous positive airway pressure in neonates. Arch Dis Child Fetal Neonatal Ed. 2010;95:F447-51.
5. Lund CH, Osborne JW. Validity and reliability of the neonatal skin condition score. J Obstet Gynecol Neonatal Nurs. 2004;33(3):320-7.
6. Mihatsch WA, Braegger C, Bronsky J, Cai W, Campoy C, Carnielli V. ESPGHAN/ESPEN/ESPR/CSPEN Guidelines on Pediatric Parenteral Nutrition. Clin Nutr. 2018;37:2303-05.
7. National Institute for Health and Care Excellence. (2020). Neonatal parenteral nutrition. NICE guideline [NG 154]. [online] Available from nice.org.uk/guidance/ng154 [Last accessed February, 2025].

CHAPTER

Respiratory Care of Neonate on Noninvasive and Invasive Ventilation

Usha Devi R

INTRODUCTION

The provision of respiratory support is a critical component of neonatal care, addressing the unique challenges posed by the immature respiratory systems of neonates. This is especially true for preterm infants, whose underdeveloped lungs and lack of adequate surfactant can result in severe respiratory compromise. The neonatal population frequently encounters conditions such as respiratory distress syndrome (RDS), transient tachypnea of the newborn (TTN), bronchopulmonary dysplasia (BPD), and apnea of prematurity, all of which require timely and effective respiratory support.

Ventilation, both noninvasive and invasive, plays a pivotal role in ensuring adequate gas exchange, supporting lung development, and preventing secondary complications. Noninvasive ventilation techniques, including nasal continuous positive airway pressure (nCPAP) and nasal intermittent positive pressure ventilation (NIPPV), aim to minimize the risks of lung injury while providing adequate respiratory support. In contrast, invasive ventilation, involving endotracheal intubation, remains essential for neonates with severe respiratory failure or when noninvasive methods are insufficient.

This chapter delves into a tailored approach to respiratory care, emphasizing strategies that balance effective support with the minimization of iatrogenic harm. By understanding these, clinicians can optimize outcomes and reduce the burden of respiratory morbidity in this vulnerable population as shown in **Figure 1**.

Care of a neonate on respiratory support is not only restricted to respiratory care but also includes:
- Thermoregulation
- Skincare
- Developmentally supportive care
- Bundle approach

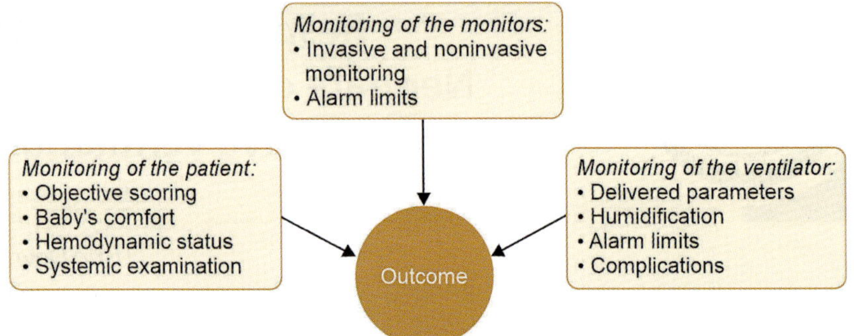

Fig. 1: Different components of monitoring of a neonate on noninvasive and invasive ventilation.

TABLE 1: Downe Vidhyasagar Respiratory distress scoring.

Respiratory rate	*Cyanosis*	*Air entry*	*Grunting*	*Retractions*	*Score*
<60 breaths/min	Nil	Normal	None	Nil	0
60–80 breaths/ min	In-room air	Mild reduction	Audible with stethoscope	Mild	1
>80 breaths/min	In ≥40% FiO_2	Markedly reduced	Audible with the naked ear	Moderate	2

Source: Downes JJ, Vidyasagar D, Boggs TR, Morrow GM. Respiratory distress syndrome of newborn infants. I. New clinical scoring system (RDS score) with acid–base and blood-gas correlations. Clin Pediatr. 1970;9:325-31.

CLINICAL PARAMETERS AND MONITORING THE MONITORS

Clinical Parameters to be Assessed

- *Chest rise/wiggle:*
    - Excessive chest rise on conventional ventilation might indicate inadvertent/high pressures beyond the requirement. Poor chest rise might be due to inadequate pressure. Titration of ventilator settings should be done accordingly.
    - In high-frequency ventilation, the chest wiggle should typically be visible up to the level of the umbilicus. Amplitude needs to be decreased if the wiggle is beyond the umbilicus and extending to the legs and vice versa.
    - The clinical assessment should be correlated with adequate lung expansion on X-rays (8 ribs in conventional ventilation, and 8–10 ribs in high-frequency ventilation).
    - Objective scoring of respiratory distress: The severity of respiratory distress is assessed by Downes' Score **(Table 1)** and Silverman-Anderson score **(Fig. 2)**. The Silverman-Anderson score is more

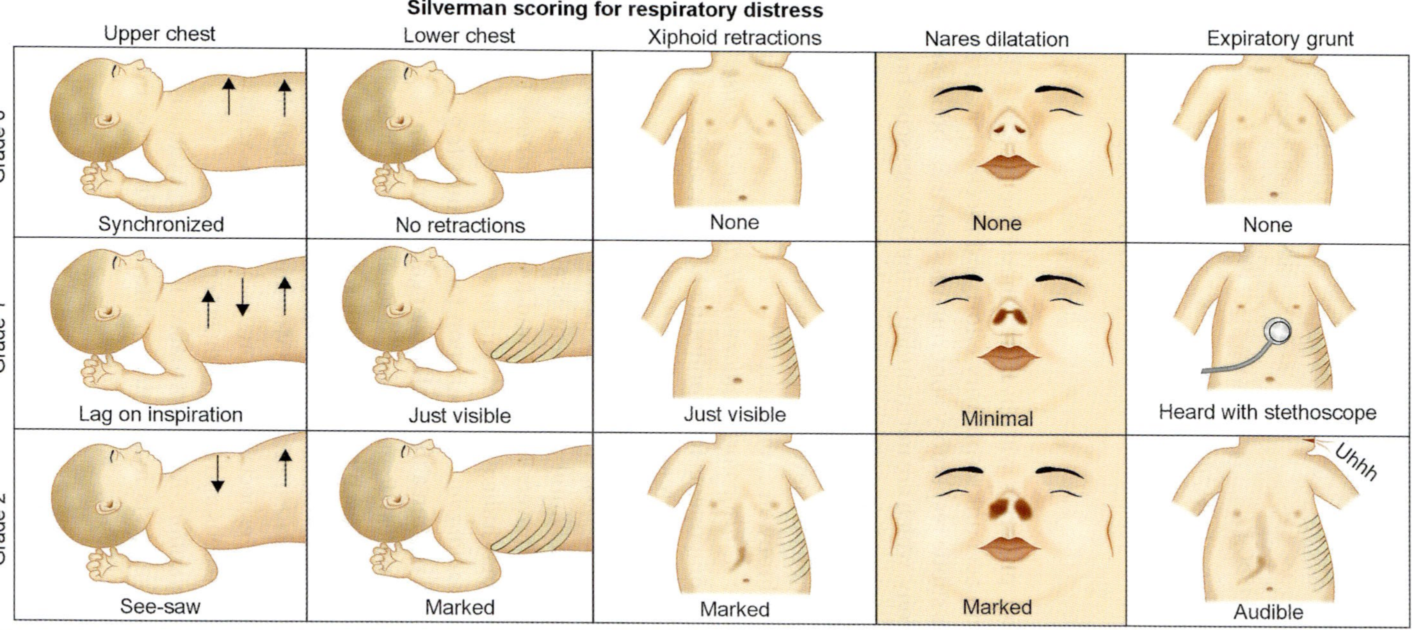

Fig. 2: Silverman Anderson scoring.

Source: Silverman WA, Andersen DA. A controlled clinical trial of effects of water mist on obstructive respiratory signs, death rate and necropsy findings among premature infants. Pediatrics 1956;17(1):1-10.

TABLE 2: Vital signs and perfusion monitoring—normative values.

Parameter	*Normal range*
Heart rate	120–160 beats/min
Respiratory rate	30–60 breaths/min
Oxygen saturation (SpO_2)	90–95%
Blood pressure [mean arterial pressure (MAP)]	~Gestational age (in weeks)
Temperature	36.5–37.5°C
Capillary refill time	<2–3 seconds
Urine output	>1 mL/kg/h

suited for preterms with hyaline membrane disease (HMD) as it takes into account respiratory effort and mechanical function and captures subtle respiratory abnormalities, such as thoracoabdominal asynchrony, which are not included in the Downes score but the latter is more comprehensive and can be applied to any gestational age (i.e., both term and preterm newborn) and disease condition.

A score of >6 indicates severe respiratory distress or respiratory failure.

- Comfort/synchrony on a ventilator
- *Hemodynamic status [color, capillary refill time (CFT), pulse, and urine output]:* The components for monitoring hemodynamic status and their normative values are shown in **Table 2**.
- *Systemic clinical examination:*
  - *Neurological status:* Regular assessment using scales such as the Neonatal Behavioral Assessment Scale (NBAS) or observing for spontaneous movements, tone, and level of alertness. Hypotonia or irritability may indicate hypoxemia or evolving sepsis.
  - *Cardiac examination:* Auscultation for murmurs (e.g., patent ductus arteriosus), rhythm abnormalities, or gallop sounds.
  - *Respiratory system:* Regularly assess for chest retractions, nasal flaring, and grunting. Auscultate for breath sounds to detect asymmetry or adventitious sounds (e.g., wheezing or crackles).
  - *Gastrointestinal examination:* Monitor abdominal distension and bowel sounds, especially in neonates on invasive ventilation, as they are prone to ileus and necrotizing enterocolitis.
  - *Skin examination:* Assess for pallor, mottling, cyanosis, or jaundice. Cyanosis suggests hypoxemia, while mottling may indicate poor perfusion.

Monitoring the Monitors

Appropriate alarm limits are needed to identify clinical deterioration and titrate settings, and thus, to decrease the risk of ventilation-induced lung

TABLE 3: Different methods for monitoring a neonate on invasive ventilation.

Invasive monitoring	*Noninvasive monitoring*	
Blood gas analysis: Frequency as per unit protocol and neonate's clinical status	Oxygenation	Pulse oximetry
		Transcutaneous oxygen monitoring
	Carbon dioxide monitoring	Transcutaneous CO_2 monitoring
		$EtCO_2$
	Tissue oxygen saturation monitoring	NIRS
	Others	*Imaging:* ECHO and USG
		Pulmonary graphics

(ECHO: echocardiogram; $EtCO_2$: end-tidal carbon dioxide; USG: ultrasonography)

injury. The different methods of monitoring a neonate on invasive ventilation are shown in **Table 3**.

Monitoring of Neonate on Invasive Ventilation

A typical monitoring chart of a neonate on conventional ventilation is shown in **Table 4**.

Ventilator Parameters

- *Set parameters:* Peak inspiratory pressure (PIP), positive end-expiratory pressure (PEEP), rate, inspiratory-to-expiratory (I:E) ratio, volume guarantee (VG)/tidal volume (TV), the fraction of inspired oxygen (FiO_2), continuous positive airway pressure (CPAP)
- *Delivered/displayed parameters:*
  - Tidal volume, minute ventilation, and baby's rate
  - PIP required to deliver set VG/TV and mean arterial pressure (MAP) required
  - Bubbling in the bubble chamber of bubble CPAP
  - Displayed temperature in the humidifier and water in the humidifier.

Ventilator Screen/Monitor

Compliance: The normal compliance for neonates on mechanical ventilation varies but typically ranges from 1–3 mL/cmH_2O in very preterm neonates and 3–7 mL/cmH_2O in term neonates. Lower values suggest stiff lungs, while higher values indicate more compliant lungs.

Resistance: Normal airway resistance for neonates typically ranges between 0.5 and 1.5 cmH_2O/L/sec. Increased resistance (e.g., in airway obstruction

TABLE 4: Monitoring chart for a neonate on invasive respiratory support.

Name:____________________CrNo.______________ Date____________ Date of ventilation_____________ ET change on __________________

ET tube size______ET mark________

Mode of ventilation																							
	Clinical parameters								***Ventilator setting***						***ABG***							***ET suction***	***Remark/ physiotherapy***
Time	Temp	HR	RR	RBS	Color	CFT	BP	SpO_2	PIP	PEEP	Ti	Rate	FiO_2	Tidal volume	pH	PO_2	pCO_2	HCO_3^-	BE	$AaDO_2$	OI		

due to mucus, bronchospasm, or pulmonary edema) may require an increase in PIP to overcome resistance and deliver the set tidal volume.

Ventilator graphics:

- *Scalar graphics*:
    - Has time on the X-axis and volume/pressure/flow on the Y-axis
    - PT scalar—only positive waves, never comes to zero
    - VT scalar—only positive waves, comes to zero
    - FT scalar—has positive and negative waves
- *Loops*:
    - *Pressure-volume loop*:
        - Sleeping loop—slope <45'—poor compliance
        - Figure of 8—Flow is not enough.
        - Beaking—pressures are too high (C20/C, normal-1, <0.8 means high PIP)
        - Set PEEP at or above the upper inflection point—normally, LIP (and UIP) should not be seen.
        - Air leak
        - Air-trapping
        - *How to find the nature of breath*:
            - Fully positive—control breath
            - Has a negative deflection initially (pressure, X-axis), followed by positive curve—assisted breath
            - Vertical loop completely around zero (inspiration negative and expiration positive)—Spontaneous, unassisted breath
    - *Flow-volume loop:*
        - Volume on X-axis, flow on Y-axis
        - May be clockwise (inspiration above baseline) or anticlockwise (inspiration below baseline)
        - Serrations in the expiratory loop—secretions
        - Cigar loop—Both peak inspiratory flow rate and peak expiratory flow rate are low—tube block
        - Ski slope pattern—initial peak followed by low expiratory flow rate—increased expiratory resistance
        - Air leak
        - Air-trapping
    - *Findings in leak:*
        - Volume time scalar: Expiratory volume will not come to zero.
        - Flow time scalar: Expiration ends fast, followed by a longer pause before the next inspiration. If auto-cycling, short expiration followed by next inspiration immediately
        - PV loop: Leak prevents closure of the PV loop. Expiratory volume just hangs

- FV loop: Volume will not come to zero (Volume is on X-axis), stops before reaching the origin

Features in Air-trapping:

- Flow time scalar: Expiratory flow will not come to zero. Inspiration for the next breath starts before that.
- PV loop: Lifted up—volume does not come to zero, but the loop is completed (volume on Y-axis).
- FV loop: Expiratory flow will not come to zero (Flow is on the Y-axis).

Monitoring of Neonate on Noninvasive Ventilation

A typical monitoring chart of a neonate on CPAP is as shown in **Table 5**.

Selection of Appropriate Interface (Nasal Prongs or Mask/Nasal Cannula)

Nasal prongs: For CPAP, the prongs should be snuggling fitting into the nostrils without putting pressure on the septum. The different types of nasal prongs and their selection criteria are shown in **Figures 3 and 4**.

Nasal mask: Small, medium, large, and extra-large sizes are available and appropriate size needs to be selected as shown in **Figure 5**.

Nasal cannula: Snuggly fitting cannulas such as Ram cannula (diameter >80% of the nares) can be used as an interface for noninvasive respiratory support as shown in **Figure 6**.

However, for high-flow oxygen therapy, the cross-sectional area of the cannula is no more than 50% that of the nares because of the risk of unexpected elevations in airway pressure. Thus, the appropriate outer diameter of the cannula is no more than two-thirds that of the nares.

Monitoring for nasal injury by the interface: This should be done at least once in every shift. The components of a typical CPAP nasal injury score are shown in **Table 6**.

This injury can be avoided by selecting nasal interface of appropriate size and proper application of barriers such as hydrocolloid/tegaderm in the areas where the interface would come into contact.

Suction

Suctioning should be performed by two persons since maintaining a sterile technique is more difficult with one person.

Routine suction should be avoided and endotracheal suction is done only when signs of tracheal secretion are present which include deteriorating oxygen saturation levels or arterial blood gases, absent or decreased chest

TABLE 5: Monitoring chart for a neonate on CPAP.

Time	*Temp*	*HR*	*RR*	*BP*	*CFT*	*SpO_2*	*CP/PP*	*Rd Score*						*FiO_2*	*PEEP*	*Flow*	*Bubble*	*Humidifier temp*	*Nasal injury score*
								UC	*LC*	*XR*	*Grn.*	*NF*	*Tot*						

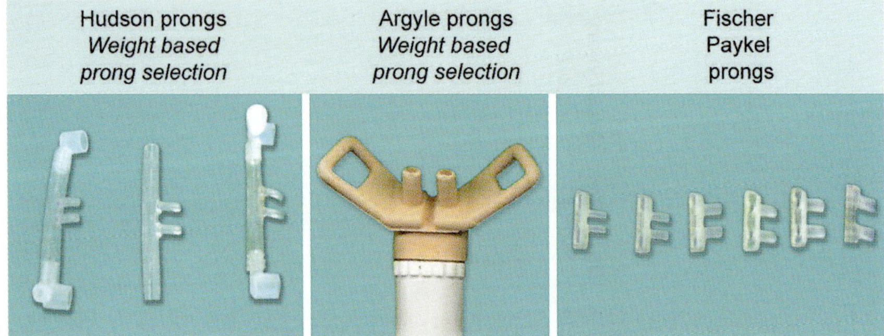

Fig. 3: Selection of appropriate size prongs by assessing the nares diameter and septal space.

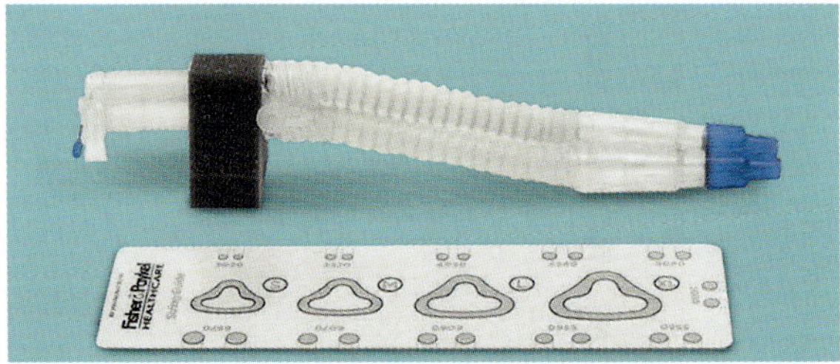

Fig. 4: Selection of Fischer Paykel prongs based on nasal septum thickness and diameter of the nasal orifice.

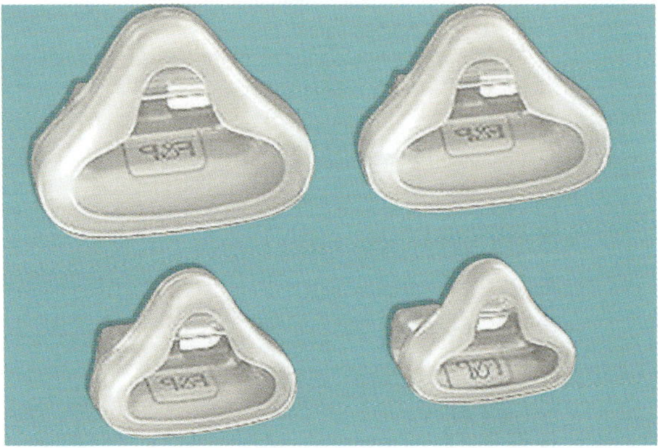

Fig. 5: Fischer and Paykel nasal masks of various sizes.

movement, reduced chest wall vibration for patients on high-frequency oscillatory ventilation (HFOV), audible or visible secretions in the endotracheal tube (ETT), increased $EtCO_2$ or transcutaneous CO_2, coarse or decreased breath sounds, increased work of breathing and irritability, saw

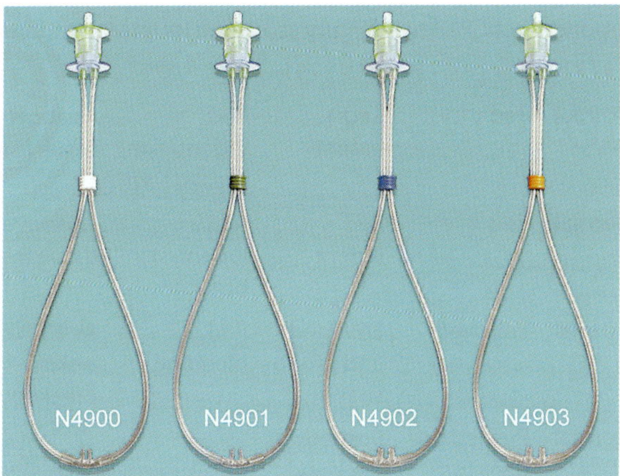

Fig. 6: Nasal cannula of different sizes based on gestational age and birth weight.

tooth pattern on the expiratory limb of flow-volume loop on the monitor screen of the ventilator, increased PIP during volume-controlled mechanical ventilation, or decreased tidal volume during pressure-controlled ventilation in the absence of known cause. No routine saline instillation should be done during suction. A suction catheter is inserted without applying a vacuum and inserted only till the tip of ETT. The choice of the size of the suction catheter is based on the internal diameter of the endotracheal tube as shown in **Table 7**. The depth can be determined by noting the length of the tube and adding the length of the ET adapter. This depth of insertion should be mentioned in the ETT card kept bedside for future reference. Suction should be applied only on withdrawal. Application of suction should be for <10 seconds to avoid hypoxemia, bradycardia, and airway trauma, and the baby should be ventilated to achieve target saturation before resuctioning. Suctioning of oral and pharyngeal secretions, especially after ETT suctioning, is very useful in preventing microaspirations and ventilator-associated pneumonia (VAP).

Position Change

The head end is elevated by 30–45°. Preterm infants should lie with their heads in a midline position, especially during the first 3 days of life, to reduce the risk of germinal matrix-intraventricular hemorrhage.

The position of the neonate should be changed periodically to prevent secretions from pooling at the base of the lungs.

Postural drainage is a therapeutic technique used to facilitate the removal of secretions from the lungs by positioning the neonate in specific postures that allow gravity to assist in clearing mucus from different lung segments.

TABLE 6: Components of CPAP nasal injury score and its interpretation.

Score	*0*	*1*	*2*	*3*	*4*	*Score*
Tip of nose	Normal	Red	Red + indent	Red/ indent/skin breakdown	As above + tissue loss	
Nasal septum	Normal	Red	Red + indent	Red/ indent/skin breakdown	As above + tissue loss	
Nostrils	Normal	Enlarged	Enlarged and prong shape	Red, bleeding	As above + skin breakdown	
Nose shape	Normal	Pushed up/ back but normal	Pushed back and shortened			
Bridge of the nose	Normal	Red	Red + indent	Red/ indent/skin breakdown	As above + tissue loss	
Upper lip	Normal	Red	Red + indent	Red/ indent/skin breakdown	As above + tissue loss	
Total score						

Nasal injury scoring: 0 = No injury, 1–4 = mild injury, 5–6 = moderate injury, >7 = severe injury

TABLE 7: Size of suction catheter for endotracheal tubes of various sizes.

ETT size	*Suction catheter size*
2.0 mm	5 Fr
2.5 mm	5–6 Fr
3.0 mm	5–6 Fr
3.5 mm	8 Fr
4.0 mm	8 Fr

(ETT: endotracheal tube)

Indications:
- Retention of pulmonary secretions
- Atelectasis caused by mucus plugging
- Postextubation respiratory support
- Neonates with chronic lung conditions, such as cystic fibrosis

Steps for performing postural drainage include:
- *Assessment:* Evaluate the neonate's respiratory status and identify areas of secretion retention.

- *Positioning:* Place the neonate in the appropriate posture based on the affected lung segment.
- *Suctioning (if necessary):* Perform gentle suctioning to remove loosened secretions following drainage.
- *Monitoring:* Observe for signs of distress, desaturation, or discomfort during and after the procedure.

Contraindications: Neonates with unstable cardiovascular status, recent surgery. Head-down tilt should be avoided in preterm babies.

Humidification

It is a natural process of the naso/oropharynx and the upper airway during natural/spontaneous breathing. During normal environmental conditions, when one inhales, the atmospheric air enters at a temperature of 24–26°C and at a relative humidity of 50%. In the upper airway, this gas is warmed to a temperature of 37°C and at a relative humidity of 50% by the time it reaches the bronchi and respiratory bronchioles. Optimal warming and humidification of the inspired gases maintain the mucus clearing, ciliary function, and the cellular integrity of the respiratory tract.

Bypassing the upper airway as in intubated neonates, high flows and use of cold medical gases as in CPAP or ventilation compromises the humidification process. Suboptimal humidification results in mucus thickening, slowing of the mucociliary function, death of the epithelial cells, and growth of bacteria. Greater the time of suboptimal humidification, worse are the effects on respiratory passage. Every effort should be made to deliver the respiratory gases at body temperature and relative humidity of 100%.

Optimal humidity: Even when the neonate is on noninvasive respiratory support, the neonatal airway is not capable of warming/humidifying cold medical gases administered at high flow rates. Hence, irrespective of respiratory support, the inspired gas should be warmed to 37°C and be fully saturated (100% RH or 44 mg/L of vapor) when it reaches the airway.

The medical gases are cold and dry. They are at a temperature of 20°C with RH as low as 5%. Hence, compressed air and oxygen should be warmed and humidified before delivering them to the infant's airway. Optimal humidity is achieved by active humidification. These humidifiers actively warm and add water vapor to the inspired gas. The gas exiting the humidification chamber should be at body temperature and with 100% RH. Avoid raining out in the inspiratory limb. It is ideal to have minimal beading (dew drops) in the inspiratory limb and some condensation in the expiratory limb.

Condensation in an inspiratory limb is avoided by:

- Heater wire circuit in inspiratory limb.
- By placing the distal segment of the inspiratory limb inside the radiant warmer or incubator.
- Keeping the room temperature at 26–28°C.

BUNDLE APPROACH

Ventilator-associated Pneumonia Bundle

- Hand hygiene
- *Head end elevation to an angle of 30–45°:* Prevents gastric reflux and subsequent aspiration, which are risk factors for VAP.
- *Suction only when required:* Inline suction reduces the risk of environmental contamination and minimizes circuit disconnection. However, there is no strong evidence to recommend this routinely over open suction.
- Two persons for suction
- No role for acid suppressants
- No sedation/paralysis for ventilation
- Optimal humidification
- *Oral colostrum swabbing:* Evidence has shown that oropharyngeal colostrum painting significantly reduces the occurrence of VAP in very low birth weight (VLBW) infants.
- Extubation readiness during each round/early extubation.

Central Line-associated Bloodstream Infection Bundle

- Hand hygiene
- Preparation for insertion—trays, persons
- Adequate disinfection
- Hub care during each handling
- Readiness to remove the central line during each round

Intraventricular Hemorrhage Bundle

- Head end elevation
- Minimal handling
- Clustering of investigations
- Pain management
- Avoid hypercapnia
- Avoid fluctuation in blood pressure
- Correction of coagulation abnormalities

CONCLUSION

Respiratory care of neonates on noninvasive and invasive ventilation requires a meticulous, holistic, and evidence-based approach. Beyond optimizing ventilator settings, comprehensive monitoring of clinical parameters, device interfaces, and humidification is vital to prevent complications such as volutrauma, air leaks, and infection. Equally important are supportive strategies including thermoregulation, developmental care, skin care, and bundle approaches aimed at reducing risks of ventilator-associated pneumonia, intraventricular hemorrhage, and central line-associated infections. By integrating vigilant clinical observation, judicious use of technology, and adherence to preventive bundles, neonatal teams can significantly enhance survival, minimize iatrogenic harm, and promote long-term respiratory and neurodevelopmental outcomes in this vulnerable population.

SUGGESTED READING

1. Donn SM, Mammel MC, van Kaam AHLC (Eds). Manual of Neonatal Respiratory Care. Cham: Springer International Publishing; 2022.
2. Keszler M, Suresh GK, Goldsmith JP, (Eds). Goldsmith's Assisted Ventilation of the Neonate: An Evidence-based Approach to Newborn Respiratory Care, 7th edition. Philadelphia: Elsevier; 2021.
3. Ma A, Yang J, Li Y, Zhang X, Kang Y. Oropharyngeal colostrum therapy reduces the incidence of ventilator-associated pneumonia in very low birth weight infants: a systematic review and meta-analysis. Pediatr Res. 2021;89(1):54-62.

CHAPTER

Transportation of Neonate on Invasive and Noninvasive Respiratory Support

Naveen Parkash Gupta, Pinaki Dutta

INTRODUCTION

Many neonates may need to be transported from one facility to another because of the nonavailability of required infrastructure or personnel. Sometimes transport can be intrahospital, i.e., from one department to another or it may be interhospital, i.e., from one hospital to another. Transport of a neonate from one facility to another in a safe manner is important to minimize the stress and provide a safe environment during the transit period, optimizing the chances of positive outcomes in these neonates.

Newborns with breathing difficulty secondary to prematurity, meconium aspiration syndrome (MAS), persistent pulmonary hypertension of neonate (PPHN), pneumothorax, etc. constitute the common causes behind the neonatal transport.

Oxygen, noninvasive ventilation [continuous positive airway pressure (CPAP) nasal intermittent mandatory ventilation (IMV)], and elective intubation are the common modes of respiratory support during neonatal transport.

Over the past few years, CPAP has been increasingly used during neonatal transport in babies with respiratory distress. In a systematic review of the use of noninvasive respiratory support during transportation in pediatric patients, 60.4% of noninvasive ventilation (NIV) transports were done in neonates and 39.6% of NIV transports were done in older children.

IMPORTANCE OF RESPIRATORY SUPPORT IN NEONATAL TRANSPORT

Neonates with respiratory distress born at primary or secondary levels need to be transported in stable condition to a tertiary-level neonatal intensive care unit (NICU), where respiratory distress can be managed on either CPAP or ventilation.

If they are not provided with adequate respiratory support during the transit, there is a possibility of deterioration in their respiratory status which may increase the risk of mortality and developing morbidities.

Providing appropriate respiratory support to neonates with respiratory distress improves the outcomes substantially in the form of decreased mortality, decreased need for intubation, and mechanical ventilation.

PHYSIOLOGY OF RESPIRATION AND IMPLICATIONS DURING TRANSPORT

The transport team should keep in mind a few things about respiratory physiology while transporting babies with respiratory distress, especially during air transport.

- Entrapped air expands as altitude increases. As per Boyles's law entrapped gas expands by 3% for every increase in altitude of 1,000 ft. This principle should be kept in mind while transporting a neonate with pneumothorax, especially which is either not drained or incompletely drained before transportation.
- As altitude increases, the partial pressure of oxygen in alveoli (PAO_2) decreases at the same level of fraction of inspired oxygen (FiO_2) compared to ground or sea level. This may lead to a decrease in PaO_2 and tissue hypoxemia. So, if we are transporting a baby with respiratory distress requiring ventilation, the baby may desaturate as we go to a higher altitude, and we need to increase FiO_2 to maintain his saturations in the target range. Pretransport stabilization is the key in such babies.

PRINCIPLES OF NEONATAL RESPIRATORY SUPPORT DURING TRANSPORT

- Oxygenation should be maintained.
- Work of breathing should be the least.
- Ventilation should be appropriate by the least invasive method.

GOALS OF RESPIRATORY SUPPORT DURING TRANSPORT

- Maintain target saturation in the right upper limb (91–95%).
- Maintain partial pressure of carbon dioxide ($PaCO_2$) between 45 and 60 mm Hg.
- Work of breathing should be minimal.
- Baby should remain hemodynamically stable—vital parameters should be maintained within the normal range as per the gestational and postnatal age.
- The baby should be comfortable. The pain score should be within the acceptable range.

HOW CAN WE ACHIEVE THESE GOALS?

Pretransport stabilization is one of the essential key components before the transport of a neonate.

Case Scenario

A preterm neonate is born at 32 weeks' gestation to a primigravida mother who came into active labor in the emergency room. The baby cried immediately after birth but started having respiratory distress immediately after birth. The baby was started on nasal prong oxygen and the clinician decided to transport the baby as there was no facility for providing ventilation in the index hospital.

The present hospital where the baby is admitted currently becomes the referring hospital. The doctor on duty makes a call to a consultant in another hospital (referral hospital). He explains the condition of the baby and asks him to transport the baby in stable condition.

The stepwise management in the transportation of the index case is discussed in **Table 1**.

As pertinent to our case, let us discuss *steps 4 and 5 (pretransport stabilization and continuum of care during transport)* which are key steps in achieving the goals of respiratory support during transport.

Pretransport Stabilization

Evidence suggests that pretransport stabilization leads to better neonatal outcomes. Hypoglycemia, hypothermia, poor perfusion, and poor respiratory status before transportation have been shown to be associated with high mortality in transported neonates. Prior stabilization and adequate continuum of care during transport result in decreased risk of mortality and morbidities. The general pretransportation stabilization checklist is shown in **Table 2**. The pretransportation stabilization checklist for neonates with respiratory distress with different etiologies is shown in **Flowchart 1**. Commonly used models for pretransport stabilization and care during transport are:

TABLE 1: Steps in neonatal transport.

Step 1	Team formation and journey to the referring hospital
Step 2	*Preparation for transport:* • Call for ambulance • Checking transport kit **(Table 1)** • Checking transport incubator and cylinders • Checking monitor, infusion pumps • Checking ventilation device
Step 3	Communication with the referring doctor and parent before leaving for transport
Step 4	Pretransport stabilization of baby on arrival at the referring hospital
Step 5	Continuum of care during transport
Step 6	Care on arrival at the referral hospital

TABLE 2: Important points in pretransport stabilization.

Sugar	• Check random blood glucose. Correct hypoglycemia (blood glucose values <45 mg/dL) if present • Start dextrose infusion and continue it during transport
Temperature	• More preterm the baby, the greater the risk of hypothermia. Cold stress increases oxygen requirement, leading to hypoxia, acidosis and worsening of respiratory status, and overall deterioration of the clinical condition. It is very crucial to avoid hypothermia pre and during tranסportation • Check the temperature of the baby, if hypothermic, correct hls temperature by putting it under a radiant warmer. Check baby's temperature every 15 minutes till it reaches the target range (36.5–37.5°C) • Once stable the baby should be shifted to the transport incubator The aim is to maintain neonate axillary temperature in the target range • In case warmer is not available, adequately cover the baby, start kangaroo mother care, and use EMBRACE depending upon its availability
Airway and breathing	• Clear the airway if there are any visible secretions • Assess the respiratory status of the baby. Check oxygen saturations • If the baby is having respiratory distress, assess oxygen needs. Start on continuous positive airway pressure (CPAP) if needed based on respiratory distress scoring • It is better to intubate and ventilate babies, with respiratory distress and impending respiratory failure rather than bringing on nasal prong oxygen as it is difficult to intubate the babies in an ambulance • If the fraction of inspired oxygen (FiO_2) requirement is <50% and the baby is not in shock, CPAP can be an alternative to ventilation • Always do a transillumination test (cold light test) or check with a torch with a sharp beam of light after creating a dark environment in case a transillumination source is not available. It is important to rule out pneumothorax pretransportation. In case transillumination is positive, get an urgent X-ray (if facilities are available), and put a chest tube before transport
Circulation	• Assess pulses (peripheral and central), blood pressure, and perfusion. Baby should have a patent intravenous access • Once hemodynamic assessment is done and if needed, start inotropes before leaving for transport if required based on clinical assessment
Laboratory parameters	• Collect blood culture before starting antibiotics. Check arterial blood gas (ABG) and electrolytes if feasible
Emotional support	• Introduce your team to parents and counsel about the clinical condition and plan of action • Show to parents before you leave the referring hospital. Let one of the parents/relatives accompany you for the transport. They can be made to sit along with the ambulance driver in front

Flowchart 1: Pretransport stabilization of neonates with respiratory distress as per the etiology.

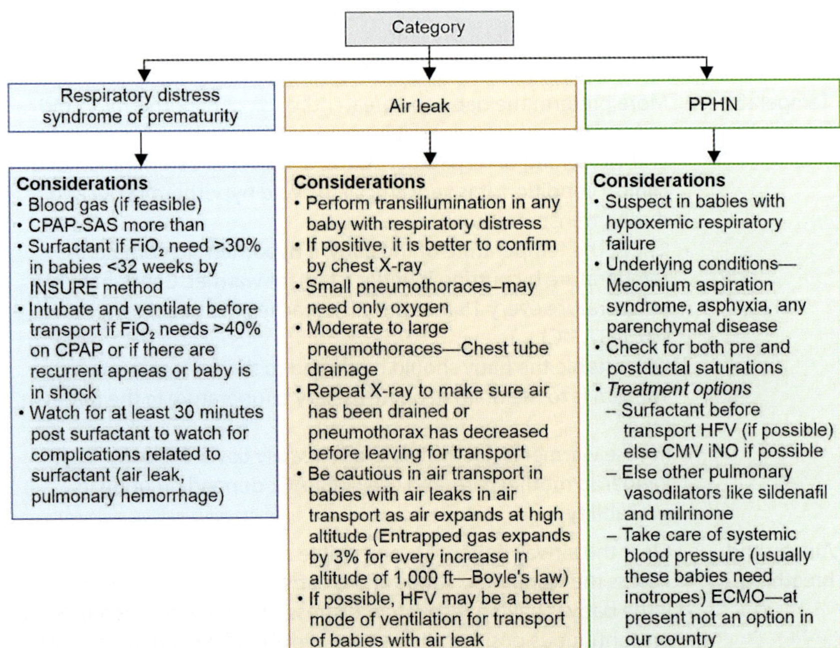

(CMV: conventional mechanical ventilation; CPAP: continuous positive airway pressure; ECMO: extracorporeal membrane oxygenation; FiO_2: fraction of inspired oxygen HFV: high-frequency ventilation; PPHN: persistent pulmonary hypertension of neonate; SAS: Silverman-Anderson score)

- *Stable:* Sugar, temperature, artificial breathing, blood pressure, laboratory work, and emotional support
- *Safer:* Sugar, arterial circulatory support, family support, environment, and respiratory support
- *Tops:* Temperature, oxygenation (airway and breathing), perfusion, and sugar.

Do a minimum number of procedures necessary for transportation. It is important not to rush to the referring hospital but at the same time be time efficient. Take all aseptic precautions during the transport.

Coming back to the case, the baby had an axillary temperature of 35°C which settled after warming inside the incubator. The baby was kept on oxygen by nasal prongs maintaining target saturation (91–95%), but since the Downes score was 6, the baby was started on nasal CPAP with a RAM cannula as interface. His requirements on CPAP were positive end-expiratory pressure (PEEP) of 7 cmH_2O with FiO_2 of 80% with preductal oxygen saturations of 87%. The transport team decided to intubate the baby and give it surfactant. Postsurfactant the baby was observed for 30 minutes.

The baby was transported in a transport ventilator with settings of peak inspiratory pressure (PIP)/PEEP of 20/5 cmH_2O, rate of 45, and FiO_2 of 50%. The infant was monitored with a multipara monitor, and oxygen saturations were targeted between 90% and 95%. The infant required one fluid bolus of 10 mL/kg of normal saline because of poor perfusion. Subsequently, the BP and perfusion were normal. The blood sugar was also normal.

Few important points to remember before we start the transportation from the referring hospital to the referral hospital:

- The starting time and the expected time of arrival to the referral hospital along with the baby's condition and the need and type of respiratory support should be conveyed a priori to the referral hospital so that necessary arrangements can be made at the arrival of the baby.
- Always talk to the parents or concerned caregivers regarding the condition of the baby, need for the transport, risk involved during transport, prognosis, cost, and possible duration of stay in the referral hospital.

Continuum of Care During Transport

The transport team should ensure that the baby remains stable during the transport. Hence, the continuity of care during transport is utmost important and critical for the baby's well-being.

Equipment for Respiratory Support During Transport

Different modes of respiratory support and the equipment available in our country for providing them during neonatal transport are shown in **Tables 3 and 4**. The interfaces available for providing noninvasive ventilation during transport are shown in **Table 5**.

TROUBLESHOOTING DURING NEONATAL TRANSPORT (ACUTE RESPIRATORY DECOMPENSATION)

Although interfacility transport by a transport team has been shown to improve outcomes, issues can occur during the transport of sick neonates, and hence, the transport team should be aware of these problems and their troubleshooting as shown in **Flowchart 2**.

Coming back to the case, the baby was transported on a transport ventilator (IMV PIP 20 PEEP 5 rate 45 FiO_2 50%) and has reached the referral hospital. The referral hospital was informed regarding the need for a ventilator and the possible need for a second dose of surfactant. The baby was immediately transferred to the NICU and started on conventional ventilation [synchronized intermittent positive pressure ventilation (SIPPV)/ synchronized intermittent mandatory ventilation (SIMV)] as per the unit protocol targeting tidal volume (4–6 mL/kg), and baseline vitals parameters

TABLE 3: Modes of respiratory support during transport.

Category	*Type of support*	*Scope*
Noninvasive respiratory support	Oxygen hood or free-flow oxygen	Babies with mild respiratory distress requiring oxygen to maintain target saturations
	Low flow nasal cannula	Babies with mild respiratory distress requiring oxygen to maintain target saturations
	Heated humidified high flow nasal cannula	Babies with moderate respiratory distress with Silverman-Anderson score (SAS) <6 or Downes score <7
	Continuous positive airway pressure (CPAP)	Babies with moderate respiratory distress with Silverman-Anderson score (SAS) <6 or Downes score <7
	Nasal intermittent positive pressure ventilation (NIPPV)	Babies who failed CPAP but not qualifying the criteria for intubation
Invasive respiratory support	Conventional mechanical ventilation (CMV)	• Babies with respiratory distress with SAS >6 or Downes score >7 • Babies on CPAP/NIPPV whose fraction of inspired oxygen (FiO_2) requirement exceeds 50% should be intubated and then transported
	High frequency oscillatory ventilation (HFOV) with or without nitric oxide	Babies with hypoxemic respiratory failure and not maintaining saturation even on conventional ventilation have been tried on HFOV during transportation by one of the centers in southern India
	Extracorporeal membrane oxygenation (ECMO)	• Babies with OI >40 or hypoxemic respiratory failure not responding to surfactant and ventilation and inhaled nitric oxide • This has not yet been tried in neonates in our country although many reports of transportation of adults and children while receiving ECMO have been reported from developed countries

were assessed (HR/BP/SPO_2/RBS). Parents were counseled regarding the condition of the baby, and further courses of management and requisite consent were also taken. X-ray chest was done, and pneumothorax was ruled out. The baby was provided with the second dose of surfactant and continued on mechanical ventilation as the FiO_2 requirement exceeded 30% after clinically ruling out shock and all relevant investigations were sent. In the

TABLE 4: Equipment available for respiratory support during transport.

Device	*Remarks*
Transport ventilator inbuilt in transport incubator (e.g., Drager Ti 500 Globe Trotter)	• Robust functioning • Expensive
Stand-alone transport ventilators: • T S 50 (Mindray) • Oxymag (Magnamed) • Hamilton T1 neonatal ventilator	• Provides both invasive and noninvasive ventilation • Less expensive than an inbuilt transport ventilator in incubator • More expensive than stand-alone nasal IMV or CPAP
Stand-alone nasal IMV or CPAP: • T-piece resuscitator • Murk's precise air oxy flow (T-piece and CPAP device) • Breath.ei Device (CPAP and auto T piece)	• T-piece resuscitator is a cost-effective device which can provide both PIP and PEEP. • *Drawback:* Rate and Ti are manually controlled • Multimodality • Built in air source and battery backup of up to 2 hours • Built-in PIP and PEEP control *Disadvantages:* • Has not been tested for invasive ventilation • If the baby requires invasive ventilation, not suitable

(CPAP: continuous positive airway pressure; IMV: intermittent mandatory ventilation; PEEP: positive end-expiratory pressure; PIP: peak inspiratory pressure)

TABLE 5: Interfaces used for providing noninvasive ventilation during transport.

Interphase	*Remarks*
Low-flow nasal cannula	• Provide low-flow oxygen (<2 L/min) • Ease of fixation present • *Disadvantage:* It cannot provide high flow oxygen or air and oxygen mixture
High-flow nasal cannula (e.g., optiflow and RAM cannula)	• Provide HHHFNC (flows > 2 L/min) • RAM cannula is good for providing CPAP and nasal IMV also • Ease of fixation • Comfortable for the child • *Disadvantage:* Delivered distending pressure may be less
Nasal mask and CPAP prongs	• Provide adequate distending pressure • Problems • Fixation while transport can be an issue • Uncomfortable for the child during transport

(CPAP: continuous positive airway pressure; HHHFNC: heated humidified high-flow nasal cannula; IMV: intermittent mandatory ventilation)

Flowchart 2: Troubleshooting during neonatal transport.

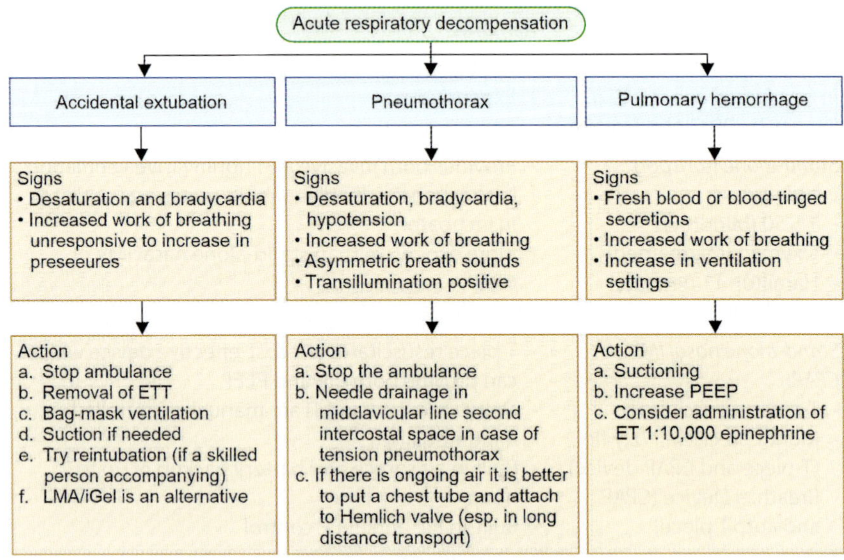

(ETT: endotracheal tube; LMA: laryngeal mask airway)

next 12 hours, baby's oxygen and pressure requirements decreased and the baby was extubated the next day to nasal CPAP and then to room air in 2 days.

NNF CPG Guidelines 2023 on Referral and Transport of Sick Neonates

We are mentioning two guidelines pertaining to the transport of babies with respiratory distress.

Recommendation 1:

Is respiratory support by intubation and ventilation superior to noninvasive respiratory support?

For neonates with respiratory distress being transferred to another health facility, en route respiratory support may be provided with nasal CPAP if respiratory distress is mild to moderate and the FiO_2 requirement is <50%.

Neonates with severe respiratory distress and FiO_2 requirement of >50% may be intubated before starting the transport.

If CPAP is used to provide respiratory support, the accompanying healthcare provider should be skilled to intubate and ventilate the neonate en route, if needed. (*Weak recommendation, very low certainty evidence*)

Recommendation 2:

Is surfactant administration before starting transport superior to surfactant administration after reaching the referral hospital?

Among preterm neonates with respiratory distress syndrome being transferred to another health facility, if indicated and if trained healthcare providers are available, surfactant may be administered before starting the transport. (*Weak recommendation, very low certainty evidence*)

CONCLUSION

Safe and effective neonatal transport requires meticulous pretransport stabilization, appropriate selection of respiratory support, and vigilant continuum of care during transit. Noninvasive modalities such as CPAP can be safely used in infants with mild to moderate respiratory distress, while intubation and invasive ventilation should be ensured for those with severe disease or high oxygen requirements. Surfactant administration prior to transport, timely management of complications like pneumothorax, and readiness to troubleshoot acute decompensation are essential to minimize morbidity and mortality. Optimal outcomes are achieved when transport teams are trained, equipped, and able to provide individualized, least-invasive support while maintaining physiological stability until definitive care is available at the referral center.

SUGGESTED READING

1. Cheema B, Welzel T, Rossouw B. Noninvasive Ventilation During Pediatric and Neonatal Critical Care Transport: A Systematic Review. Pediatr Crit Care Med. 2019;20(1):9-18.
2. Jani P, Luig M, Wall M, Berry A. Transport of very preterm infants with respiratory distress syndrome using nasal continuous positive airway pressure. J Neonatal Perinatal Med. 2014;7(3):165-72.
3. Murray PG, Stewart MJ. Use of nasal continuous positive airway pressure during retrieval of neonates with acute respiratory distress. Pediatrics. 2008;121(4):e754-8.
4. National Neonatology Forum. (2024). NNF CPG Guideline 2024. Referral and Transport of Sick Neonates. [online] Available from https://www.nnfi.org/nnf-cpg-guidelines.php [Last accessed February, 2025].
5. Resnick S, Sokol J. Impact of introducing binasal continuous positive airway pressure for acute respiratory distress in newborns during retrieval: Experience from Western Australia. J Paediatr Child Health. 2010;46(12):754-9.
6. Roy S, Alnaji F, Reddy D, Barrowman N, Sheffield H. Noninvasive ventilation of air transported infants with respiratory distress in the Canadian Arctic. Paediatr Child Health. 2022;27(5):272-7.
7. Trevisanuto D, Cavallin F, Loddo C, Brombin L, Lolli E, Doglioni N, et al. Trends in neonatal emergency transport in the last two decades. Eur J Pediatr. 2021;180(2):635-41.

SECTION

Miscellaneous Topics

CHAPTER

Pharmacological Therapies

Aakash Pandita, Priyanka Gupta

INTRODUCTION

Neonatal ventilation aims to achieve optimal cardiorespiratory status with minimal support. Pharmacological therapies can aid in achieving this goal to some extent. Dosing, frequency, duration of use, adverse effect profiles, and long-term respiratory, cardiac, and neurodevelopmental outcomes have not been studied well for most drugs used in neonates. Various pharmacological adjuncts used in neonatal respiratory care have been outlined further.

STEROIDS

Corticosteroids are potent anti-inflammatory agents that can potentially reduce the incidence and severity of inflammation-mediated lung pathologies such as bronchopulmonary dysplasia (BPD) by modulating a wide range of inflammatory pathways **(Fig. 1)**. Steroids accelerate lung maturation by

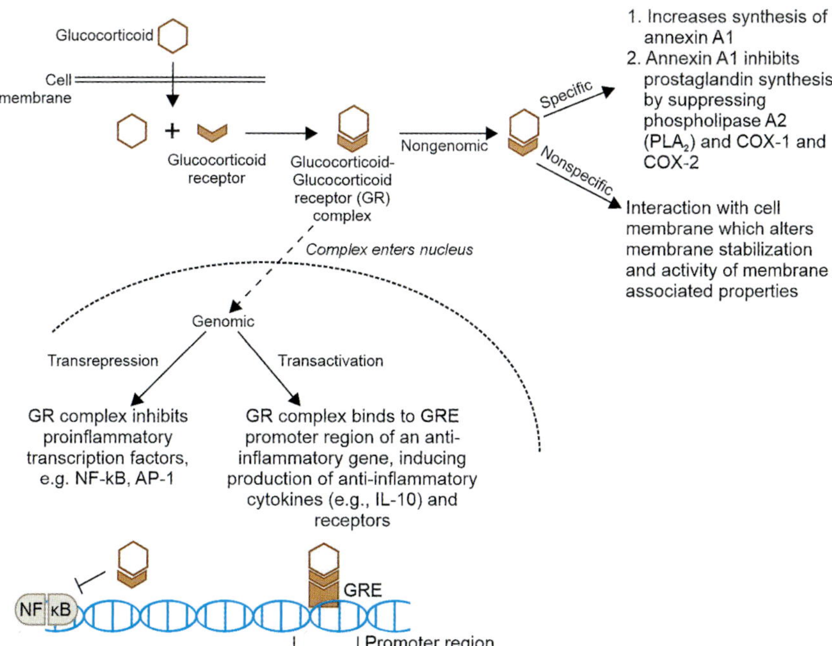

Fig. 1: Mechanism of action of corticosteroids. (COX: cyclooxygenase; IL: interleukin; NF: nuclear factor)

increasing alveolar wall thinning and microvascular maturation. They also promote surfactant production, especially when given during the first week after birth. They decrease elastase activity and collagen formation, increasing the antioxidant status in the developing lung. In addition to decreasing inflammatory molecules, corticosteroids decrease pulmonary edema and promote bronchodilation, improving pulmonary mechanics and facilitating extubation. The various steroid preparations available and their equivalent activity is shown in **Table 1**.

TABLE 1: Various steroids regimen used in BPD

Neurosis	Two puffs (200 µg per puff) of budesonide administered every 12 hours in the first 14 days of life and one puff administered every 12 hours from day 15 until the last dose till they no longer required oxygen and positive-pressure support or until they reached a postmenstrual age of 32 weeks 0 days
Premiloc Regimen	1 mg/kg of hydrocortisone hemisuccinate per day divided into two doses/day for 7 days, followed by one dose of 0·5 mg/kg per day for 3 days in the first 10 postnatal days
DART Regimen	*Dexamethasone: Cumulative dose—0.89 mg/kg* • *Day 1–3:* 0.075 mg/kg/dose 12 hourly • *Day 4–6:* 0.050 mg/kg/dose 12 hourly • *Day 7 and 8:* 0.025 mg/kg/dose 12 hourly • *Day 9 and 10:* 0.01 mg/kg/dose 12 hourly
Minidex Regimen	0.05 mg/kg × 10 days followed by alternate day doses × 6 days
STOP BPD Regimen (Hydrocortisone)	• 5 mg/kg per day in 4 doses per day for 7 days, followed by 3.75 mg/kg per day in 3 doses per day for 5 days, subsequently lowering the frequency by 1 dose every 5 days • Total 22 days, cumulative dose—72.5 mg/kg
Modified DART Regimen	*Dexamethasone 9-day course:* 0.2 mg/kg/day div q12h × 3 days 0.1 mg/kg/day div q12h × 3 days 0.05 mg/kg/day q12h × 3 days
Bhandari Regimen	Oral prednisolone 2 mg/kg/day div BID × 5 days 1 mg/kg/day QD × 3 days 1 mg/kg/day QoD × 3 doses
Linafelter Regimen	The starting dose of prednisolone is 2 mg/kg/day → weaned weekly from 2 mg/kg/day to 1 mg/kg/day to 0.5 mg/kg/day once the infant is on 0.5 mg/kg/day daily, next attempt to wean to 0.5 mg/kg/day three times a week before finally trialing to discontinue prednisolone
Steroids for Extubation	*Dexamethasone:* 3 doses of 0.25 to 0.5 mg/kg IV

Based on the period of administration:

- Prophylactic/early (<8 days)
- *Late:*
    - Early evolving BPD (7–28 days)
    - Late evolving BPD (28 days to 36 weeks)
    - Established BPD (>36 weeks)

Prophylactic/Early Postnatal Steroid Therapy

Most of the research regarding early steroid therapy has evaluated dexamethasone, which is a more potent steroid compared to hydrocortisone raising concerns for developmental sequelae. The evolution of using various forms of corticosteroids in clinical practice is as shown in **Figure 2**.

In a large trial, neonates under 30 weeks were randomized to receive dexamethasone [early short course (2 doses beginning at 12 hours of age)]. The study found that early dexamethasone reduced later prolonged usage of steroid treatment and ventilator and/or oxygen use but did not decrease death or BPD at 36 weeks of gestation. In a 2001 study by the Vermont Oxford Network, extremely premature neonates on invasive ventilation were randomized to receive dexamethasone for 12 days. Because of increased complications such as gastrointestinal perforation, and hyperglycemia, hypertension trial was stopped early. Also, early dexamethasone did not decrease BPD or death and increased the risk of periventricular leukomalacia (PVL).

The PREMILOC trial found that 60% of neonates of <28 weeks survived without BPD who were exposed to early hydrocortisone compared to infants assigned to placebo [odds ratio (OR): 1.48, 95% confidence interval (CI) 1.02–2.16, p = 0·04) with number needed to treat (NNT) of 12. There was no difference in rates of gastric perforation. However, subgroup analyses showed a higher rate only in infants born at 24–25 weeks gestational age who

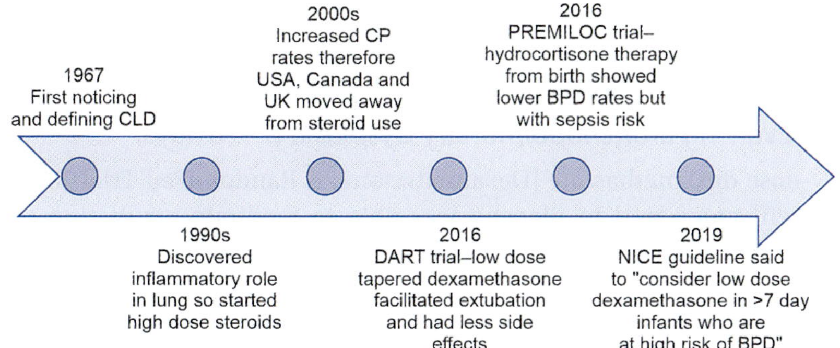

Fig. 2: Evolution of steroids in clinical practice. (BPD: bronchopulmonary dysplasia; (CLD: chronic lung disease; CP: cerebral palsy; DART: Dexamethasone: A Randomized Trial; NICE: National Institute for Health and Care Excellence)

were treated with hydrocortisone. No adrenal suppression was noted with the hydrocortisone dosage used in this trial. Follow-up at 2 years showed no significant difference in the rates of cerebral palsy (CP) or other major neurological outcomes. Also, among surviving infants born at 24–25 weeks, significant improvement in global neurological assessment was observed in the hydrocortisone group compared with the placebo group.

Cochrane review 2017 found that early postnatal steroid therapy facilitates extubation, and lowers the incidence of BPD at 28 days of life, 36 weeks of postmenstrual age (PMA), death, and BPD. However, there was no difference in neonatal mortality. There was an increase in the incidence of gastrointestinal bleeding, intestinal perforation, hyperglycemia, hypertension, growth failure, and hypertrophic cardiomyopathy. Follow-up showed an increased incidence of CP [risk ratio (RR) = 1.42, 95% CI 1.06–1.91) in the group exposed to early postnatal corticosteroids, particularly dexamethasone.

Early inhaled budesonide has been evaluated for the prevention of BPD for extreme premature babies, which found that incidence of BPD was less in the budesonide group compared to placebo. However, the mortality also increased in the budesonide-exposed group. A randomized clinical study used intratracheal budesonide administration with surfactant and found that combining budesonide with surfactant for rescue therapy of respiratory distress syndrome (RDS) in preterm infants decreases the BPD and duration of respiratory support. Based on the current evidence, inhaled steroids cannot be recommended as of now because of poor pulmonary deposition and the risk of increased mortality. Further studies are needed before recommending its routine use.

In summary, routine use of early steroids cannot be recommended because of the heterogeneity of the existing literature concerning neurodevelopmental outcomes (especially with dexamethasone) until more follow-up data is available. Hydrocortisone may have neurodevelopmental benefits, especially with 24–25-week-old babies, but routine use cannot be recommended until its impact on long-term outcomes are studied.

Late (≥8 days) Postnatal Steroid Therapy

Early Evolving Bronchopulmonary Dysplasia (7–28 days)

Low-dose dexamethasone [Dexamethasone: A Randomized Trial (DART) regimen] compared to placebo was able to facilitate extubation (day 3: 34% vs. 3%, $p < 0.01$; day 7: 51% vs. 12%, $p < 0.01$; day 10: 60% vs. 12%, $p < 0.01$). However, it did not improve survival or oxygen dependence at 36 weeks' PMA. DART follow-up showed no differences in the rate of major disability, CP, or combined death or CP at 2 years of age. Very low doses of dexamethasone in chronic lung disease (Minidex study) showed that babies treated with Minidex extubated significantly faster than controls and significantly improved ventilatory index and oxygen requirements. However, they had a similar rate of chronic lung disease at 36 weeks corrected age. Stop BPD trial infants <28 weeks' GA and on invasive ventilation >7 days, can improve short-term respiratory outcomes but no difference for death or BPD at 36 weeks' PMA.

Late Evolving Bronchopulmonary Dysplasia (28 days to 36 weeks)

An observational study from the USA analyzed the *Modified DART* protocol. It compared dexamethasone versus hydrocortisone versus methylprednisolone. The study found that by day 7, dexamethasone treatment was associated with the greatest decrease in ventilation status.

Established Bronchopulmonary Dysplasia (>36 weeks)

Bhandari et al., in an observational study assessed the effect of oral prednisolone in infants with oxygen-dependent BPD. They found that in neonates exposed to the oral prednisolone group, 63% responded to treatment. Another retrospective study by Linafelter et al., noted a significant decrease in respiratory support after 1 week of prednisolone therapy and noted no further benefits from the prolongation of therapy and significant linear growth impairment by week 4. Inhaled beclomethasone, budesonide, and fluticasone have been commonly used to treat evolving or established BPD, although there is limited supporting evidence for the use of inhalation corticosteroids.

The Cochrane systematic review on late postnatal steroid therapy concluded that steroid regimen initiated on or after 8 days reduced neonatal mortality rate at 28 days and at 36 weeks PMA. Also, it facilitated early extubation with a trend toward an increase in CP rates.

To summarize, late postnatal steroid therapy should be restricted to infants who are unable to be weaned off from mechanical ventilation with minimal dosing and duration of treatment. Therapy should be initiated after providing information on short- and long-term risks and benefits to the parents.

Steroids for facilitating extubation: Steroids have been used in attempts to facilitate and improve success rates of extubation. However, routine use is not recommended. Their use should be reserved for infants intubated for more than 7 days or repeated extubation failures. Cochrane systematic review concluded that dexamethasone use for facilitating extubation is associated with side effects such as hyperglycemia.

The various steroid regimens used in the treatment of BPD are shown in **Table 2**.

TABLE 2: Comparison of equivalent activity of different steroids.

Drug	*Approximate equivalent dose (mg)*	*Glucocorticoid potency*	*Mineralocorticoid potency*	*Duration of action (h)*
Hydrocortisone	20	1	1	Short acting 8–12
Prednisone Prednisolone	5	4	0.8	Intermediate acting 12–36
Methylpredniso-lone	4	5	0.5	Intermediate acting 12–36
Dexamethasone	0.75	25	0	Long acting >36
Betamethasone	0.75	25	0	Long acting >36
Fludrocortisone	–	10	125	Intermediate acting 12–36

RESPIRATORY STIMULANTS

Caffeine

Caffeine is a methylxanthine and acts via three mechanisms:

1. *Adenosine antagonism*: It is the main mechanism of action at therapeutic levels. It acts via inhibition of A1 and A2a receptors.
2. *Phosphodiesterase (PDE) inhibition*: Caffeine prevents the breakdown of cyclic adenosine monophosphate (cAMP) leading to central nervous system (CNS) stimulation.
3. *Intracellular calcium mobilization*: It inhibits voltage-sensitive calcium channels leading to inhibition of neurotransmission.

Caffeine acts centrally as well as peripherally and prevents apnea of prematurity by stimulation of the respiratory center in the medulla, increased sensitivity to carbon dioxide in the respiratory center, increased skeletal muscle tone, enhanced diaphragmatic contractility, increased minute ventilation, bronchodilatation [by increasing cAMP, cyclic guanosine monophosphate (cGMP)], and enhanced peripheral chemoreceptors activity.

Caffeine has a plasma half-life of approximately 100 hours. It is rapidly and completely absorbed with no first-pass metabolism. Peak plasma concentration of both oral and intravenous routes is almost the same. It is metabolized by liver enzymes, microsomal cytochrome P450 mono-oxygenase and xanthine oxidase, therefore most of the drug is excreted unchanged in the urine. In premature neonates, the predominant process of caffeine metabolism is N7 demethylation, which is postnatal age-dependent, regardless of gestational age and/or birth weight.

The loading dose of caffeine is 10 mg/kg, with a maintenance dose of 2.5–5 mg/kg. The therapeutic range of caffeine for apnea in preterm neonates is 8 to 20 mg/L. The usual form of caffeine, the citrate in 20 mg/mL, is equivalent to a 10 mg/mL solution of the base and may be administered intravenously or orally. Caffeine offers several advantages over theophylline—better enteral absorption, a longer half-life leading to once-daily dosing, lesser adverse effects like tachycardia and feed intolerance greater CNS penetration.

There has been considerable variation regarding the timing of initiation, dosing, and duration of caffeine. Many studies concluded that early caffeine (within 3 days) decreases the incidence of composite outcomes of death or BPD. However, Cynthia et al., in a randomized controlled trial, found a trend toward increased mortality in the early caffeine group. Though the trend was not statistically significant, the trial was stopped in between. In a randomized control trial comparing high doses (10 mg/kg/day) versus low doses (2.5 mg/kg/day) of caffeine, a significantly lower risk of extubation failure and disability at 12 months was noted in the high-dose group. However, there was no difference in the BPD rates. Loading doses up to 80 mg/kg have been used in various trials. The current recommendation is to continue caffeine therapy until preterm infants are 34–36 weeks corrected gestational age and free of any apnea episodes for at least 8 days. However, a recent randomized control trial in India included 26–32 weeks of neonates and studied the recurrence of apnea using two protocols. First protocol stopped caffeine after a 7-day apnea-free interval and second protocol continued caffeine till 34 weeks of PMA. The trial concluded that continuing caffeine till 34 weeks does not decrease the risk of recurrence of apnea.

The CAP ("Caffeine for Apnea of Prematurity") trial was a large international, randomized placebo-controlled trial, designed to clarify possible risks and benefits of methylxanthine treatment. Infants could be included if they were (1) born with a birth weight of 500 to 1,250 g, and (2) less than 10 days old. The short-term outcomes of the CAP trial showed a significant reduction in the incidence of BPD. Mortality and incidence of brain lesions detected by sonography or necrotizing enterocolitis did not differ between the two groups. Weight gain during the first 3 weeks of life was lower in the caffeine group, but no sustained growth restriction could be observed between 4–6 weeks after randomization. Mortality, deafness, and blindness did not differ between both groups, yet there was a significant reduction in the incidence of CP and cognitive delay at 18 months in the caffeine-treated group. It showed a sustained improvement in motor function at the ages of 5 and 11 years, as well as a reduction in developmental coordination disorder.

Theophylline/aminophylline: They are methylated xanthine alkaloids with half-life of 30 hours. Compared to caffeine, theophylline has a more potent inotropic, vasodilator, bronchodilator, and diuretic action with a higher propensity of side effects. Apart from PDE inhibition and adenosine

TABLE 3: Comparison of caffeine and aminophylline.

	Caffeine	*Aminophyliine*
Cardiac stimulation	Less	More
CNS stimulation	Less	More
Loading dose	20 mg/kg	6 mg/kg
Maintenance dose	5–8 mg/kg OD	2 mg/kg/dose 8–12 hourly
Plasma half-life	100 hours	30 hours
Therapeutic level	5–25 mg/L	8–12 mg/L
Toxicity	>40–60 mg/L	>20 mg/L
Metabolism	Excreted unchanged or N demethylation	Excreted unchanged or 8-hydroxylation
Elimination	86% unchanged in urine	50% unchanged in urine
Route of administration	IV/PO	IV/PO
Therapeutic range	Wide	Narrow

antagonism, it is also an inhibitor of lymphocyte function as well as mast cell histamine release, thereby helpful in reducing airway inflammation. The therapeutic plasma concentration is about 7–20 mg/L. Toxicity signs include tachycardia, irritability, diaphoresis, diarrhea, seizures, vomiting, and gastroesophageal reflux. The usual intravenous (IV) dose of theophylline is 4–6 mg/kg loading with a maintenance dose of 1 mg/kg every 8 hours or 2 mg/kg every 12 hours.

The pharmacokinetic, pharmacodynamic, and dosing comparison between caffeine and aminophylline is shown in **Table 3**.

Doxapram: It is a pyrrolidinone derivative that stimulates central and peripheral chemoreceptors, leading to the stimulation of ventral brainstem nuclei. Currently, there is insufficient data on the use of doxapram in premature neonates to reduce apneic spells. It can be used as a second-line agent in addition to methylxanthines for refractory apnea of prematurity. The dose is 2.5–3 mg/kg loading followed by a maintenance infusion of 0.5–2.5 mg/kg/h. Side effects include hypertension, vomiting, feed intolerance, hypokalemia, jitteriness, hyperglycemia, and glycosuria.

DIURETICS

Diuretics decrease the work of breathing and help in mechanical ventilation by decreasing pulmonary fluid and improving lung compliance.

Furosemide: It is most commonly used diuretic in neonates. It acts by blocking the NaCl reabsorption by the Na/K/2Cl symporter in the thick ascending loop of Henle. Also, it increases prostaglandin E2 (PGE2) synthesis by renal cyclooxygenase 2. Through its diuretic action, it decreases intravascular volume and increases systemic venous capacitance. PGE2-mediated effects lead to pulmonary vasodilation, decrease pulmonary interstitial fluid accumulation, and decrease the closure of ductus arteriosus. The usual dosage is 1–2 mg/kg IV.

Side effects include hypotension, hypokalemia, hypocalcemia, hypercalciuria, nephrocalcinosis, hypomagnesemia, hyponatremia, hypochloremic alkalosis, and ototoxicity. Hearing loss caused by furosemide is often transient and reversible.

Various studies have found that furosemide has the potential to improve lung compliance, and functional residual capacity, and facilitate quicker extubation in neonates with RDS. The Cochrane systematic review on diuretic use in preterms with RDS recommends against the use of furosemide for infants with RDS. The Cochrane review of loop diuretics in infants with BPD concluded that despite long-term administration of furosemide improved oxygenation and lung compliance, routine use of furosemide is not recommended to prevent or treat BPD. When administered as an aerosol, furosemide has been shown to decrease bronchospasm. However, routine use is not recommended.

Thiazides and potassium-sparing diuretics: Thiazides act at the distal tubule to inhibit reabsorption of NaCl through the apical luminal transporter. They are less potent than loop diuretics. Spironolactone is a potassium-sparing diuretic that blocks aldosterone activity by competitive inhibition. Side effects profile of thiazides include hyponatremia, hypokalemia, hypomagnesemia, and hypophosphatemia. They do not cause hypercalciuria. The usual dosage of chlorothiazide and spironolactone is 10–20 and 1–2 mg/kg, respectively. The use of thiazide and spironolactone together has been shown to decrease airway resistance and improve lung compliance. The Cochrane systematic review on the use of these diuretics on neonates with BPD concluded that there is no strong evidence of benefit from routine use of thiazide diuretics.

The various diuretics available, and their mechanism of action, dosing, and route of administration are shown in **Table 4**.

TABLE 4: Diuretics.

Drug	*Mode of action*	*Route*	*Onset of action*	*Dose*
Furosemide	Loop diuretic	IV	15–30 min	1 mg/kg/dose
		PO	30–60 min	1–3 mg/kg/dose
Hydrochlorothiazide	Distal tubule	PO	1–2 hours	2–4 mg/kg/dose
Spironolactone	Competitive aldosterone antagonist	PO	3–5 days	1.5–3 mg/kg/dose

SEDATION AND ANALGESIA

Sedation and analgesia are important in managing pain in the neonates receiving respiratory support. Acute pain can lead to hypoxemia, pulmonary and systemic hypertension, an increase in the release of stress hormones, increased intracranial pressures, and intraventricular hemorrhage (IVH). Safety data on pharmacological measures for pain is scarce. The American Academy of Pediatrics (AAP) guidelines 2010 recommends routine administration of premedication for neonates undergoing nonemergent intubation. Acute and chronic pain responses can lead to long-term neurodevelopmental consequences. Nonpharmacological measures like oral sucrose, kangaroo mother care, containment, swaddling, facilitated tucking, and reducing noise, light, and music therapy have been shown to decrease the stress response in neonates.

Opioids: Their analgesic effect is attributed to their activation of the endorphin m, k, and/or d receptors in the CNS. This initiates signal transduction and activation of inhibitory G proteins and reduces cAMP levels, leading to reduced neuronal excitability and decreased neurotransmitter release.

Morphine: It is a strong agonist of the μ-opioid receptor (MOR) through which it mediates effects such as analgesia and respiratory depression. Intravenous administration is the most common route of use for premature infants. Morphine has a quick onset of action and peaks at about 1 hour after injection. Its duration of action is between 2 and 4 hours. The loading dose is 100 μg/kg over the first hour, with a continuous infusion dose range between 5 and 15 μg/kg/h. Morphine does not provide sedation at doses that are used to provide analgesia.

Vasodilation, hypotension, and bradycardia are common side effects of morphine. The metabolism of morphine matures with increasing gestational age (GA). A weaning regimen that reduces the dose by 10–20% per day is recommended to prevent withdrawal symptoms after prolonged use. Morphine effects can be reversed by a naloxone dose of 0.1 mg/kg.

NEOPAIN trial showed a reduction in pain score and smaller increases in heart rate and respiratory rate were noted in the morphine group. However, these infants took longer to tolerate full enteral feeds, had significant hypotension more often, and required mechanical ventilation for a longer duration. Mortality rates and morbidities related to prematurity such as IVH and PVL were similar. Neurologic outcomes also did not differ between the infants given morphine. Currently, there is insufficient evidence to recommend the routine use of continuous morphine infusions for infants undergoing mechanical ventilation.

Fentanyl: It is a synthetic opioid. Fentanyl crosses the blood-cerebrospinal fluid barrier more rapidly and produces analgesic effects more quickly than morphine due to its higher lipid solubility. Fentanyl has a shorter duration of action (30–40 minutes) than morphine, making it suitable for short procedures like intubation that require rapid induction and recovery from sedation and analgesia. The onset of action is 1–2 min with peak effects in 10 minutes. Prolonged use can lead to the development of tolerance, tachyphylaxis, and withdrawal symptoms on discontinuation. Dosage—sedation/analgesia: 1–4 μg/kg/dose (maximum dose: 100 μg/dose) IV Q2-4 hourly and for continuous IV infusion: 1–5 μg/kg/h. It should be used with caution in bradycardia, respiratory depression, and increased intracranial pressure. Some studies showed that fentanyl use prolongs the duration of mechanical ventilation possibly due to decreased chest compliance because of fentanyl-induced chest wall rigidity. Long-term data regarding neurodevelopmental outcomes is scarce.

The pharmacokinetic, pharmacodynamic, and dosing comparison between fentanyl and morphine is shown in **Table 5**.

Dexmedetomidine: It is an analgesic agent with additional anxiolytic and sedative properties with the advantage of minimal respiratory depression. Dexmedetomidine is an imidazole derivative and a selective central a2-adrenergic receptor agonist. It has high specificity for the a2A subtype of

TABLE 5: Fentanyl and morphine.

	Fentanyl	***Morphine***
	Lipophilic	***Hydrophilic***
Onset	Fast (10–20 minutes)	Slow (60 minutes)
Duration of action	30–40 minutes	2 to 4 hours
Blood-brain barrier	Crosses more rapidly	Less rapidly
Analgesic efficacy	80–100 times more potent than morphine	Less potent
Metabolism	Hepatic microsomal P450	Hepatic UDP—glucoronosyl transferase 2B7
Excretion	Renal clearance	Renal and hepatic
Histamine release	Less	More
Therapeutic effects	More predictable	Less predictable
GI side effects	Less	More
Hypotension/ bronchoconstriction	Less	More
Chest wall rigidity	Yes	No
Tachyphylaxis	More severe	Less
Dosage (loading)	1–4 μg/kg/dose (max –100 μg)	100 μg/kg over 1 hour
Infusion dosage	1–5 μg/kg/h	5–15 μg/kg/h
Antagonist		Naloxone (0.1 mg/kg)

this receptor. Dexmedetomidine is increasingly being used in the postoperative cardiac intensive care environment. Dexmedetomidine use has been associated with less need for adjunctive sedation, shorter duration of mechanical ventilation, and lower incidence of culture-positive sepsis episodes compared with fentanyl use. Dexmedetomidine also promotes macrophage activity and reduction of inflammatory mediators. Advantages include minimal withdrawal signs, respiratory depression, and gastrointestinal dysmotility. Adverse effects associated with dexmedetomidine include hypotension, bradycardia, decreased secretion, bowel motility, and excessive diuresis.

Midazolam: It has a rapid onset of action (3 minutes) and time to peak sedative effects (20 minutes) compared with other benzodiazepines, making it a preferred drug for use in short procedures. It is also frequently used as a continuous infusion for sedation of mechanically ventilated neonates. Midazolam clearance increases with postnatal age and is decreased by critical illness. It is highly protein-bound. The adverse effects are respiratory depression, hypotension, hypotonia, hypertonia, dyskinetic movements, myoclonus, and paradoxic agitation. A randomized trial of the use of continuous midazolam infusion found that it is associated with prolonged neonatal intensive care unit (NICU) stay, and tended to increase the incidence of hypotension and bradycardia in preterm infants when its use was continued beyond 48 hours. One of the trials also found that midazolam use led to an increased incidence of neurologic adverse effects such as IVH and PVL compared with morphine or placebo use. So, routine prolonged usage of midazolam should be avoided, especially in preterm neonates. Dosage 0.05–0.15 mg/kg per dose, initial IV infusion dosage—<32-weeks' gestation: 0.5 μg/kg/min, ≥32-weeks' gestation: 1 μg/kg/min, and infant and child: 1–2 μg/kg/min.

MUSCLE RELAXANTS

The use of muscle relaxants is not routinely indicated during mechanical ventilation of neonates, but muscle relaxants are sometimes used as part of premedication regimens and in certain patient populations such as infants with PPHN. Paralysis may improve oxygenation and ventilation of severely hypoxemic term infants. However, data regarding the use of muscle relaxants is extremely limited and they should be used with caution, especially in preterm neonates. The various muscle relaxants available and their dosing are shown in **Table 6**.

TABLE 6: Muscle relaxants.

Drug	*Initial dose*	*Dose frequency*
Vecuronium	0.03–0.15 mg/kg	1–2 hours
Pancuronium	0.04–0.15 mg/kg	1–4 hours
Rocuronium	0.3–0.6 mg/kg	0.5–1 hour

BRONCHODILATOR AND MUCOLYTIC THERAPY

Mechanically ventilated infants with BPD have airway smooth muscle hypertrophy that leads to an increase in airway resistance. Also, the tracheobronchial tree of preterm infants harbors a relatively higher number of goblet cells that express mucus and fewer ciliated airway cells to assist in the mobilization of airway secretions and mucus. Bronchodilators decrease airway resistance and mucolytic agents that promote mucin breakdown and can be of help in mechanical ventilation of the neonate.

Salbutamol: Albuterol is a selective b2-adrenergic agonist that causes bronchodilation by enhancing cAMP production, and decreasing intracellular calcium in smooth muscle cells. At high doses, inhaled albuterol loses such bronchial b2 selectivity and leads to adverse effects such as vasodilation, hypotension, reflex tachycardia, hyperglycemia, and hypokalemia, secondary to its effects on other b2-adrenergic receptor systems. A 2016 Cochrane collaboration systematic review identified only two trials of albuterol that met the criteria for inclusion and concluded that available data are insufficient to reliably assess the effectiveness of albuterol in improving clinical outcomes for infants with BPD.

Epinephrine: It stimulates both a- and b-adrenergic receptors. It acts on vascular smooth muscle to produce vasoconstriction. This shrinks upper respiratory mucosa and reduces edema. It is useful in neonates with established postextubation stridor. It may also be considered as an adjunct to therapy for pulmonary hemorrhage. Side effects include tachycardia, arrhythmias, hypertension, peripheral vasoconstriction, hyperglycemia, hyperkalemia, and metabolic acidosis.

N-acetylcysteine (NAC): NAC is a thiol compound that possesses a free sulfhydryl group through which it reduces disulfide bonds present in mucoproteins, thereby reducing the elasticity and viscosity of mucus. Data on the use of NAC in neonates is limited. The use of NAC in preterm infants should be undertaken cautiously, and when used, NAC should be administered along with bronchodilators.

The various bronchodilators, anticholinergics, and mucolytic drugs available for clinical use, and their dosing is are shown in **Table 7**.

TABLE 7: Bronchodilators, anticholinergic, and mucolytic therapy.

Drug	*Dose*	*Dose frequency*
Salbutamol	0.2 mg/kg	Every 3–6 hours
Ipratropium bromide	0.025 mg/kg	Every 8 hours
N-acetylcysteine	10–20 mg	Every 6–8 hours
Cromoglycic acid	10 mg	Every 6 hours

CONCLUSION

The aim of mechanical ventilation for neonates should be to provide the least support required for optimal cardiorespiratory status minimizing lung injury such as volutrauma and barotrauma. Pharmacologic therapies should be used sparingly and wisely to prevent prolonged mechanical ventilation. Except for caffeine and, to a limited extent, late administration of corticosteroids and thiazide diuretics, none of the other drug classes has proven effective in reducing ventilator-associated lung injury or BPD to date.

SUGGESTED READING

1. Bhandari A, Schramm CM, Kimble C, Pappagallo M, Hussain N. Effect of a short course of prednisolone in infants with oxygen-dependent bronchopulmonary dysplasia. Pediatrics. 2008;121(2):e344–9. doi: 10.1542/peds.2006-3668.
2. Barrington KJ. Premedication for endotracheal intubation in the newborn infant. Paediatr Child Health. 2011;16:159-64.
3. Baud O, Maury L, Lebail F, Ramful D, El Moussawi F, Nicaise C, et al. Effect of early low-dose hydrocortisone on survival without bronchopulmonary dysplasia in extremely preterm infants (PREMILOC): a double-blind, placebo-controlled, multicentre, randomized trial. Lancet. 2016;387(10030):1827-36.
4. Doyle LW, Cheong JL, Hay S, Manley BJ, Halliday HL. Late (≥7 days) systemic postnatal corticosteroids for prevention of bronchopulmonary dysplasia in preterm infants. Cochrane Database Syst Rev. 2021;11(11):CD001145.
5. Doyle LW, Davis PG, Morley CJ, McPhee A, Carlin JB; DART Study Investigators. Low-dose dexamethasone facilitates extubation among chronically ventilator-dependent infants: a multicenter, international, randomized, controlled trial. Pediatrics. 2006;117(1):75-83.
6. Linafelter A, Cuna A, Liu C, Quigley A, Truog WE, Sampath V, et al. Extended course of prednisolone in infants with severe bronchopulmonary dysplasia. Early Hum Dev. 2019;136:1-6. doi: 10.1016/j.earlhumdev.2019.06.007. Epub 2019 Jun 29. PMID: 31265946.
7. Schmidt B, Anderson PJ, Doyle LW, Dewey D, Grunau RE, Asztalos EV, et al. Survival without disability to age 5 years after neonatal caffeine therapy for apnea of prematurity. JAMA. 2012;307:275-82.
8. Schmidt B, Roberts RS, Davis P, Doyle LW, Barrington KJ, Ohlsson A, et al. Caffeine therapy for apnea of prematurity. N Engl J Med. 2006;354:2112-21.
9. Schmidt B, Roberts RS, Davis P, Doyle LW, Barrington KJ, Ohlsson A, et al. Long-term effects of caffeine therapy for apnea of prematurity. N Engl J Med. 2007;357:1893-902.

SECTION

Case Scenarios

CHAPTER

Case Scenarios

Gunjana Kumar

CASE SCENARIO 1

A preterm infant of 28 + 4 weeks of gestation with a birth weight of 1,000 grams was born to a 25-year-old primigravida mother with a history of preterm premature rupture of the membrane. The baby is born via spontaneous vaginal delivery with no antenatal steroid coverage. The baby was born limp and needed tactile stimulation followed by positive pressure ventilation via a T-piece resuscitator for 30 seconds with 30% oxygen. Apgar scores recorded are 5 and 7 at 1 and 5 minutes, respectively. Later, the baby had spontaneous breathing efforts with respiratory distress (Silverman–Anderson score of 6/10).

Cord blood gas analysis was performed **(Table 1)**.

TABLE 1: Cord blood gas analysis of case 1.

pH	*$PaCO_2$*	*PaO_2*	*HCO_3*	*BE*	*Lactate*
7.25	66	38.9	20.1	–2.6	4.8

Q. What immediate action do you think should be taken?

Receive the baby in a polythene bag/wrap without drying and maintain ambient room temperature between 23 and 25°C, delivery room continuous positive airway pressure (DR CPAP) is to be initiated immediately. Maintain minute-specific target oxygen saturation. Shift the baby after initial stabilization to neonatal intensive care unit (NICU) in the incubator.

Q. What are the diagnostic possibilities? What next intervention is to be performed in the NICU?

- Case of respiratory distress syndrome (RDS)
- The baby in NICU is shifted to CPAP support with humidification.
- *Initial settings:* Positive end-expiratory pressure (PEEP) 5, fraction of inspired oxygen (FiO_2)—50%, flow of 5 L/min with oxygen saturation (SpO_2) of 92%.
- In view of persistent retractions, PEEP is increased to 6.

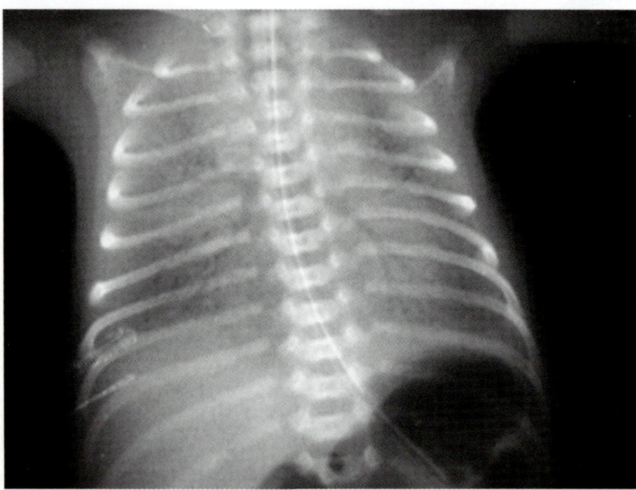

Fig. 1: Chest X-ray suggestive of respiratory distress syndrome (RDS): Uniform ground-glass opacity and under aeration with air bronchogram.

- For a high FiO_2 requirement of >30%, the baby is given surfactant via less invasive surfactant administration (LISA) technique [INtubation-SURfactant-Extubation (INSURE) technique could also be considered where expertise in LISA technique is not there].
- Adequacy of CPAP is monitored by monitoring vitals, looking at signs of respiratory distress (increase PEEP if there were any retractions, FiO_2 based on target saturation level—91–95%) and monitoring for complications. X-ray could be considered for lung expansion **(Fig. 1)**.

Q. After administrating surfactant, the FiO_2 requirement gradually tapered and decreased to 25% over the next 24 hours with target saturation maintained within the range of 91–95%, how would you plan weaning of such neonates?

For a baby on FiO_2 >50% and CPAP pressure >5 cm, wean FiO_2 till it reaches 50% and then wean the pressure to 5 cm. Once the FiO_2 is at 50%, wean it to a level <30% before reducing CPAP pressure from 5 to 4 cm. When a baby is on a pressure of 4 cm with FiO_2 <30% with saturation between 91 and 95% and minimal retractions, CPAP could be removed. One may use heated humidified high-flow nasal cannula (HHHFNC) when weaning a baby from CPAP.

Learning Points

- Antenatal steroid coverage and magnesium sulfate to the mother prior to the delivery are important perinatal interventions for preterm birth.
- In utero transfer and delivery at tertiary care centers are of utmost importance in high-risk deliveries.
- A noninvasive ventilation strategy prevents lung injury.

CASE SCENARIO 2

A 26-week, 700-gram neonate is born to a gravida two 38-year-old mother via in vitro fertilization (IVF) conception. The mother was given a course of antenatal steroid (dexamethasone) completed 48 hours prior to the delivery. Later the mother underwent emergency lower segment cesarean section (LSCS) for grade 3 placenta previa with bleeding per vagina. Cardiotocogram (CTG) was suggestive of absent baseline fetal heart rate (HR) variability along with recurrent late decelerations. The mother received antenatal magnesium sulfate with antenatal antibiotics for 24 hours.

The baby did not cry immediately after birth, requiring intubation. The baby was shifted to NICU on a T-piece resuscitator with PEEP—5, peak inspiratory pressure (PIP)—20, and FiO_2—60%.

Cord blood gas was performed in the labor room **(Table 2)**.

TABLE 2: Cord blood gas analysis of case 2.

pH	*$PaCO_2$*	*PaO_2*	*HCO_3*	*BE*	*Lactate*
7.15	50	30	14.5	–9.2	6.1

Q. How would you proceed with the management of this case?

- *Respiratory management:* Pressure synchronized intermittent mandatory ventilation (PSIMV) + volume guarantee (VG) + pressure support ventilation (PSV) mode:
  - PEEP—6, Pmax—20, respiratory rate (RR)—60 breaths/min, Ti—0.33, tidal volume (TV)—5 mL/kg, FiO_2—60%
  - Administered surfactant within 2 hours of birth.
  - Repeat arterial blood gas (ABG) done at 12 hours of life **(Table 3)**.

TABLE 3: Repeat arterial blood gas (ABG) at 12 hours of life of case 2.

pH	*$PaCO_2$*	*PaO_2*	*HCO_3*	*BE*	*Lactate*
7.28	37	50	18.1	–4.8	4

  - Thermoregulatory and circulatory monitoring
  - Minimal enteral feeding was initiated
  - Chest X-ray performed **(Fig. 2)**

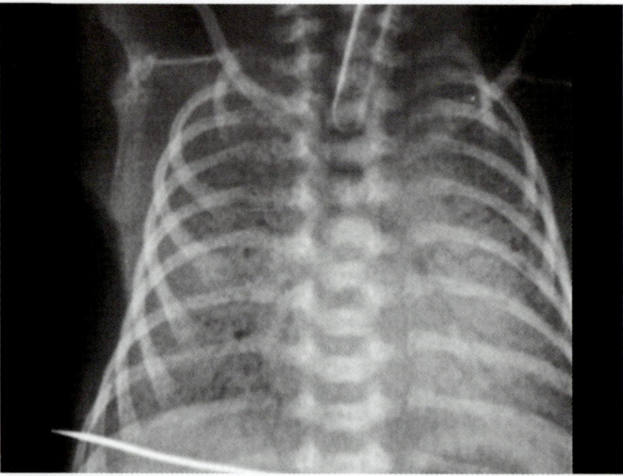

Fig. 2: Chest X-ray suggestive of respiratory distress syndrome (RDS): Decreased aeration, air bronchograms, uniform ground-glass opacity, and indistinct heart borders.

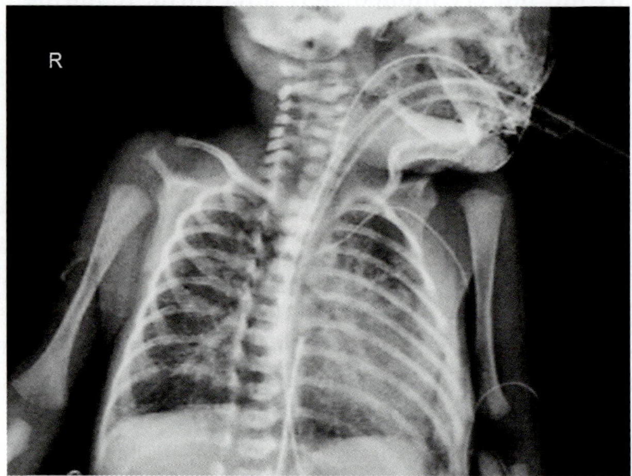

Fig. 3: Chest X-ray taken at 36 hours of life showing bilateral plethoric lung field.

Q. After administrating the surfactant, the FiO_2 was gradually tapered to 30% in the next 12 hours. The baby was hemodynamically stable till 36 hours of life. At 36 hours of life, the baby had hemodynamic instability in the form of tachycardia HR—180 beats/min, capillary refill time (CFT) >3 seconds, and bounding pulses. Also, the baby had an increasing FiO_2 requirement of up to 50%. How will you proceed next?

- DOPE was ruled out: *D*isplacement, *O*bstruction, *P*neumothorax, *E*quipment failure
- Repeat chest X-ray performed **(Fig. 3)**
- Repeat ABG done at 36 hours of life **(Table 4)**

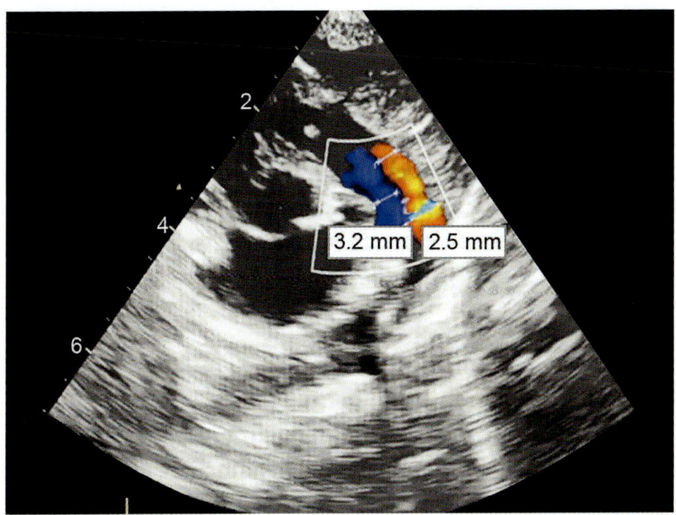

Fig. 4: 2D echocardiography: Parasternal short axis view representing patent ductus arteriosus (PDA) with left to right shunt of diameter 2.5 mm. PDA/left pulmonary artery (LPA) ratio—0.8.

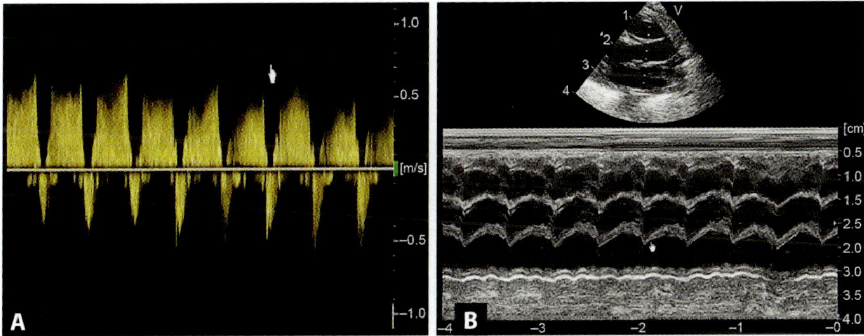

Figs. 5A and B: (A) The pulse wave (PW) Doppler representing growing pattern of patent ductus arteriosus (PDA); (B) Parasternal long axis view showing left atria (LA)/aorta (AO) ratio 1.2.

TABLE 4: Repeat arterial blood gas (ABG) at 36 hours of life of case 2.

pH	*$PaCO_2$*	*PaO_2*	*HCO_3*	*BE*	*Lactate*
7.20	35	55	16.2	–9.9	6.5

- 2D echocardiography is planned immediately **(Figs. 4 and 5)**

  For hemodynamically significant PDA causing systemic hypotension with increasing FiO_2 requirement, the baby is planned to be initiated on injection ibuprofen for 3 days.

- Ultrasonography (USG) cranium was performed—no intraventricular and cerebral Doppler
  Resistive index (RI)—0.71 in anterior cerebral artery (ACA)

Q. On day 5 of life, the baby's FiO_2 requirement gradually decreased to 25% with settings on PSIMV + VG + PSV mode as PEEP—5, Pmax—20, Rate 50, Ti 0.35, and TV 5 mL/kg. When will you plan to extubate this baby?

Assess the baby:

- Monitor respiratory status—breathing comfortably without any retractions or tachypnea.
- Reduce the TV to 4 mL/kg, assess working PIP is <12–15 cmH_2O, FiO_2 <30%.
- Assess the readiness of the baby based on the spontaneous breath test
- Extubate the baby to CPAP/noninvasive positive pressure ventilation (NIPPV) (PEEP—5–6, PIP—2 cmH_2O above the working PIP on invasive ventilation, FiO_2—titrated based on oxygen saturation level).
- Once extubated, assess daily to wean the baby to room air/HHHFNC depending on respiratory status of the neonate.
- Hike the feeds based on the tolerance of the baby by 20–30 mL/kg/day till the baby reaches full feeds of 150 mL/kg/day. Consider fortification once the baby is at 100 mL/kg/day of feeds.

Learning Points

- Excessive volume, not pressure is the key element in ventilator-associated lung injury.
- Volume-targeted ventilation reduces lung and brain injury, and being an autoweaning modality allows faster weaning from mechanical ventilation.
- Excessive leak around the endotracheal (ET) tube (>35–40%) may affect the accuracy of TV measurement, potentially resulting in inadvertent hypocapnia, unless the ventilator has a good leak compensation.
- Care of the flow sensor is of utmost importance while using VG.

CASE SCENARIO 3

A 38-week, 3,300-gram baby born via vaginal delivery to a primigravida mother was referred from the peripheral hospital to a tertiary care center at 2 hours of life with a history of meconium-stained amniotic fluid (MSAF) liquor.

As per the history and documents available, the baby required advanced resuscitation at the time of birth, requiring chest compression for 60 second. Apgar score is not known. On receiving in the emergency, the baby was imp, intubated on bag and tube ventilation with 100% oxygen with saturation of 88%.

The baby was shifted immediately to the NICU for further management.

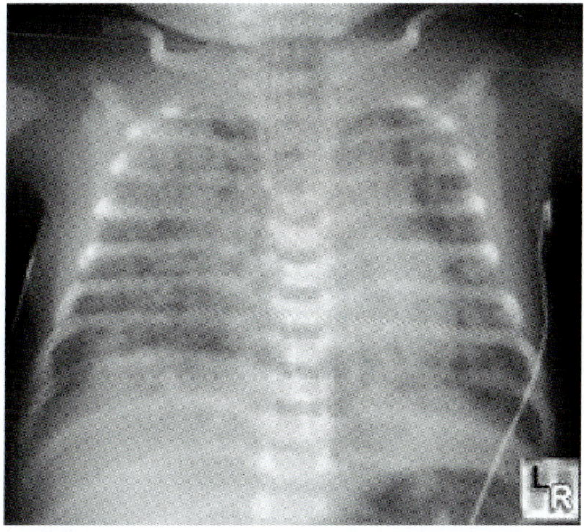

Fig. 6: Chest X-ray suggestive of MAS: Heterogeneous bilateral coarse patchy nodular opacities.

Q. What are your concerns at this stage? What would you do?

- Baby born through MSAF liquor with perinatal asphyxia, likely possibility of meconium aspiration syndrome (MAS).
- Secure airway and breathing, the baby was taken on PSIMV + VG + PSV mode of ventilation—TV 6 mL/kg (higher TV required), PEEP—5, Pmax—25, Ti—0.4 second, FiO_2—100% (saturation is 90% at this settings). In view of the high FiO_2 requirement, surfactant was administered.
- Blood gas analysis was done to monitor the ventilation **(Table 5)**.

TABLE 5: Blood gas analysis of case scenario 3.

pH	*$PaCO_2$*	*PaO_2*	*HCO_3*	*BE*	*Lactate*
7.10	50	45	14.2	–12	10.2

- Circulatory status is to be assessed regularly.
- The risk of complications associated with MAS, such as air leaks, progressive respiratory failure, and pulmonary hypertension, is assessed.
- Chest X-ray performed **(Fig. 6)**.

Q. After giving surfactant, the FiO_2 requirement was reduced to 40% with saturation of 93%. At 26 hours of life, the baby had desaturation episodes with increasing FiO_2 requirement up to 100% with SpO_2 of 88%. What should you do now?

- DOPE approach
- Transillumination of the chest was done **(Fig. 7)**.
- Ultrasonography chest was done: Absence of lung sliding, no B lines. M mode suggestive of barcode sign **(Fig. 8)**.
- A repeat chest X-ray was requested **(Fig. 9)**.

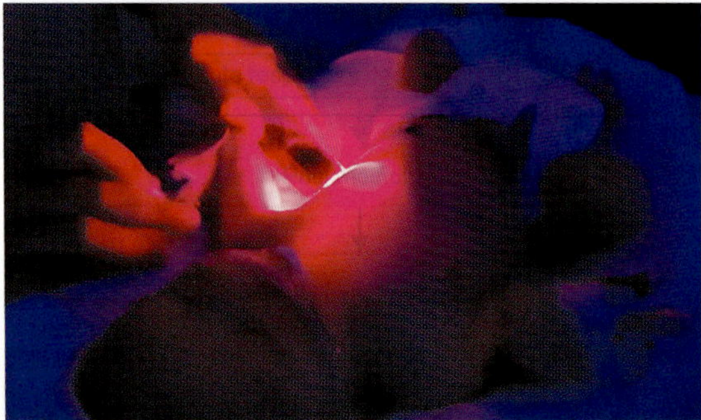

Fig. 7: Transillumination test showing large halo suggestive of pneumothorax.

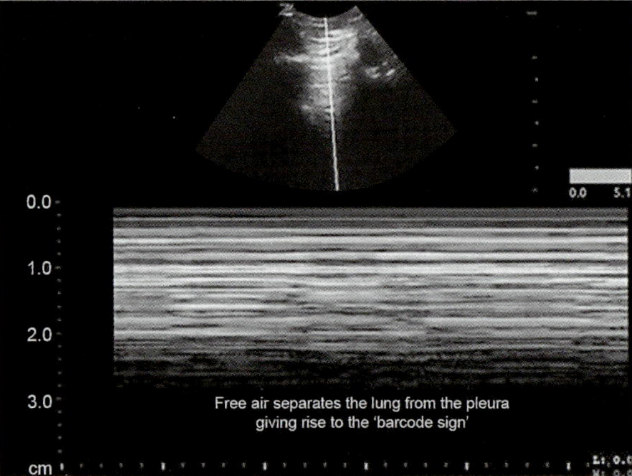

Fig. 8: Ultrasonography (USG) lung: M-mode suggestive of barcode sign suggestive of pneumothorax.

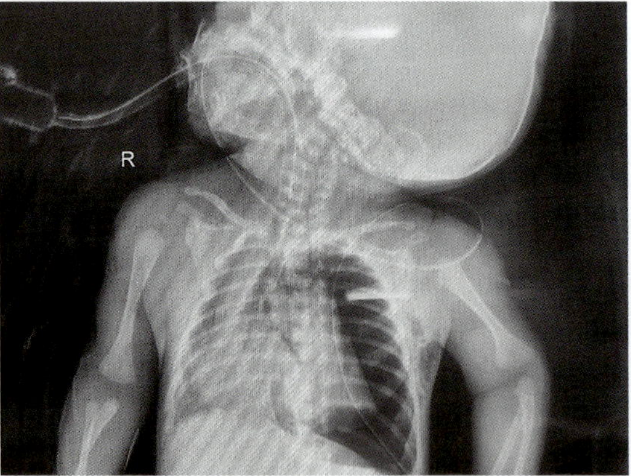

Fig. 9: Chest X-ray showing findings of increased radiolucency of left-sided lung area, with clear border of a collapsed lung, absent lung markings beyond the collapsed lung border, Mediastinal shift and herniation of pneumothorax bounder by parietal pleura into the contralateral side.

Q. How would you proceed with this case now? How to adjust ventilation settings now?

- Needle drainage followed by intercostal drainage (ICD) insertion was done.
- After draining the pneumothorax observe for the improvement in the oxygenation.

Q. Immediately after ICD insertion, there was a transient improvement in the oxygen saturation to 92% on 100% oxygen with no improvement in the respiratory status of the baby. The current ventilatory setting has a TV of 6 mL/kg with blood gas as shown in Table 6. What steps would you take next?

TABLE 6: Repeat blood gas analysis of case scenario 3 after intercostal drainage (ICD) insertion.

pH	*$PaCO_2$*	*PaO_2*	*HCO_3*	*BE*	*Lactate*
7.11	66	48	16	−10	8.7

- *Perform 2D echocardiography* ***(Figs. 10 and 11)****:* Echocardiography suggestive of pulmonary hypertension (PH)
- In view of pneumothorax and high TV requirement of >6 mL/kg [mean airway pressure (MAP) of 10 cmH_2O], the preferred ventilation mode is high-frequency oscillatory ventilation (HFOV).

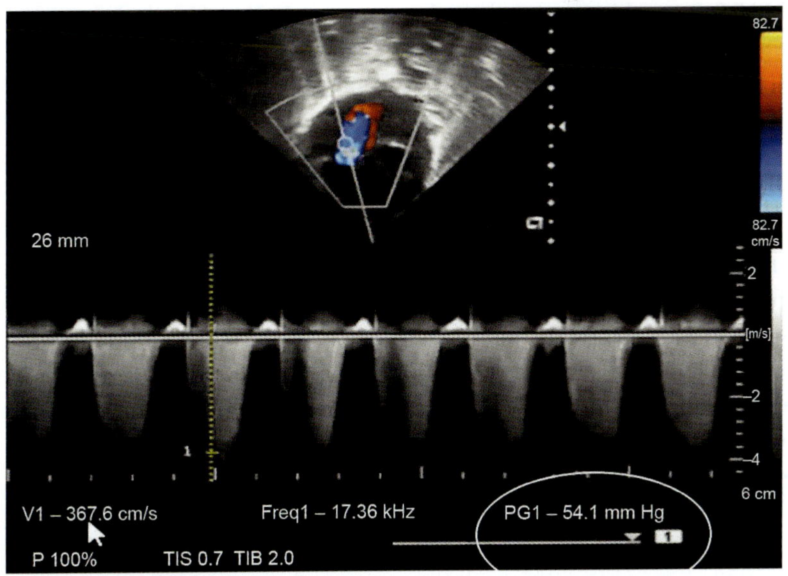

Fig. 10: 2D echocardiography suggestive of tricuspid regurgitation (TR) jet with a pressure gradient of 54 mm Hg suggestive of pulmonary hypertension (PH).

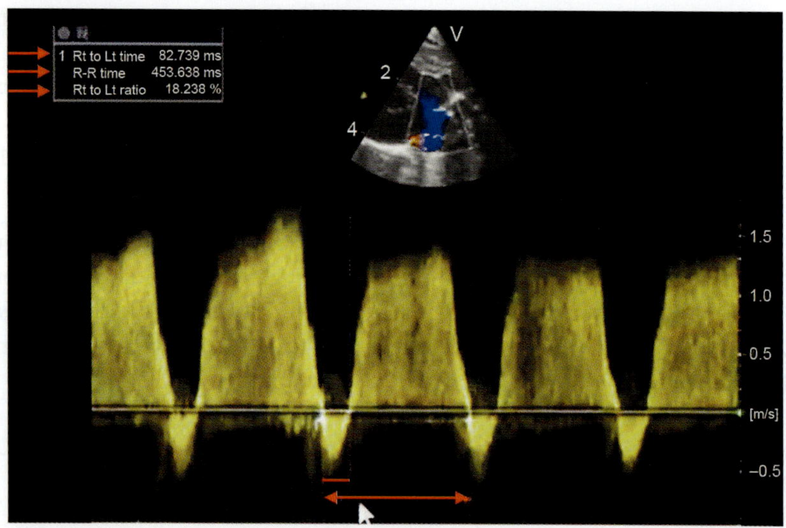

Fig. 11: 2D echocardiography showing patent ductus arteriosus (PDA) with right to left shunt.

Settings: MAP 11/amplitude 25/FiO_2 60%/frequency 10 Hz.
Oxygenation index (OI): 13.7

Gradually the oxygen requirement was decreased from 100 to 30% over the next 12 hours.

Repeat blood gas analysis was performed **(Table 7)**.

TABLE 7: Repeat blood gas analysis of case scenario 3 after taking the baby on high-frequency oscillatory (HFO) ventilation

pH	*$PaCO_2$*	*PaO_2*	*HCO_3*	*BE*	*Lactate*
7.30	40	60	20	−2	4.1

Monitor via chest X-ray, the lung expansion of eight to night posterior ribs.

Q. How would you wean such neonates from the ventilatory support?
After weaning of FiO_2 to <40% and improved systemic status, MAP being <9–10 cmH_2O, Wean the amplitude in 2–4 cmH_2O increments. Do not wean the frequency. After this, the baby can be weaned to SIMV + VG + PSV mode. Later, if the infant is stable, oxygenating well, and blood gases are satisfactory, then the infant could be extubated to CPAP.

Learning Points

- High-frequency oscillatory (HFO) provides low tidal volumes and is an effective mode of ventilation for neonates with severe lung disease.
- Gentle ventilation with optimum lung recruitment, targeting $PaCO_2$ between 50–60 mm Hg and PaO_2 between 50 and 80 mm Hg while avoiding acidosis (pH >7.25) appears to be a rationale approach in cases of pulmonary hypertension.

CASE SCENARIO 4

A 39-week 3,400 grams neonate is born to a G2P1L1 mother with an antenatal history of left congenital diaphragmatic hernia (CDH) with a mediastinal shift to the right, containing a small intestine and liver. Lung-to-head ratio (LHR) of 0.27. Amniocentesis is done at 17 + 6 weeks, depicting fluorescence in situ hybridization (FISH) and karyotyping being normal.

Baby cried immediately after birth but soon had respiratory distress.

Cord blood gas analysis was performed immediately **(Table 8)**.

TABLE 8: Cord blood gas analysis of case 4.

pH	*$PaCO_2$*	*PaO_2*	*HCO_3*	*BE*	*Lactate*
7.32	32	22	18.8	−2	3.7

Q. What delivery room practices will you recommend?

Antenatal counseling is to be performed by a senior neonatologist, and delivery is to be attended by senior consultant neonatologists, followed by immediate endotracheal intubation. Avoiding bag and mask ventilation.

Q. What ventilatory mode would you prefer?

- Initially could be started on the PSIMV + VG + PS mode of ventilation
- *Initial setting:* TV—5 mL/kg, PEEP—5, Pmax <25 cmH_2O, 40 breaths, Ti—0.3 seconds, FiO_2—100%, SpO_2 preductal 70% (target preductal saturation >85%).
- Repeat blood gas analysis was performed **(Table 9)**.

TABLE 9: Blood gas analysis of case 4 after initial stabilization.

pH	*$PaCO_2$*	*PaO_2*	*HCO_3*	*BE*	*Lactate*
7.229	74	45	18	−7	2.9

- Chest X-ray performed **(Fig. 12)**

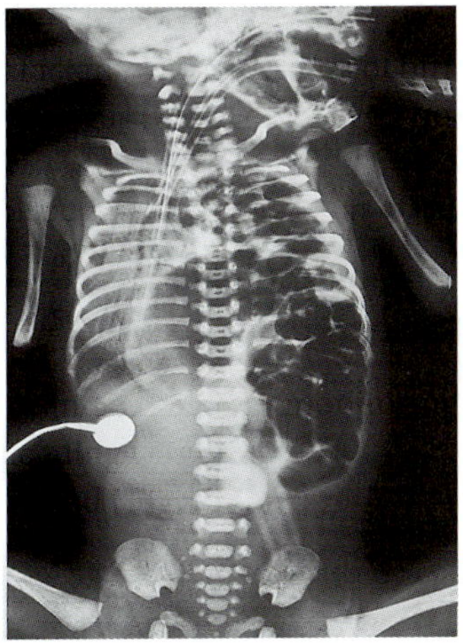

Fig. 12: Chest X-ray suggestive of left-sided diaphragmatic hernia.

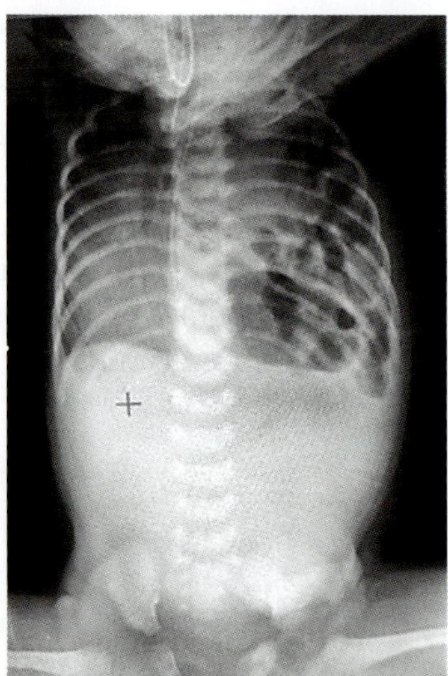

Fig. 13: Chest X-ray of the baby of high-frequency oscillatory ventilation (HFOV) showing 8–9 posterior ribs.

- The baby was further shifted to HFOV as the target goal is $PaCO_2$ of 45–55 mm Hg and preductal SpO_2 >85%.
- *Initial setting on HFOV:* MAP—10–12 cmH_2O, frequency—8–10 Hz, I:E ratio—1:2, FiO_2—50% with SpO_2—87%.
- *Target in neonates with CDH:* Supplemental oxygen should be titrated to achieve a preductal saturation of at least 85%, but not >95%.
- Target $PaCO_2$ 45–60 mm Hg and pH 7.25–7.40.
- Repeat chest X-ray performed after taking the baby on HFO to look for lung expansion **(Fig. 13)**.

Q. At 12 hours of life, the baby had increasing FiO_2 and MAP requirement as the preductal saturation decreased to 70% on 100% oxygen on HFO with MAP of 13. 2D echocardiography: Large PDA 3 mm, apical muscular ventricular septal defect (VSD) with bidirectional shunt, with dilated right atrium (RA)/right ventricle (RV), RV systolic pressure (RVSP)—40 mm Hg, mild RV dysfunction. Left arch, no coenzyme A (CoA). How would you proceed?

- Repeat ABG was performed at 12 hours of life **(Table 10)**

TABLE 10: Blood gas analysis of case 4 at 12 hours of life.

pH	*$PaCO_2$*	*PaO_2*	*HCO_3*	*BE*	*Lactate*
7.20	50	45	16	–9	5.1

- OI—28.8
- Start the baby on inhaled nitric oxide (iNO) at 20 ppm.

Q. After initiating iNO, the oxygen requirement decreased to 30%, and then gradually, iNO was weaned off. After stabilization for persistent pulmonary hypertension of the newborn (PPHN), how would you proceed in this case?

- Repeat ABG was performed after stabilizing the baby on iNO **(Table 11)**.

TABLE 11: Blood gas analysis of case 4 after stabilizing the baby on inhaled nitric oxide (iNO).

pH	*$PaCO_2$*	*PaO_2*	*HCO_3*	*BE*	*Lactate*
7.22	55	60	20	–3	2.8

- FiO_2 requirement is 30%
- *Order of tapering in HFOV:* Amplitude first, then MAP and lastly frequency
- Wean the baby to conventional ventilation
- *PSMIV + VG + PSV mode:* TV 4 mL/kg, PEEP 5, Pmax 20, rate 40/min, FiO_2 30%.
- Planned for surgery.

Q. Surgical findings:

- **Most small bowel, large bowel loops, spleen, and stomach are in left thoracic cavity.**
- **Posterolateral diaphragmatic defect with deficient lateral aspect of posterior lip.**
- **Left lung tissue partially expanding.**
- **Repair without patch done**

How would you manage this neonate postoperatively?

- Repeat chest X-ray performed postoperatively **(Fig. 14)**.
- Taken on conventional ventilation (PSIMV + VG + PSV), TV 5 mL/kg, PEEP 5, Pmax 20, rate 40, FiO_2 70%.

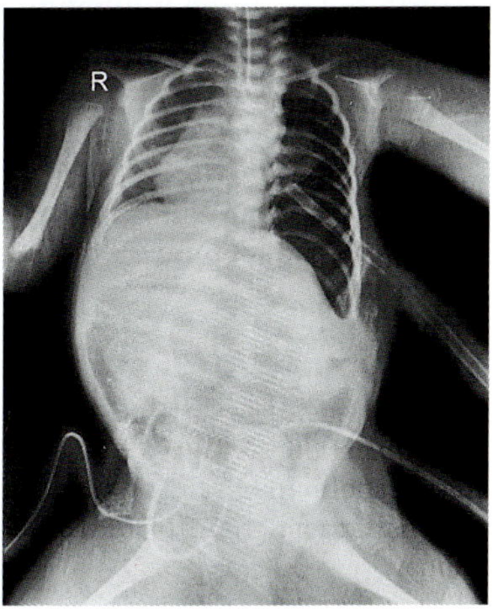

Fig. 14: Postoperative chest X-ray of the baby.

- Gradually FiO_2 tapering to 30%
- Repeat blood gas was planned **(Table 12)**.

TABLE 12: Blood gas values of case 4 during the phase of recovery on conventional **(Fig. 12)** and heated humidified high-flow nasal cannula (HHHFNC) mode of ventilation **(Fig. 12)**.

Ventilation	*Ph*	*$PaCO_2$*	*PaO_2*	*HCO_3*	*BE*	*Lactate*
PSIMV + VG + PSV	7.284	42	60	23.9	0.7	2.0
Extubated HHHFNC at 6 L/min at 30% FiO_2	7.48	39	62	22.4	1	1.7

(FiO_2: fraction of inspired oxygen; HHHFNC: heated humidified high-flow nasal cannula; PSIMV: pressure synchronized intermittent mandatory ventilation; PSV: pressure support ventilation; VG: volume guarantee)

Baby is extubated to HHHFNC (6 L/min, 30% FiO_2); flow is reduced further to 2 L/min, titrating FiO_2 based on the oxygen saturation target level. Monitored based on clinical parameters and blood gas analysis **(Table 12)**.

At 2L/min and FiO_2 of 21%, baby weaned off to room air.

Learning Points

- Immediate intubation with "gentle ventilation", reduced oxygen exposure and judicious use of pulmonary vasodilators and vasopressors are the cornerstone in management of CDH.
- Preductal saturation of 85–95% is acceptable, if the baby appears well perfused with pH >7.2 and PCO2 <65 mm Hg.

CASE SCENARIO 5

A 26-week, 700 grams neonate outborn baby is referred at day 28 of life in view of the failure of extubation. As per the previous records available, the baby cried immediately after birth but required intubation in view of respiratory distress. Required two doses of surfactant. Extubation was tried thrice but failed, and the baby was continued on mechanical ventilation.

Q. What ventilatory settings would you plan for this baby?

Chest X-ray performed to know the lung condition **(Fig. 15)**.

Taken on PSIMV + VG + PSV mode: PEEP 5 cmH_2O, TV 4–6 mL/kg, rate: 30/min, Ti 0.45

Target saturation: 91–95%

Blood gas analysis was planned ***(Table 13)****:* Target values: $PaCO_2$ 45–55 mm Hg, pH 7.25–7.35

TABLE 13: Blood gas analysis of case 5.

pH	*$PaCO_2$*	*PaO_2*	*HCO_3*	*BE*	*Lactate*
7.30	50	50	21	–2.5	2.0

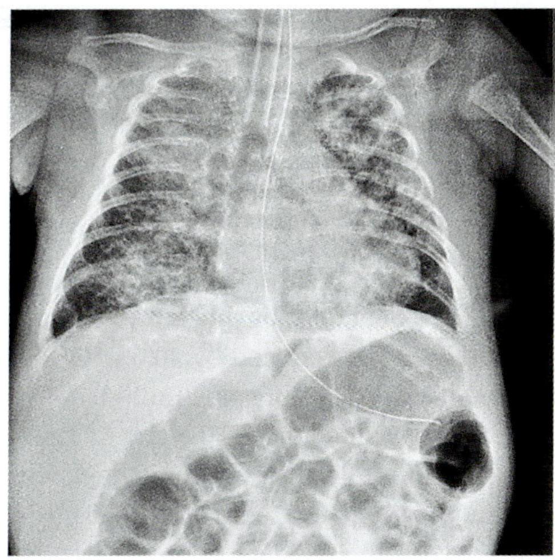

Fig. 15: Chest X-ray suggestive of bronchopulmonary dysplasia: Bilateral heterogeneous opacities, dense fibrotic strands with generalized cystic areas.

Q. Baby is continued to be intubated at 6 weeks of life. What ventilatory changes would you make?

PSMIV + VG + PSV mode: PEEP 6–8 cmH_2O, TV 6–8 mL/kg, Ti 0.5 second, rate 30/min

Target SpO_2 92–98%, $PaCO_2$ 45–60 mm Hg, pH >7.25

Q. How would you plan the extubation of such neonates?

- At 8 weeks, the baby is given a trial of extubation once the baby is on minimum ventilatory settings (TV 5 mL/kg, PEEP 5 cmH_2O, rate 30/min, Ti 0.45, FiO_2 30%) with normal blood gas analysis **(Table 14)**.

TABLE 14: Blood gas analysis of case 5.

pH	*$PaCO_2$*	*PaO_2*	*HCO_3*	*BE*	*Lactate*
7.35	48	55	23	2	1.2

- Taken on NIPPV mode of ventilation
- PEEP 6, PIP 20, FiO_2 40%, rate 40/min, Ti 0.5 second

Q. The baby maintained the saturation for 6 hours, after 6 hours of extubation, the baby started to have worsening respiratory distress with increasing FiO_2 requirement 60%. How would you manage this baby next?

- A rescue mode of nasal HFO (nHFO) ventilation trial can be given
- Switched to nHFOV
- *Settings:* Paw (MAP): 8–10 cmH_2O, amplitude (ΔP): <25 cmH_2O, frequency: 10–12 Hz, I:E ratio: 1:2, FiO_2: 50%

Q. The baby remained on nHFOV for 7 days, how would you plan further weaning?

- Gradual tapering with reducing FiO_2 <30% and then MAP to around 8 cmH_2O
- Once the MAP—8, amplitude—20, FiO_2—30%, I:E ratio: 1:2, frequency—10, baby was weaned to NIPPV mode
- PEEP—6, PIP—20, FiO_2—40%, rate—40, Ti—0.5 second

Q. What is the further plan of action for this baby?

On NIPPV support, the FiO_2 was reduced by 30% with PEEP—6, and PIP—14, the baby was weaned to CPAP support to PEEP—6 cmH_2O, FiO_2—30%.

Further, the baby can be weaned to HHHFNC at 6 L/min with FiO_2—30%. Later, as the baby was comfortable at this setting, the flow can be reduced to 2 L/min and then a trial of weaning to room air can be given.

In case of failure to wean the neonate to room air, the baby is kept on a low-flow nasal cannula flow at 1 L/min at 25% oxygen.

Learning Points

- The key to managing bronchopulmonary dysplasia is to avoid excessive tidal volumes and ensure adequate lung volume recruitment to maintain gas exchange with minimal support.
- Slow rates, with long Ti are needed as the disease progress.

SUGGESTED READING

1. El Shahed AI, Dargaville PA, Soll R. Surfactant for meconium aspiration syndrome in term and late preterm infants. Cochrane Database Syst Rev. 2014;2014(12):CD002054.
2. Klingenberg C, Wheeler KI, McCallion N, Morley CJ, Davis PG. Volume-targeted versus pressure-limited ventilation in neonates. Cochrane Database Syst Rev. 2017;10(10):CD003666.
3. Puligandla P, Skarsgard E, Baird R, Guadagno E, Dimmer A, Ganescu O, et al. Diagnosis and management of congenital diaphragmatic hernia: a 2023 update from the Canadian congenital diaphragmatic hernia collaborative. Arch Dis Child Fetal Neonatal Ed. 2024;109(3):239-52.
4. Ramaswamy VV, Abiramalatha T, Bandyopadhyay T, Shaik NB, Pullattayil S AK, Cavallin F, et al. Delivery room CPAP in improving outcomes of preterm neonates in low-and middle-income countries: A systematic review and network meta-analysis. Resuscitation. 2022;170:250-63.
5. Sweet DG, Carnielli VP, Greisen G, Hallman M, Klebermass-Schrehof K, Ozek E, et al. European consensus guidelines on the management of respiratory distress syndrome: 2022 update. Neonatology. 2023;120(1):3-23.
6. Wyckoff MH, Wyllie J, Aziz K, de Almeida MF, Fabres J, Fawke J, et al. Neonatal life support: 2020 international consensus on cardiopulmonary resuscitation and emergency cardiovascular care science with treatment recommendations. Circulation. 2020;142(16_suppl_1):S185-221.

Index

Page numbers followed by *b* refer to box, *f* refer to figure, *fc* refer to flowchart, and *t* refer to table.

A

I

N

S

T